PHYSIOLOGY OF
THE KIDNEY
AND
BODY FLUIDS

PHYSIOLOGY of the

ROBERT F. PITTS, Ph.D., M.D.

*Professor of Physiology, Maxwell M. Upson Department of Physiology
and Biophysics, Cornell University Medical College*

KIDNEY and BODY FLUIDS

An

Introductory Text

THIRD EDITION

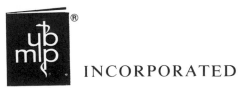

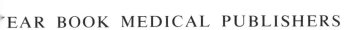

YEAR BOOK MEDICAL PUBLISHERS INCORPORATED

35 EAST WACKER DRIVE, CHICAGO

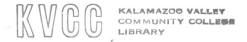

Reprinted, May 1964

Reprinted, March 1965

Reprinted, January 1966

Reprinted, January 1967

Second Edition, 1968

Reprinted, February 1969

Reprinted, February, 1970

Reprinted, February, 1971

Reprinted, January 1972

Third Edition, 1974

Library of Congress Catalog Card Number: 73-94395

Cloth: 0-8151-6702-4   Paper: 0-8151-6703-2

Preface to the Third Edition

THE RESPONSE of medical students and graduate students in the medical sciences to the first and second editions of this monograph has been gratifying to the author. Moreover, the book seems to have found a receptive audience abroad, for it has now been translated into Italian, French, German, Japanese and Spanish. In Madison Avenue jargon, "It seems we have been doing something right." This third edition continues in the tradition of the first two. Some errors have been corrected and some material has been added, most notably on glomerular hemodynamics, on the site of the glomerular filtration barrier, on the mechanism of amino acid reabsorption, on the buffering of acid by bone, on renal tubular acidosis, and on the mechanism and control of ammonia secretion. Two sections have been added on clinical problems: the intact nephron hypothesis and the trade-off hypothesis; I have done so not because I consider myself at all qualified as a clinical nephrologist, but because of my interest in the physiologic implications. Finally, a new chapter on renal metabolism—a somewhat neglected field—has been added, in the hope that it will stimulate future work in this area. As in the second edition, Erich E. Windhager has revised Chapter 7, Mechanisms of Reabsorption and Excretion of Ions and Water.

I would advise the beginning student to read the following Preface to the First Edition, because it contains factual material not covered elsewhere in the text and because it more or less sets the stage for the ensuing discussion of renal functions.

R.F.P.

Preface to the First Edition

MORE THAN 100 years ago, Claude Bernard pointed out that the medium in which we exist is not the atmosphere which surrounds us but the blood and tissue fluids which bathe our muscles, glands and brain. He described this internal environment as a cosmos, elaborately isolated from and protected from the vicissitudes of the external world by a variety of physiological devices which operate to preserve and stabilize its physical properties, chemical constitution and volume. The partial pressures of oxygen and carbon dioxide, the concentrations of nutrients and wastes, the temperature, the hydrogen ion concentration, the osmotic pressure, the concentrations of the several cations and anions, and the volume of this internal fluid environment are all precisely maintained within narrow limits of normal.

The kidneys play a prominent role in regulating the concentration of metabolic wastes, and the osmotic pressure, the volume and the ionic composition of our internal environment. Claude Bernard argued that we have achieved a free and independent life, mentally and physically, by becoming relatively independent of our external environment. It may therefore be claimed, with some justification, that our present high station in the animal kingdom ultimately depends on our kidneys.

The kidneys are commonly described as excretory organs, but the assignment of such a limited role scarcely does them justice. They are primarily organs which regulate volume and composition of the internal fluid environment; their excretory function is incidental to their regulatory function. Primacy of regulatory function may be illustrated as follows: Consider two persons—one with normal renal function, the other a patient with long-standing, chronic, bilateral renal disease. Suppose both individuals ingest identical diets, containing 70 Gm of protein, 250 Gm of carbohydrate and 100 Gm of fat (2,200 Cal). Suppose each diet contains 5 Gm of sodium chloride, 2 Gm of potassium and 1 Gm each of phosphorus and sulfur; suppose fluid intakes are equal and generous. How, then, will the compositions of the urine of these two individuals differ? The answer is: they will not differ.

Each person will excrete per day 12 Gm of nitrogen, 5 Gm of sodium chloride, 2 Gm of potassium and 1 Gm each of phosphorus and sulfur. If fluid intake is high, the urine volumes will be the same. True, the patient with chronic renal disease may excrete a little protein, some red blood cells and casts, but the major excretory products will be the same.

Why, then, is the physician concerned about the patient with chronic renal disease? The answer is: the diseased kidney is deficient in its capacity to regulate the composition and, to a lesser extent, the volume of the internal fluid environment. The patient with renal disease will excrete each day 12 Gm of urea nitrogen derived from the 70 Gm of dietary protein exactly as does the normal individual, but the plasma urea nitrogen concentration may be 100–150 mg per 100 ml, rather than the normal 10–15 mg per 100 ml. The patient will excrete 2 Gm (51 mEq) of potassium, but the plasma concentration may be 5–8 mEq per liter, instead of the normal 4 mEq per liter. The plasma concentrations of phosphate and sulfate may increase some 3–6 fold; that of calcium may be low. If salt or fluid intake is restricted, continued excretion may rapidly deplete salt and water reserves, leading to a far greater reduction in volume and to a much greater distortion of composition of the internal fluid environment than that suffered by a normal person. Salt restriction alone may lead to hyponatremia (reduced sodium concentration of the blood) and to a reduction in osmotic pressure of the body fluids. Metabolic acidosis gradually develops as a consequence of progressive failure of the mechanisms which regulate the bicarbonate concentration of extracellular fluid.

When, as a consequence of the inexorable progress of renal disease, of some added regulatory burden or of some intercurrent infection which precipitates renal failure, the regulatory capacities of the kidneys become so compromised that the composition and volume of the internal fluid environment deviate markedly from normal, vital organs fail and the individual succumbs. The success of the physician in prolonging the life and useful existence of the patient with chronic renal disease is in proportion to his ability to stay the progress of the disease and to his skill in helping the patient compensate for his renal regulatory deficiencies. Unfortunately, at present no specific therapy is available for the treatment of bilateral chronic renal disease. Regeneration of damaged renal tissue does not occur, and restoration of function by renal transplantation is successful only when the donor and recipient are immunologically similar.

The purpose of this volume is to describe the basic renal mechanisms of glomerular ultrafiltration, tubular reabsorption and tubular secretion; to clarify the operation of these mechanisms in the regulation of volume and composition of the internal fluid environment; and to provide a basis for an appreciation of the consequences of renal diseases and of the principles involved in therapy.

I am indebted to Miss Michelena Perrotta and Miss Sally Aleks for typing the manuscript, to Miss Jeannette de Haas and Mrs. Martha MacLeod for assistance in preparing the figures, and to Drs. Gerhard Giebisch and Richard Kessler for criticizing portions of the manuscript. I am also indebted to authors and publishers who permitted the reproduction of figures and data.

R.F.P.

Table of Contents

1

Anatomy of the Kidney

Gross Morphology of the Kidney

THE KIDNEYS are paired, somewhat flattened, bean-shaped organs, which lie retroperitoneally on either side of the vertebral column against the posterior abdominal wall. Together they weigh about 300 Gm and thus constitute 0.4% of the weight of the body. They are embedded in a mass of fat and loose areolar tissue. The upper pole of the right kidney rests on the 12th rib; that of the left kidney, on the 11th and 12th ribs. Each kidney lies posteriorly against the diaphragm, lateral lumbocostal arch, psoas major, quadratus lumborum and the tendon of the transversus abdominis (1).

The renal artery and nerves enter, and the renal vein, lymphatics and ureter leave, the kidney through the hilus, a longitudinal slit occupying somewhat less than the middle third of the medial border of the organ. The hilus opens into a more extensive but shallow and flattened C-shaped space, the renal sinus (Fig. 1–1), completely surrounded by kidney tissue. The renal sinus is largely occupied by the renal pelvis and its connecting major and minor calices. The chinks are filled with loose areolar and adipose tissue, through which course the renal vessels and nerves. The kidney is invested by a tough, collagenous and nearly indistensible capsule, loosely adherent to the underlying glandular tissue, from which it can be easily stripped. The capsule is reflected into the sinus through the hilus. The outer layer of this reflected area is anchored to blood vessels and the pelvis, and the inner layer forms a lining for the sinus.

The walls of the sinus are studded with

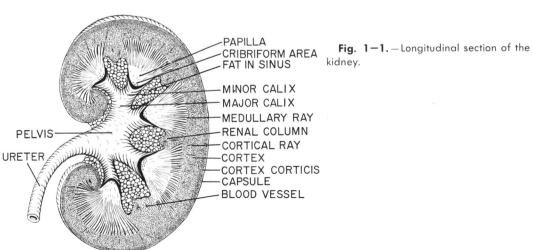

PAPILLA
CRIBRIFORM AREA
FAT IN SINUS

MINOR CALIX
MAJOR CALIX
MEDULLARY RAY
RENAL COLUMN
CORTICAL RAY
CORTEX
CORTEX CORTICIS
CAPSULE
BLOOD VESSEL

PELVIS
URETER

Fig. 1–1. — Longitudinal section of the kidney.

1

conical elevations, the renal papillae, which average 8–10 in number, although as many as 18 may be present. The papillae are flattened cones, 7–10 mm in height, with elliptical bases. The apex of each papilla—the cribriform area—is pierced by 18–24 minute orifices, barely visible to the naked eye; these are the openings of the papillary ducts of Bellini, which in turn are formed by the terminal fusion of many collecting ducts.

Each papilla is thrust into a terminal extension of the renal pelvis, a minor calix (Gr. *kalyx* = cup). Urine flowing from the orifices of the ducts of Bellini enters a minor calix, flows on into either the superior or the inferior major calix, and then flows into the renal pelvis and finally out, via the ureter, to the urinary bladder. The walls of the calices, pelvis and ureter contain smooth muscle, which contracts rhythmically and propels the urine along its course in peristaltic spurts.

The kidney of man is a multilobed organ. Each renal lobe is a pyramidal mass of tissue, the base forming the surface of the kidney, the apex forming the papilla. In the fetal kidney, lobulation is evident on the surface; but, in the adult kidney, fusion is so complete that no traces of external lobular markings persist. In insectivores and rodents, the entire kidney can be considered to be a single lobe, ending in a single papilla. The kidney of the dog is much like that of man, giving, on the surface, no evidence of its lobular structure. However, many mammals retain in their adult form the surface lobulation seen in the fetal human kidney.

The cortex, which is reddish brown in color, not only forms the shell of the kidney but also dips down between adjacent pyramids toward the renal sinus; these inward extensions are known as the columns of Bertin. The outermost layer of the cortex is finely granular, whereas the deeper portions are marked by radially arranged columns—medullary rays—extending outward from the pyramids. The uniform granularity of the outer cortex corticis is attributable to the fact that it is made up solely of highly convoluted proximal and distal tubules, which lie randomly in all planes. The radial columns of the deeper cortex are composed of straight segments of proximal and distal tubules, collecting ducts and blood vessels. Glomeruli are scattered throughout the granular cortex between the medullary rays but are absent from the outermost cortex corticis.

The medullary pyramids exhibit a fanlike striation, the rays of the fan spreading outward from the tips of the papillae, through the medulla proper, to penetrate the deeper layers of the cortex. The striation is attributable to the parallel course of loops of Henle and blood vessels. The color of the pyramids shades from reddish brown at the corticomedullary junction to gray-brown at the tips of the papillae. Often an outer zone of the medulla, made up of an outer and an inner stripe, and an inner zone, the papilla proper, can be distinguished. The differentiation of outer and inner stripe depends on the relative proportions of thick and thin limbs of Henle's loops. The only tubular elements of the inner zone are thin limbs of Henle's loops.

Gross Vascular Supply of the Kidney

Commonly, each kidney is supplied with blood by a single renal artery (Fig. 1–2), which arises from the abdominal aorta just below the superior mesenteric and middle suprarenal arteries. Either just before or just after entering the hilus, each renal artery divides into a series of branches, which pass dorsal and ventral to the pelvis through the arcolar and adiposc tissue of the sinus. The branches in the anterior group are the more numerous and supply some two thirds of the kidney. These arterial branches pass between the calices and penetrate the parenchyma between the pyramids. Within the parenchyma, these arteries are called interlobar, because they course between the lobes or pyramids.

At the junction of cortex and medulla, the interlobar arteries bend over the bases of the pyramids to form a series of incomplete arches, the arciform arteries. Interlobular arteries arise at right angles from the arciform arteries and run radially toward the periphery in the cortical medullary rays. In their course

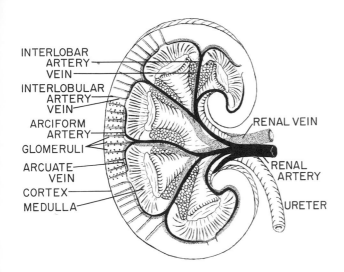

INTERLOBAR
ARTERY
VEIN
INTERLOBULAR
ARTERY
VEIN
ARCIFORM
ARTERY
GLOMERULI
ARCUATE
VEIN
CORTEX
MEDULLA
RENAL VEIN
RENAL
ARTERY
URETER

Fig. 1—2.—Gross morphology of the renal circulation.

through the cortex, they give rise to short lateral branches, the afferent arterioles, each of which supplies a glomerulus. Certain of these interlobular arteries continue through the cortex corticis to supply the capsule; some anastomose with the arterial supply of the perirenal fat and areolar tissue.

The pattern of the major venous drainage of the kidney corresponds in general to that of the arterial supply. Interlobular veins arise on the surface in stellate sinuses, which receive capillaries from the cortex corticis. These veins penetrate the cortex, receive additional cortical venules and the ascending venae rectae from the medulla, and join the arcuate veins, which arch over the bases of the pyramids. The arcuate veins form complete, or true, arches and anastomose freely. Interlobar veins drain the arcuate veins and emerge from the renal parenchyma in the columns of Bertin. In the sinus, they assemble to form the renal veins, which join the vena cava.

The details of the glomerular and peritubular capillary circulations are best considered along with the morphology of the nephron.

Microscopic Structure, Vascular Supply and Innervation of the Nephron

NEPHRON.—In man, each kidney is composed of 1–1¼ million units, all basically similar in structure and presumably also grossly similar in function. Each unit, which is termed a nephron (Fig. 1–3), consists of a renal, or malpighian, corpuscle (glomerulus and Bowman's capsule), a proximal convoluted tubule, a loop of Henle and a distal convoluted tubule (all described below). Many nephrons deliver their contents into each collecting duct, and in turn several collecting ducts join to empty through a duct of Bellini into a renal calix.

By definition, the morphologic unit, the nephron, excludes the collecting duct, for its embryologic origin differs from that of the remainder of the tubule. Until recently, the collecting duct was thought to play a passive role in urine formation; i.e., it was considered to serve only as a urinary conduit. Now it is known that it is involved in the processes of concentrating the urine, regulating acid-base balance, secreting potassium ions and salvaging sodium ions more or less completely from the urine in states of sodium depletion. Thus, because its role is allied with and complementary to that of the remainder of the tubule, the collecting duct should be included as a part of the nephron in a functional definition of the renal unit.

BOWMAN'S CAPSULE.—The nephron has its origin in the expanded blind end of the uriniferous tubule, termed Bowman's capsule, which together with its contained capillary tuft constitutes the renal corpuscle. The outer, fibrous layer of Bowman's capsule is

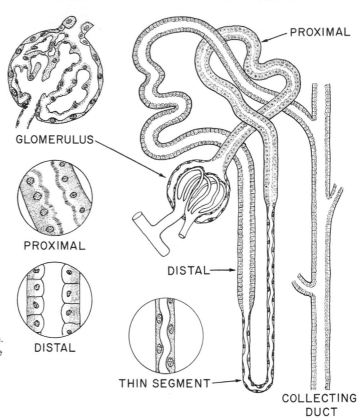

GLOMERULUS

PROXIMAL

DISTAL

PROXIMAL

DISTAL

THIN SEGMENT

COLLECTING DUCT

Fig. 1—3. — Relationship of component parts of the nephron. (Adapted from Smith, H. W.: *The Kidney* [New York: Oxford University Press, 1935].)

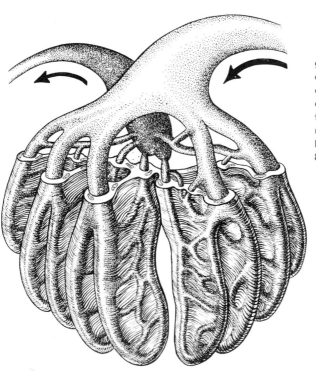

Fig. 1—4. — Anatomy of the glomerulus, illustrating the arrangement of capillary lobules derived from the expanded chamber of the afferent arteriole. The lower section illustrates the foldings of the glomerular basement membrane. (From Elias, H., Hossman, A., Barth, I. B., and Solmar, A. J.. Urology 83:790, 1960.)

continuous with the basement membrane of the tubule. Similarly, the flattened epithelial lining of Bowman's capsule is continuous with the cuboidal epithelium of the tubule. The renal corpuscles of man have an average diameter of 100 μ and, when engorged with blood, are just visible to the naked eye.

GLOMERULUS. – On the side opposite its attachment to the proximal convoluted tubule, Bowman's capsule is invaginated by a lobulated tuft of capillaries, the glomerulus* (Fig. 1–4). The basement membrane of the capsule is reflected over the capillary loops to form the much attenuated capillary basement membrane. It is also fused with the adventitia of the afferent arteriole supplying the glomerulus and of the efferent arteriole draining it. The epithelial lining of the capsule, where it is reflected over the capillary loops, forms the highly specialized podocyte layer of the capillary wall (see p. 55). The glomerulus nearly fills Bowman's capsule. Only small clefts remain, through which the filtrate expressed through the capillary walls flows into the tubular lumen (2).

As the afferent arteriole enters Bowman's capsule, it expands into a relatively wide chamber, which branches into 5–8 trunks. Each of these trunks subdivides, the subdivisions of each trunk constituting a separate glomerular lobule. In all, some 20–40 capillary loops are grouped into 5–8 or more lobules. Numerous anastomoses join the loops within a given lobule. The loops successively recombine to form the emergent efferent arteriole. The afferent and efferent arterioles, by virtue of the contractility of the smooth muscle elements encircling their lumens, constitute variable resistances to the flow of blood through the glomerular tuft and through the postglomerular peritubular capillaries. The cellular elements of the media and adventitia of the afferent arteriole become more numerous and modified in form and in staining properties as the vessel enters

Bowman's capsule. These juxtaglomerular cells form a thickened cuff around the afferent arteriole known as the polar cuff or polkissen (Ger. *Polkissen* = pole cushion). A specialized segment of the distal tubule of that same nephron, known as the macula densa, is closely applied to the polkissen. Together, these two structures are termed the juxtaglomerular apparatus. The granular cells of the polkissen probably play an endocrine role, in that they appear to be the source of renin, an enzyme that splits an α_2 globulin of plasma to produce a powerful blood-borne vasoconstrictor. According to some, the macula densa is a sensing organ that responds to the sodium concentration of the urine in the distal tubule and controls the output of renin from its associated polar cuff (see section, Autoregulation of Renal Circulation, p. 167).

PROXIMAL TUBULE. – The proximal tubule is joined to Bowman's capsule by a short connecting segment. The tubule coils extensively in the neighborhood of the parent renal corpuscle, as the pars convoluta, and then enters a cortical medulla ray to penetrate the deeper layers of the cortex and outer medulla to a variable depth, as the pars recta. Throughout its length, the proximal tubule is composed of a single layer of cuboidal or truncated pyramidal cells resting on an enveloping basement membrane. The basement membrane is, no doubt, largely a supporting structure, although it is necessary for the proper organization of regenerating tubular cells following chemical or ischemic damage. This membrane must be permeable to water and solutes, for they traverse it in the course of reabsorption from tubular lumen into peritubular capillaries.

The proximal tubular cells are coarsely granular; their nuclei are large and basally located. The apical surfaces of the cells bulge into the tubular lumen, nearly obliterating its cavity and giving it an irregular contour. These surfaces are covered with numerous cytoplasmic filaments about 1 μ in length, which form the nonmotile brush border. The basal aspects of the cells exhibit a striated

---

*The term glomerulus is often used interchangeably with "renal corpuscle" to include the capillary tuft and Bowman's capsule. Properly, it refers only to the capillary tuft.

appearance, owing to the linear disposition of the mitochondria in narrow channels between multiple infoldings of the cell membrane. Adjacent cells are held together by basal trabecular projections, which interlock, and by terminal bars, which seal the chinks between adjacent luminal surfaces. The brush border, the coarse granularity of the cytoplasm and the basal striations, although present throughout the proximal segment, are less evident in the pars recta than in the pars convoluta.

HENLE'S LOOP. — The loop of Henle includes the descending thick limb, already described as the pars recta of the proximal tubule; the descending and ascending thin limbs; and the ascending thick limb, to be described below as a part of the pars recta of the distal tubule. The extent of loop development varies with the position of the renal corpuscle in the cortex. The nephrons that have renal corpuscles lying in the outer two thirds of the cortex (cortical nephrons) have relatively short loops. Some of these nephrons lie entirely within the cortex and have no thin segments at all. Others have loops that penetrate the medulla to varying depths; these generally have short thin segments. The nephrons that have renal corpuscles lying in the inner third of the cortex (juxtamedullary nephrons) have relatively long loops. The thin segments of some of these loops extend to the tips of the papillae. All intergrades of loop length are to be found in the human kidney, although cortical nephrons are much more numerous than juxtamedullary nephrons (ratio approximately 7:1).

In various species of mammals, the numbers of nephrons with long loops and the lengths of loop in proportion to total nephron length correlate well with capacity to form concentrated urine. Certain desert rodents that complete their life span without water, other than that present in relatively dry seeds and derived from the metabolism of fat, protein and carbohydrate, have only nephrons with loops that are very long in proportion to nephron length.

The hairpin configuration of the loop of Henle (i.e., descending and ascending limbs lying in close approximation) was once considered to be solely of morphogenic significance. The two ends of the tubule are fixed early in development — one end by its vascular attachment at the glomerulus, the other by its junction with the collecting duct. Growth at the two ends gives rise to the proximal and distal convolutions. Growth in the middle, along the axis of the pyramid, forms the hairpin loop of Henle. Although a morphogenic significance is not denied, a functional significance related to the concentration of urine is now accorded the hairpin configuration and the resultant countercurrent flow of fluid — toward the papilla in the descending limb, away from the papilla in the ascending limb (see pp. 124–135).

The thin segment of the loop of Henle arises abruptly from the descending thick segment of the loop, the pars recta of the proximal tubule. The diameter of its lumen is less than that of either the proximal or the distal segment. The cells are flattened and thin except in the nuclear region, which bulges into the lumen. The cytoplasm is clear, with only a few scattered mitochondria and granules. The cell borders are serrated and interdigitated, meshing together as the cogs of gear wheels. The thin segment may be confined to the descending limb of Henle's loop or may form the bend of the loop and continue for a variable distance up the ascending limb. As noted above, some nephrons of the human kidney have no thin segments at all.

DISTAL TUBULE. — The distal tubule arises abruptly from the thin segment as the thick ascending limb of Henle's loop. It continues in a nearly straight course to the region of the parent renal corpuscle, in the neighborhood of which it convolutes. The cells of the pars recta are cuboidal; those of the cortical convolutions are more columnar. In the region where the distal tubule makes contact with the afferent arteriole of the parent renal corpuscle, the cells are high, columnar and densely packed, forming a plaque called the macula densa. The cells of the distal tubule lack a brush border, but they exhibit basal striation similar to that of the proximal tubular cells and due, as in the case of the proximal cells, to the accumulation of mitochondria in channels created by the infolding of the cell membrane. The distal tubule is shorter than the proximal tubule, and its convolutions are less complex. The distal tubule connects with a collecting duct through an arcade or transition segment made up of dark granular cells, presumably of distal tubular origin, intermixed with clear duct cells.

COLLECTING DUCT. — The collecting duct, formed in the outer cortex by the junction of two or more transition segments of distal tubules, receives additional contributions in its course through the outer and inner cortex. In the medulla, several collecting ducts fuse to form one of the many papillary ducts that drain into a minor calix. The cells making up the collecting ducts are cuboidal, sparsely granular and regular in size. The nuclei are round and uniformly placed within the cells. Cell boundaries are definite.

DIMENSIONS OF RENAL TUBULES IN MAN. — The proximal segments are 12–24 mm long; the thin limbs of Henle's loops, 0–14 mm; the ascending thick limbs of Henle's loops, 6–18 mm; and the distal convoluted segments, 2–9 mm. The total lengths of nephrons, excluding the collecting ducts, are 20–44 mm. The average length of the collecting ducts is 22 mm.

The external diameters of the proximal tubules are 50–65 μ; of the thin limbs of Henle's loops, 14–22 μ; of the distal tubules, 20–50 μ; and of the collecting ducts, as much as 200 μ in their terminal portions, the ducts of Bellini. Proximal tubules make up the bulk of the renal parenchyma (3, 4).

VASCULAR SUPPLY OF TUBULES. — The vascular supply of the tubules is essentially portal, the blood that perfuses the peritubular capillaries having initially traversed the glomerular capillaries. However, branches of afferent arterioles of cortical glomeruli feeding directly into the cortical capillary net are occasionally observed; and, similarly, direct connections between afferent arterioles of juxtamedullary glomeruli and the vascular loops descending into the medulla and papilla have been described. Nevertheless, any direct arteriolar supply of peritubular capillaries is insignificant in the normal kidney. In aged persons, and especially in patients with chronic renal disease, the number of anastomotic connections between preglomerular arterioles and peritubular capillaries is increased. Many of these connections result from the persistence of a single capillary loop in an otherwise degenerate glomerulus, the loop undergoing transformation into an arteriolar-like structure.

VASCULAR SUPPLY OF CORTICAL NEPHRONS. — The vascular supply of the cortical nephrons is quite different from that of the juxtamedullary nephrons (Fig. 1–5). In the cortical nephrons, the efferent glomerular arteriole, which is slightly smaller than the afferent, breaks up immediately into a rich, freely anastomosing network of capillaries that envelops the convolutions of proximal and distal tubules, and the cortical reaches of the ascending and descending thick limbs of Henle's loops and collecting ducts. The capillary net derived from one glomerulus communicates so freely with that of adjacent nephrons that no distinction is possible. The postglomerular blood is therefore widely disseminated among a group of nephrons. The capillary net recombines into venules that enter the interlobular veins.

VASCULAR SUPPLY OF JUXTAMEDULLARY NEPHRONS. — The juxtamedullary nephrons have a more complex vascular supply than that of the cortical nephrons. In the juxtamedullary nephrons, the diameter of the efferent glomerular arteriole is equal to or larger than that of the afferent arteriole. It gives off one or more side branches, which supply a capillary net enveloping the cortical convolutions of proximal and distal tubules — a net entirely analogous to that of the above-described network of cortical nephrons. The unique feature of the juxtamedullary circulation is the medullary blood supply, derived from the repeated branching of the descending efferent arteriole in the py-

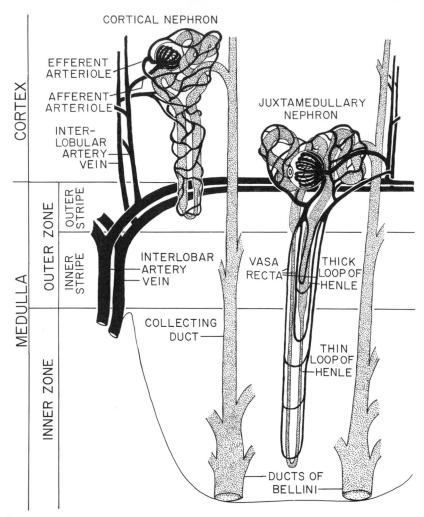

Fig. 1—5.—Comparison of the blood supplies of cortical and juxtamedullary nephrons.

ramid. These vessels are straight-bore tubes that follow the descending limbs of Henle's loops through the medulla and papilla, turn at the bend of the loop and return to reassemble into a venule that enters an interlobular vein close to its junction with an arcuate vein. The arrangement of descending and ascending limbs of these vasa recta (arteriolae rectae) is that of a countercurrent hairpin loop. The function of the medullary vascular loops as countercurrent exchangers is described on pages 130–131.

Lymphatic network.—A rich lymphatic network drains the cortex; no such network is found in the medulla and papilla. Two basic plexuses exist. One, subcapsular, drains the outer cortex and freely anastomoses with a perinephric system in the fat and areolar tissue surrounding the kidney. The other drains the deeper cortex through a series of channels, which follow the interlobular, arcuate and interlobar vessels and leave the kidney at the hilus. Both systems drain into lateral aortic nodes. Renal lymph from the subcapsular plexus has been studied; that from the hilar lymphatics has received less attention. The role of the lymphatic system in renal function is largely undetermined, but it is probably of minor significance.

Nerve supply.—The kidney is richly

supplied with thoracolumbar sympathetic nerve fibers derived from the fourth dorsal segment to the fourth lumbar segment. No vagal innervation has been demonstrated. Afferent fibers from the capsule, from the renal pelvis and perhaps also from the renal parenchyma have been identified. Afferent and efferent fibers course through the splanchnic nerves and the aortic and renal plexuses and follow the renal vessels to their terminations in smooth muscle of afferent and efferent arterioles and between renal tubular cells. These latter terminations are most numerous in the proximal tubules. The sympathetic vasomotor supply is largely, if not entirely, vasoconstrictor in function. The role of the parenchymal innervation is uncertain, but some investigators believe that sympathetic impulses to tubular cells enhance the reabsorption of sodium and water. Because of the very significant vasomotor responses that result from excitation of renal nerves and from renal denervation in anesthetized animals, direct tubular responses to nerve impulses have not been clearly demonstrated. Many believe them to be nonexistent — a view which the author shares.

Summary

The kidney is a compound tubular organ made up of a large number of similar units — nephrons — operating in parallel. Each nephron is functionally defined as consisting of a renal corpuscle, a proximal convoluted tubule, a loop of Henle, a distal convoluted tubule and a multibranched collecting duct that is common to and drains a number of units. Although embryologically not a part of the nephron, the collecting duct is involved in the elaboration of urine; hence, functionally it must be considered the terminal part of the nephron. The blood that perfuses the glomerular capillary tuft is distributed to the tubules of the cortex by a richly anastomosing capillary net and to the tubules of the medulla and papilla by elongated recurrent capillary loops, the vasa recta. The tubular supply is portal in nature, for essentially all blood perfusing tubular capillaries is of postglomerular origin.

The features of renal architecture that are considered to have special functional significance* include the following:

1. Each segment of the renal tubule is long in proportion to its diameter. Diffusion from the center of the fluid stream to the luminal membrane, therefore, is not a factor that, ordinarily, limits tubular reabsorption.

2. The luminal surface area of the proximal tubule is greatly increased by the filamentous projections making up the brush border. Similarly, the basal surface area of both the proximal and the distal tubular cells is increased by infoldings of the basal cell membrane. Mitochondria are lodged in the channels between these infoldings, in intimate contact with the basal membrane. Processes depending on diffusion, as well as those depending on active secretory and reabsorptive transport by membrane carriers, are facilitated by the greatly expanded surfaces of the cells. The location of mitochondria between infoldings of the basal membrane suggests that they may provide energy for active transfers occurring in this region.

3. The loop of Henle, with countercurrent flow along opposed descending and ascending limbs, is a tubular segment specialized for multiplication of osmolar concentration in the medullary and papillary interstitium.

4. The collecting duct serves as an osmotic exchanger to translate hypertonicity of the medullary and papillary interstitium into urinary hypertonicity. (See pp. 125–129 for a discussion of the functions of loop and collecting duct in concentrating the urine.)

5. Blood is supplied to the glomerular capillary tufts by way of short, direct, wide-bore vessels, insuring a high filtration pressure.

6. The peritubular capillary system is a portal one, operating at low pressure. Because the proteins of blood plasma have been

---

*The author does not wish to imply that all structural features do not have functional significance. Rather, he wishes to point out that, with present knowledge, one can make only limited structural and functional correlations.

concentrated by expression of fluid in the glomerulus, the colloid osmotic pressure of peritubular blood is increased. Both factors favor the entry of reabsorbed fluid and solutes into the vascular system from the peritubular interstitial fluid. The loops of Henle are supplied by recurrent vascular loops, the vasa recta. Their countercurrent arrangement facilitates passive osmotic exchange and reduces the rate of loss of osmotically active particles from the medulla and papilla (see pp. 130–132).

7. The kidneys receive the greatest blood flow, in proportion to weight, of any organ of the body. At rest, renal blood flow amounts to 20–25% of cardiac output, yet the weight of the kidneys amounts to only 0.4% of the body weight. High flow is obviously related to the function of regulating the composition of the body fluids.

REFERENCES

1. Huber, G. C.: *Piersol's Human Anatomy* (9th ed.; Philadelphia: J. B. Lippincott Company, 1930).
2. Mueller, C. B., Mason, A. D., Jr., and Stout, D. G.: Anatomy of the glomerulus, Am. J. Med. 18:267, 1955.
3. Pai, H. C.: Dissections of nephrons from the human kidney, J. Anat. 69:344, 1935.
4. Maximow, A. A., and Bloom, W.: *A Textbook of Histology* (Philadelphia: W. B. Saunders Company, 1930).

2

Volume and Composition
of the Body Fluids

Body Water

WATER is, by far, the most abundant component of the human body, constituting 45–75% of body weight (1–6). Such a wide range among a number of persons might suggest that the water content of any one person is also variable. Actually, nothing could be further from the truth. Body weight, and hence water content, remains constant from day to day in the normal adult in caloric balance, despite marked fluctuations in water intake. The ingestion of an extra liter or more of water induces a brisk diuresis, and the excess fluid is eliminated within the brief span of 2–3 hours. Variability of body water in relation to body weight among a number of persons is largely a function of the amount of adipose tissue. Leanness is associated with a high fraction of body water; obesity, with a low fraction. Schloerb *et al.* (7), in a study of young adults, observed averages of 63% water in males and 52% in females—findings that are in accord with the greater development of subcutaneous adipose tissue in women. The highest proportion of water in relation to body weight is found in the infant—a fact that will come as no surprise to any mother.

Table 2–1 summarizes the percentage of water in various tissues, the proportion of the total weight of the body represented by each tissue and the total volume of water

TABLE 2–1.—DISTRIBUTION OF WATER AND PERCENTAGE OF BODY WEIGHT IN VARIOUS TISSUES OF A 70-KG MAN*

TISSUE	% WATER	% BODY WEIGHT	LITERS OF WATER PER 70 KG
Skin	72	18	9.07
Muscle	75.6	41.7	22.10
Skeleton	22	15.9	2.45
Brain	74.8	2.0	1.05
Liver	68.3	2.3	1.03
Heart	79.2	0.5	0.28
Lungs	79.0	0.7	0.39
Kidneys	82.7	0.4	0.25
Spleen	75.8	0.2	0.10
Blood	83.0	8.0	4.65
Intestine	74.5	1.8	0.94
Adipose tissue	10	±10.0	0.70

*From Skelton, H.: Arch. Int. Med. 40:140, 1927.

contained in each tissue in a relatively lean 70-kg man (8). As the table indicates, most of the water of the body is present in skin and muscle, and the skeleton and adipose tissue contain the least in relation to weight. Because progressive expansion of the fat stores of the body results in little increase in water content, the percentage of water decreases with gain in weight.

Body Fluid Compartments

DISTRIBUTION

The water of the body can be considered as distributed among three compartments: an extracellular, an intracellular and a trans-

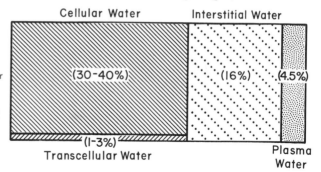

TOTAL BODY WATER
(50 – 70 % of Body Weight)

Fig. 2–1. — Distribution of water in the body. (From Pitts, R. F.: *The Physiological Basis of Diuretic Therapy* [Springfield, Ill.: Charles C Thomas, Publisher, 1959].)

cellular compartment (depicted diagrammatically in Fig. 2–1).

EXTRACELLULAR FLUID. — The extracellular fluid includes the blood plasma, 4.5% of body weight; the interstitial fluid, 16% of body weight; and the lymph, about 2% of body weight. Plasma circulates rapidly in the vascular compartment, whereas interstitial fluid seeps more slowly through tissue interstices. Plasma proteins that leak through capillary walls and excess interstitial fluid are returned to the vascular compartment by lymphatic vessels. Flow is sluggish, and the volume of the lymphatic compartment given above is only a rough estimate.

More than a century ago, Claude Bernard (9) pointed out that interstitial fluid constitutes the true environment of the body, in that it bathes all tissue cells, supplies their nutriments and removes their wastes. Water and solutes, with the exception of proteins and lipids, exchange rapidly across the single-layered endothelium that makes up the capillary wall and separates the vascular from the interstitial compartment. Because diffusion distances are small, minor concentration gradients between blood plasma and interstitial fluid are adequate to supply the nutrients used and to remove the wastes produced by cells.

INTRACELLULAR FLUID. — Intracellular fluid is neither a continuous nor a homogeneous phase; rather, it represents the sum of the fluid contents of all of the cells of the body. Because such diverse cells as erythrocytes, muscle cells and renal tubular cells vary in water content and chemical constitution scarcely less than they do in structure, it is evident that representation of a single cellular compartment, such as that depicted in Figure 2–1, not only is a gross oversimplification but is quite misleading. Somewhat more than half of the total body water is contained in cells, and intracellular water constitutes 30–40% of body weight.

TRANSCELLULAR FLUID. — The transcellular fluid is a specialized fraction of extracellular fluid. It includes cerebrospinal, intraocular, pleural, peritoneal and synovial fluids and the digestive secretions. (The last-named could, in fact, be considered extracorporeal fluid, insofar as these secretions are contained in the open-ended digestive tract.) The common factor that sets the transcellular fluids apart from extracellular fluid is that each of the several discontinuous fractions is separated from blood plasma not only by the capillary endothelium but also by a continuous layer of epithelial cells. These epithelial cell layers modify the composition of the transcellular fluids with respect to extracellular fluid in varying degree. With the exception of the digestive secretions, their volumes are insignificant fractions of body weight. In man, digestive secretions in the fasting state represent only 1–3% of body weight; in herbivorous animals, they may amount to as much as 6%.

MEASUREMENT OF BODY FLUID COMPARTMENTS

The total body water and the volumes of the plasma and extracellular fluid compartments can be measured in man with varying degrees of precision by dilution technics. Interstitial water is calculated as the difference between extracellular water and plasma water. Intracellular water is calculated as the difference between total body water and extracellular water. The latter two calculated volumes are subject to the sum of the errors and uncertainties of the measurements of the component volumes. The principles of measurement of all volumes are the same. However, the properties of the substance used in measuring a specific volume must be such as to insure uniform distribution of the substance throughout, and its confinement within, that volume.

If one had a large beaker containing an unknown volume of water and wished to measure it without resorting to the simple expedient of pouring it into a graduated cylinder, one could proceed as follows: Add 10 mg of a dye, such as Evans blue; stir well to insure thorough mixing; remove a few milliliters; and measure the concentration colorimetrically. If the concentration is 0.0015 mg/ml, then

measuring fluid compartments are excreted; some are slowly destroyed, whereas others are incorporated into body constituents. Under any circumstance, it is necessary to subtract from the amount administered that which is removed, in one way or another, from the equilibrium mixture.

TOTAL BODY WATER. – The drug antipyrine can be used in the measurement of total body water. It is distributed evenly throughout all of the water of the body; i.e., it diffuses readily across cell membranes, is not specifically bound to any cellular or extracellular component and is present in the same concentration in all of the water of the body. Antipyrine is, however, slowly excreted and also slowly metabolized. Two isotopes of water – deuterium oxide (D_2O) and tritiated water (HTO) – are also used in the measurement of total body water. In body fluids, D_2O is quantified in terms of its effect on the specific gravity of water, using an extremely sensitive method involving the rate of fall of a precisely measured drop through an organic solvent. HTO is quantified by measuring the radioactivity of tritium. Because tritium is an extremely weak beta-emitter, it is commonly measured by liquid scintillation methods. Within limits, D_2O and HTO become distributed in the body exactly like

$$\text{Volume} = \frac{\text{Quantity of dye}}{\text{Concentration of dye}} = \frac{10 \text{ mg}}{0.0015 \text{ mg/ml}} = 6,666 \text{ ml}$$

It is evident that the measurement will be valid only if the dye is thoroughly mixed and only if all of it remains within the volume to be measured. Accordingly, the general equation applicable to in vivo measurements of volume is as follows:

water. Both isotopes are excreted in urine, feces and expired air, and they are evaporated through the skin in proportion to their concentrations relative to the concentration of water. Deuterium and tritium also replace hydrogen in certain compounds that contain

$$\text{Volume of distribution} = \frac{\text{Quantity administered} - \text{Quantity excreted}}{\text{Concentration}}$$

Various modifications of procedure enable one to correct for excretion or metabolism, or for both. All of the substances used in

exchangeable hydrogen atoms. Both isotopes are incorporated into newly synthesized body constituents. However, over the interval required for the equilibration of D_2O or HTO with body water, these errors are insignificant.

As an example of the use of such methods in measuring total body water, let us inject 100 ml of D_2O as isotonic saline solution intravenously into a normal man weighing 90 kg. After an equilibration period of 2 hours, a blood sample is drawn and the plasma is separated and analyzed. The D_2O concentration is found to be 0.2 volumes per cent (vol%) of the plasma water; i.e., 0.200 ml/100 ml, or 0.002 ml/ml. During the equilibration period, urinary, respiratory and cutaneous losses have been found to average 0.4% of the administered dose. Substituting these values in the general equation,

$$\text{Volume of distribution} = \frac{(100 - 0.4)}{0.002} = \frac{99.6}{0.002} = 49,800 \text{ ml}$$

Our subject weighs 90 kg; therefore body water constitutes $49.8/90 \times 100 = 55.3\%$ of body weight.

Although the analysis of D_2O or HTO is accurate within $\pm 1 - 2\%$, the over-all accuracy of the determination of total body water is appreciably less. Accordingly, changes in water content are most precisely and most easily measured in terms of changes in body weight. An accurate set of bed scales is an extremely useful and precise instrument with which to follow the state of hydration of a patient during therapy.

PLASMA VOLUME. — The plasma volume is measured as the volume of distribution of a substance confined within the vascular bed. For such measurement, Evans blue and radioiodinated human serum albumin (RISA) are in common use today. Evans blue binds tightly to the subject's own plasma albumin, whereas iodine-131 is administered precombined with albumin. In either instance, the volume of distribution of the administered substance is that of plasma albumin. To whatever degree albumin escapes from the vascular bed or is metabolized during the course of equilibration, the plasma volume will be overestimated.

Two procedures are in common use.

1. Dye or RISA is injected intravenously at zero time; after 10 minutes, a blood sample is drawn, and the separated plasma is analyzed for the tag — colorimetrically for Evans blue or by scintillation methods for RISA. During this interval, the tag is uniformly distributed throughout the vascular compartment, and loss from the compartment is negligible.

2. Actually, if one follows the plasma concentration of Evans blue or RISA at intervals for a period of 1 hour or more, concentration is observed to decrease at first sharply and then more slowly. Plotted semilogarithmically, the relationship between concentration and time becomes linear after 10 – 15 minutes (Fig. 2 – 2). The slope of the curve is such as to indicate a clearance from the plasma of 4 – 6% of the remaining tag per hour. If one extrapolates the linear segment of the curve to zero time, one obtains the volume of distribution, provided mixing occurred instantaneously and there has been no loss from the vascular bed. The second method is a bit more precise, although the 10-minute sample method is satisfactory. Plasma volume amounts, on an average, to 4.5% of body weight. Results with Evans blue and RISA are comparable, and a choice between the two tags depends solely on personal preference and the availability of equipment for measurement (10).

The plasma volume can also be estimated by measuring the volume of distribution of red cells tagged with radioactive phosphorus

Fig. 2–2. — Plasma concentration of dye as a function of time, following intravenous administration of Evans blue.

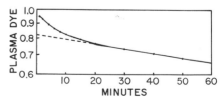

(^{32}P) or chromium (^{51}Cr). From the hematocrit, the plasma volume can be calculated. Strangely, the two methods do not agree precisely: the estimate of volume based on tagged red cells is less than that based on tagged albumin. The reason for the difference is this: The hematocrit of blood drawn from an artery or vein is higher than that of the blood in minute peripheral vessels. Because red cells and plasma must enter and leave tissues at the same rate, it follows that the volume of plasma in peripheral vessels must be greater than the volume of red cells and that the transit time of plasma from artery to vein must exceed that of red cells; i.e., plasma circulates slowly through tissue capillaries, and red cells circulate rapidly. The products of transit time and volume for plasma and for red cells must, of course, be equal. Direct microscopic observation of minute vessels indicates that red cells move rapidly in a narrow axial stream, whereas plasma flows slowly in a relatively wide peripheral cuff. The differences between plasma volumes measured by the two methods are not large; so, for practical purposes, either is satisfactory.

EXTRACELLULAR FLUID VOLUME.—The extracellular fluid volume is less precisely determinable than is total body water or plasma volume. A substance whose distribution is to be used to measure extracellular fluid must be sufficiently diffusible to cross capillary walls readily and enter the most distant reaches of cell interstices, and yet it must be absolutely excluded from cells. As a practical matter, the substance should be excreted slowly in comparison with the rate at which it distributes throughout the extracellular compartment. It must, of course, be nontoxic and must not itself alter the distribution of fluid. No such ideal substance is known. As a matter of fact, there is no exact agreement as to what should be included under the heading of extracellular volume. Should it include the water of bone, cerebrospinal fluid and other transcellular fluids, such as digestive secretions? Certain substances used in measuring extracellular fluid enter digestive secretions;

a fraction of some, including sodium and chloride, enters cells and is adsorbed on solids, such as bone and collagen.

The volumes of distribution of several substances that have been proposed as measures of extracellular fluid rank, in increasing order, as follows: inulin, raffinose, sucrose, mannitol, thiosulfate, radiosulfate, thiocyanate, radiochloride and radiosodium. Volumes of distribution range from 16% of body weight for inulin to more than 30% for radiosodium. However, according to Swan *et al.* (11), the volumes of distribution of mannitol, radiosulfate and thiosulfate are equal when measured simultaneously in nephrectomized dogs, and they average 22–23% of body weight. In dogs with normal renal function, the rates of excretion of mannitol and thiosulfate are so rapid in comparison with the rates of distribution that special technics are required if they are to be used in measuring extracellular fluid volume. In contrast, radiosulfate, when administered in tracer amounts, is slowly excreted, and its properties approach those of an ideal measuring substance. Sulfate enters cells, and is incorporated into cell constituents, very slowly. It does not enter transcellular fluids in significant amounts. Furthermore, it diffuses more rapidly and attains a more nearly complete distribution through tissue interstices than does inulin. The volume of distribution of radiosulfate is believed to equal plasma volume plus that fraction of the interstitial volume that is in ready diffusion equilibrium with plasma; but whether this volume is equal to the true anatomic extracellular space is unknown.

For measurement, a tracer dose of radiosulfate (^{35}SO$_4$) is administered intravenously. Blood samples are drawn at frequent intervals over a period of several hours, and the plasma is separated. Carrier sulfate is added; sulfate is precipitated as the barium salt; and ^{35}S is determined by means of a Geiger-Müller counter in a gas-flow chamber. Plasma concentrations are plotted semilogarithmically, as in Figure 2–2, and the linear portion of the curve is extrapolated back to zero time to obtain the plasma concentration that would have existed had mixing been instantaneous. Dividing this value into the dose administered gives the volume of distribution. Volume of distribution must be corrected for differences in water concentration of plasma ($\pm 6\%$ protein) and of interstitial fluid ($\pm 1\%$ protein) and for Donnan distribution of sulfate between fluids of differing protein content.

Figure 2–3 illustrates the method that must be employed to measure the volume of distribution of a substance, such as inulin, that is rapidly excreted (12). A priming dose of inulin is administered intravenously in an amount sufficient to raise plasma concentration to about 20 mg/100 ml. Inulin is infused to maintain constancy of plasma concentration. After an equilibration period of several hours, a series of blood samples is drawn and plasma concentration is measured precisely. When constancy of concentration is achieved, the bladder is evacuated and the infusion is stopped. All urine is collected for a period of 4–6 hours. During this interval, all of the inulin that was present in the body

at the time the infusion was stopped is excreted. Dividing the plasma concentration just prior to stopping the infusion into the quantity of inulin present in the body at that time (quantity excreted) gives the volume of distribution. Again, corrections must be applied for differences in protein content of plasma and interstitial fluids.

The volume of distribution of inulin is the lowest of any of the substances commonly employed in measuring extracellular fluid. Because of high molecular weight and the fact that the compound is not significantly metabolized in the body, inulin most probably does not enter cells. However, because the rate of diffusion is low, inulin may well be excluded from a fraction of the extracellular fluid measured by $^{35}SO_4$.

INTRACELLULAR FLUID VOLUME.—The volume of intracellular fluid cannot be measured directly; rather, it must be calculated as the difference between total body water and the volume of extracellular fluid. The uncertainties of both measurements, and especially that of extracellular volume, render any estimate of intracellular volume un-

Fig. 2–3. —Measurement of extracellular fluid volume by use of inulin.

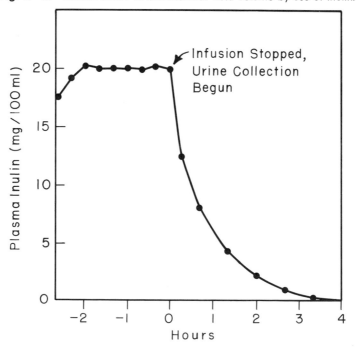

certain. The measurement of total body water includes extracellular, transcellular and intracellular water. That of extracellular volume may include all, some fraction of or none of the transcellular volume. Accordingly, the intracellular volume may be overestimated by whatever amount of transcellular fluid is excluded from measured extracellular fluid. The volume of intracellular fluid amounts to 30–40% of body weight.

INTERSTITIAL FLUID VOLUME.—The volume of interstitial fluid must be calculated as the difference between the volume of extracellular fluid and that of plasma. The uncertainty of its absolute value is as great as that of intracellular fluid. However, gross changes in interstitial fluid can be estimated with sufficient accuracy to yield useful information no matter which substance is used in measuring extracellular volume.

Body Fat

In the obese person, fat is a major component of the body, second in mass only to water. Even in a slender person, it constitutes an appreciable fraction of body weight. According to Behnke (13), the human body can be considered as made up of (1) functional tissue, which is the lean body mass, and (2) a variable amount of adipose or fat-storage tissue. Several methods are available for quantifying the fat stores of the body; those based on specific gravity, gaseous nitrogen solubility and total body water will be described briefly.

SPECIFIC GRAVITY.—On average, the lean body mass consists of 15% bone, with a specific gravity of 1.56; 10% structural lipid,* with a specific gravity of 0.94; and 75% cells, with a specific gravity of 1.06. Storage fat, like structural lipid, has a specific gravity of 0.94.

The specific gravity of the body as a whole can be determined by weighing the person in air and then in water (submerged). The differ-

*Structural lipid includes myelin, lecithin, cholesterol and other lipids essential in the body economy.

ence in weight is equal to the volume of water displaced. Weight in air divided by volume of water displaced is equal to specific gravity. The weight in water must be corrected for the residual air contained in the lungs. Extremely lean persons have body specific gravities as high as 1.099. The addition of 10%, 20% and 33% of excess storage fat reduces body specific gravity to 1.08, 1.062 and 1.036, respectively (Fig. 2–4).

NITROGEN SOLUBILITY.—Behnke has verified the relationship between body fat and specific gravity by measuring the gaseous nitrogen that can be washed out of the body on prolonged breathing of pure oxygen. Nitrogen is 5–6 times as soluble in fat as in the aqueous media of the body. From total body water, total body gaseous nitrogen and solubility of nitrogen in lipid and water, fat stores can be calculated.

TOTAL BODY WATER IN PROPORTION TO BODY WEIGHT.—Pace and Rathbun (14) have observed that the total water content of the body of various laboratory animals averages 73.2% of the lean body mass. Accordingly, the following equation holds:

Percentage of excess fat
$$= \frac{100 - \text{Percentage of body water}}{0.732}.$$

Because the body fat, calculated in this fashion, agrees well with that calculated from specific gravity, it is apparent that the water

Fig. 2-4.—Relationships between body fat, specific gravity and percentage of water. (Adapted from Behnke, A. R., Jr.: Harvey Lect. 37:198, 1941–42.)

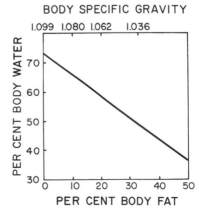

BODY SPECIFIC GRAVITY
1.099 1.080 1.062   1.036

content of the lean body mass of man must be essentially the same as that of laboratory animals. If the water content of the body is 65.9% of body weight, the body contains 10% excess fat over and above the structural lipid of Behnke. If the water content is 36.6% of body weight, the fat content is 50%, indicating extreme obesity. The equation holds only for the adult with average skeletal proportions. It does not hold for the infant nor for the edematous or dehydrated adult. The general relationships among percentage of water, percentage of fat and specific gravity of the body are summarized in Figure 2–4.

Ionic Composition of the Body Fluids

The ionic composition of the body fluids can be discussed meaningfully only in terms of chemical equivalents. When concentrations of all ionic constituents are so expressed, the sum of the concentrations of the positive ions (cations), such as sodium, potassium, calcium and magnesium, exactly equals the sum of the concentrations of the negative ions (anions), such as chloride, bicarbonate, phosphate, sulfate, protein and organic anion. Balance is obligatory, because solutions must be electrically neutral; i.e., the number of positive charges must equal the number of negative charges.

DEFINITION OF CHEMICAL EQUIVALENTS. — One equivalent of hydrogen ions consists of $6.023 \cdot 10^{23}$ separate particles, weighing 1.008 Gm. This quantity of hydrogen ions exactly balances or neutralizes 1 equivalent of hydroxyl ions, which consists of $6.023 \cdot 10^{23}$ separate particles, weighing 17.008 Gm. Neutralization results in the formation of 18.016 Gm, or 1 mole (mol), of water. One equivalent of hydrogen ions also combines with 1 equivalent of chloride ions (35.5 Gm) to form 1 mol of hydrochloric acid. Each hydrogen ion carries a unit positive charge; each chloride and hydroxyl ion carries a unit negative charge. Such ions are termed univalent and balance each other in a 1:1 ratio. Because the concentrations of

ions in the body fluids amount to fractions of an equivalent per liter, it is more convenient to express them in terms of milliequivalents (mEq) in order to handle whole numbers rather than decimal values. One milliequivalent of a univalent ion is equal to 1/1,000th of an equivalent and consists of $6.023 \cdot 10^{20}$ particles. One milliequivalent of hydrogen ions weighs 1.008 mg, and 1 mEq of hydroxyl ions weighs 17.008 mg.

Certain cations, such as calcium and magnesium, are divalent; i.e., each carries two unit positive charges. Sulfate is a divalent anion and carries two unit negative charges. Each calcium or magnesium ion can, therefore, combine with two chloride ions. Similarly, one sulfate ion can combine with two hydrogen ions. Accordingly, 1 mEq of divalent calcium ions consists of just half the number of particles ($3.012 \cdot 10^{20}$) of a milliequivalent of hydrogen ions and weighs 20 mg. One milliequivalent of sulfate ions consists of $3.012 \cdot 10^{20}$ particles and weighs 48 mg. The rule is that 1 mEq of positive cations exactly balances or neutralizes 1 mEq of negative anions. If the ion is univalent, 1 mEq consists of $6.023 \cdot 10^{20}$ particles and weighs 1/1,000th of a gram-atomic weight; if it is divalent, it consists of $3.012 \cdot 10^{20}$ particles and weighs 1/2,000th of a gram-atomic weight.

The fact that, for the most part, equivalent weights are not whole numbers (e.g., hydrogen has an equivalent weight of 1.008 Gm) is explained as follows: Oxygen was originally chosen as the standard of reference; exactly 8 Gm of oxygen was arbitrarily designated as 1 equivalent. This quantity of oxygen combines with 1.008 Gm of hydrogen. Deviations from whole numbers result from the fact that oxygen (the standard of reference), as well as many other elements, is a mixture of stable isotopes of differing atomic weights.

EXTRACELLULAR FLUID

PLASMA. — The major cation of blood plasma is sodium; the major anions are chloride, bicarbonate and protein. The average normal

TABLE 2–2.—IONIC STRUCTURE OF PLASMA
AND INTERSTITIAL FLUID*

ION SPECIES	PLASMA (mEq/L)	PLASMA WATER (mEq/L)	INTERSTITIAL FLUID (mEq/L)
Na	142	151	144
K	4	4.3	4
Ca	5	5.4	2.5
Mg	3	3.2	1.5
Cations	154	163.9	152.0
Cl	103	109.7	114
HCO$_3$	27	28.7	30
PO$_4$	2	2.1	2.0
SO$_4$	1	1.1	1.0
Organic acid	5	5.3	5.0
Protein	16	17	0.0
Anions	154	163.9	152.0

*From Pitts, R. F.: *The Physiological Basis of Diuretic Therapy* (Springfield, Ill.: Charles C Thomas, Publisher, 1959).

concentrations of the several ionic species in plasma are given in Table 2–2. The sum of the concentrations of cations exactly equals the sum of the concentrations of anions. Exact balance is obligatory; however, the concentrations shown in Table 2–2 are in no sense absolute. Thus, normal sodium concentrations are 138–146 mEq/L of plasma; chloride 98–110 mEq/L; and bicarbonate, 24–28 mEq/L. Other ions normally exhibit similar variations in concentration.

Protein occupies volume out of all proportion to the few milliequivalents of anion it represents. One liter of plasma contains only 940 ml of water; the remaining volume is occupied by 60 Gm of protein. For the most part, ions are dissolved in the aqueous phase of plasma*; concentrations in plasma water, therefore, exceed those in whole plasma by a factor of 1,000/940.

INTERSTITIAL FLUID.—Interstitial fluid is an ultrafiltrate of plasma. A simple filtrate of plasma is devoid of particulate matter, such as erythrocytes, leukocytes and platelets, whereas an ultrafiltrate is, in addition, devoid of protein. Although interstitial fluid is not

*Calcium and magnesium are in part bound to plasma proteins, in part dissolved in plasma water. In order to strike an even balance, it is necessary to include the protein anions per liter of plasma water as well as the protein-bound moieties of calcium and magnesium in the calculation.

entirely free of protein, concentration is low in comparison with that of plasma. One cannot sample normal interstitial fluid in amounts sufficient for analysis. However, edema fluid can be collected from Southey's tubes inserted into subcutaneous tissue of patients with congestive heart failure, and lymph can be collected from both peripheral and central channels. Edema fluid and lymph from peripheral channels contain less than 1% protein, whereas lymph collected from the liver may contain 2–3%. Accordingly, capillaries in different regions of the body vary in regard to their permeability to protein.

The capillary endothelium, while restraining protein more or less completely, permits free exchange of water and diffusible solutes between plasma and interstitial fluid. One might anticipate that concentrations of diffusible ions in plasma water and in interstitial fluid would be equal. Actually, small but significant differences exist, in line with those predicted by the Gibbs-Donnan rule. As shown in Table 2–2, the concentrations of cations are somewhat lower, and those of anions are somewhat higher, in interstitial fluid than in plasma water.

GIBBS-DONNAN RULE.—If a nondiffusible ion (protein anion) is present on one side of a membrane permeable to all other ion species, the diffusible ions will distribute unequally on the two sides of the membrane in such a manner as to satisfy three requirements: (1) Total cations must equal total anions on each side of the membrane. (2) On the side containing protein, the concentrations of diffusible anions must be less, and the concentrations of diffusible cations must be greater, than on the side containing no protein. (3) The osmotic pressure on the side containing protein (oncotic pressure) will be slightly greater than on the side containing no protein, and it must be balanced in some way to prevent the transfer of fluid. In the capillaries, net transfer of fluid is prevented by an outwardly directed hydrostatic pressure equal to the oncotic pressure.

The Gibbs-Donnan rule was originally

deduced from thermodynamic principles; it predicts that, under equilibrium conditions, the product of the concentrations of any pair of diffusible cations and anions on one side of a membrane will equal the product of the same pair of ions on the other side. Expressed mathematically, the relationship is the following: $(B^+)_1 \cdot (A^-)_1 = (B^+)_2 \cdot (A^-)_2$. If only $B \cdot A$ is present on the two sides, then $(B^+)_1 = (B^+)_2$ and $(A^-)_1 = (A^-)_2$; i.e., the ions are distributed equally. However, if a nondiffusible anion is present on one side, conditions are altered. Let us consider the closed system illustrated in Figure 2–5, in which two compartments of equal volume are separated by a rigid membrane permeable to Na^+ and Cl^- ions but impermeable to Pr^- (protein) ions. Initially (Fig. 2–5, *left*), 5 Na^+ and 5 Pr^- ions are placed in compartment 1 and 10 Na^+ ions and 10 Cl^- ions in compartment 2. At equilibrium (Fig. 2–5, *right*), the diffusible ions as well as the nondiffusible ions will be unequally distributed.

The products of the concentrations of the diffusible ions, Na^+ and Cl^-, on the two sides are equal, as required by the Gibbs-Donnan law — namely, $6 \times 6 = 36$, and $9 \times 4 = 36$. Despite inequality of concentrations on the two sides, no tendency toward equalization is noted with the passage of time.

If the equation given above is rewritten as

$$\frac{(Na^+)_1}{(Na^+)_2} = \frac{(Cl^-)_2}{(Cl^-)_1}$$

then, in the example given,

$$\frac{(Na^+)_1}{(Na^+)_2} = \frac{9}{6} = \frac{3}{2}$$

and

$$\frac{(Cl^-)_2}{(Cl^-)_1} = \frac{6}{4} = \frac{3}{2}$$

If a system such as the foregoing contained a variety of diffusible ions, all cations and all anions would distribute in such a manner that the ratio of the concentrations of any one on the two sides would be the same as that of any other. Hydrogen ions diffuse in the same manner as do sodium ions; hence, the protein-containing side (plasma) will be more acid than the non-protein-containing side (interstitial fluid). Furthermore, it is evident that the osmolar concentration is slightly greater on the protein-containing side, even if one disregards the nondiffusible protein anion. Thus, side 1 at equilibrium contains 13 diffusible particles, whereas side 2 contains only 12. Obviously, if the movement of water were not prevented by the closed-system conditions in the example of Figure 2–5, osmosis would occur and compartment 1 would expand at the expense of compartment 2. Colloid osmotic pressure has its origin not only in the effect of protein particles per se on the activity of water but also in the effect of the excess of diffusible ions.

The distributions of univalent cations between plasma and interstitial fluid, shown in Table 2–2, have been calculated on the basis of an average Gibbs-Donnan ratio of 100:95, whereas the distributions of univalent anions have been calculated on the basis of a ratio of 100:105. The ratios of divalent cations and anions are uncertain. However, the low calcium and magnesium values in interstitial fluid shown in Table 2–2 are related to protein-binding in plasma rather than to Gibbs-Donnan distribution.

INTRACELLULAR FLUID

As pointed out earlier, a composition of intracellular fluid applicable to all cells cannot be described. Erythrocytes, muscle cells and liver cells obviously contain quite different functional proteins. Their ionic composi-

Fig. 2—5.—The effect of nondiffusible protein anions on the distribution of diffusible cations and anions under closed-system conditions.

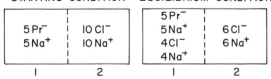

STARTING CONDITION		EQUILIBRIUM CONDITION	
5 Pr⁻ 5 Na⁺	10 Cl⁻ 10 Na⁺	5 Pr⁻ 5 Na⁺ 4 Cl⁻ 4 Na⁺	6 Cl⁻ 6 Na⁺
1	2	1	2

tions differ as well. However, certain features of all cell fluids are qualitatively similar and distinct from those of extracellular fluid. Thus, the major cations of intracellular fluid are potassium and magnesium, and the major anions are proteins and organic phosphates. The major ionic components of striated muscle are given in Table 2–3. Chloride and bicarbonate are included to emphasize differences between intra- and extracellular composition.

For many reasons, the values of intracellular ion concentrations are uncertain. It is impossible to analyze cell contents directly; tissues must be analyzed and cell composition calculated from the differences between the total quantities of ions measured and the quantities contained in interstitial fluid. Inasmuch as the volume of interstitial fluid within a tissue cannot be determined with any degree of precision, the exact quantities of extracellular ions to be subtracted are unknown. The errors are greatest for those ions, such as chloride and sodium, that are present in highest concentration in interstitial fluid and in lowest concentration in intracellular fluid. Chloride, the major anion of extracellular fluid, is present in very low concentration in muscle cells; some investigators claim that it is absent. However, certain other cells, including erythrocytes and the cells of the gastric mucosa, gonads and skin, contain significant quantities of chloride. Chloride cannot be said to be exclusively an extracellular ion. The major intracellular anions are protein and organic phos-

phates, including adenosine mono-, di- and triphosphate, glycerophosphate and creatine phosphate. The total osmolar concentration of intracellular fluid is generally considered to be essentially the same as that of extracellular fluid. However, this fact cannot be derived from the data of Table 2–3, for the osmotic activity of the polyvalent anions within cells in unknown. Furthermore, one cannot balance total cations against total anions, for concentrations and degree of dissociation are unknown. There is still no agreement on whether all cellular ions are free in solution or are in part bound; even water may be bound in some degree.

DIFFERENCES IN IONIC CONCENTRATIONS ACROSS CELL MEMBRANES. — The maintenance of differences in ionic concentrations across cell membranes derives not from absolute ionic impermeability* but from active accumulation of certain ions within cells and active extrusion of others from cells. Cells are, therefore, effectively but not actually impermeable to ions. That cell membranes are not impermeable to sodium, chloride and potassium ions is attested by the fact that the radioactive isotopes of these ions, introduced into extracellular fluid, exchange more or less rapidly with their nonradioactive counterparts within cells. One must therefore conclude that the tendency of sodium ions to diffuse from extracellular fluid, where concentration is high, into cells, where concentration is low, is opposed by their active extrusion from cells. Similarly, the tendency for potassium ions to diffuse from the interior of cells, where concentration is high, to extracellular fluid, where concentration is low, is opposed by their active accumulation in cells. The potential that exists across the cell membrane — negative inside, positive outside — opposes the loss of potassium but facilitates the entry of sodium. In general, cells are far more permeable to potassium than to sodium.

The mechanism that extrudes sodium from

TABLE 2–3. — ELECTROLYTE COMPOSITION
OF MUSCLE*

ION	mEq/L H_2O
Na	± 10
K	160
Mg	35
Cl	± 2
HCO_3	± 8
Protein	55
PO_4 (organic)	140

*Modified from Pitts, R. F.: *The Physiological Basis of Diuretic Therapy* (Springfield, Ill.: Charles C Thomas, Publisher, 1959).

*Cell membranes are undoubtedly impermeable to proteins and organic phosphate complexes but not to other intracellular ions.

cells and that accumulates potassium within cells is called an "ion pump." In most (if not all) cells, the outward pumping of sodium is linked obligatorily with the inward pumping of potassium. These ion pumps are metabolically activated. Cold, anoxia and various metabolic inhibitors inactivate the pumps; and the characteristic differences between intracellular and extracellular concentrations tend to disappear as ions diffuse unopposed down their concentration gradients. The most familiar example of change in cell composition due to failure of ion pumps is the loss of potassium and the gain of sodium, which occurs when bank blood is stored in the cold. Rewarming the blood and adding glucose reactivate the ion pumps; potassium is reaccumulated in, and sodium is extruded from, red cells, so that normal composition of plasma and intracellular fluid is restored.

No definitive description of an ion pump in any tissue is possible at the present time. However, certain properties of the pumps of erythrocytes, muscle cells and nerve axons, as described by Shaw, Glynn, Hodgkin, Keynes and others, can be explained in terms of the diagrams of Figure 2–6. The passive movements (fluxes) of sodium and potassium into and out of cells are shown by the outer straight arrows at either side of Figure 2–6, A. The heavier arrows indicate the directions of the major fluxes down gradients of concentration—potassium outward and sodium inward. If passive influx of sodium and passive efflux of potassium were to continue unopposed, concentrations of the two ion species inside and outside cells would tend to equalize. The curved arrows

connected by the circle represent the active fluxes that oppose the attainment of diffusion equilibrium. The outward pumping of sodium appears to be linked to the inward pumping of potassium; both demand a continuous supply of energy.

Figure 2–6, B, illustrates a hypothetical cyclic carrier system that explains the coupled fluxes of sodium and potassium. K^+ and Na^+ ions cross the cell membrane in combination with carriers X and Y. X is K^+-specific, and Y is Na^+-specific. The complexes KX and NaY are presumed to diffuse freely within the substance of the membrane and to be in equilibrium with K^+ and X and with Na^+ and Y, respectively, at the inner and outer surfaces of the membrane. At the inner surface, X is converted to Y by the expenditure of metabolic energy. So long as energy is supplied and so long as the concentrations of Na^+ inside and of K^+ outside are above some limiting value, the system will operate in counterclockwise direction, pumping sodium out of, and potassium into, the cell.

Much current investigative interest is centered in the relationship of a magnesium-dependent, sodium- and potassium-activated adenosine triphosphatase to the coupled sodium potassium membrane pump. This enzyme is found in the microsomal fraction of homogenates of many tissues subjected to differential centrifugation. The microsomes are, in part, fragments of the limiting plasma membrane of cells and therefore might be expected to contain the transport system. Although enzymatic splitting of adenosine triphosphate (ATP) is obligatorily dependent on the presence of magnesium ions in the

Fig. 2–6. — Mechanism of transport of sodium and potassium across cell membranes. **A,** *straight arrows,* passive diffusion of ions; *curved arrows,* active trans- port of ions. **B,** hypothetical coupled carrier mechanism. (From Glynn, I. M.: J. Physiol. 134:278, 1956.)

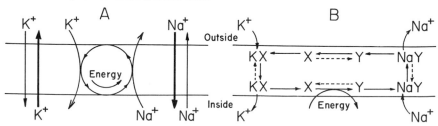

medium, full activity requires the presence of both sodium and potassium ions in proper proportions. Kinetic studies have shown that sodium and potassium are bound to the membrane fragments at different sites, possibly located on the inside and outside of the original membrane. Cardiac glycosides, which interfere with the extrusion of sodium from and the accumulation of potassium by intact cells, depress that fraction of enzyme activity that is dependent on the presence of sodium and potassium. Whether enzymatic binding and splitting of ATP power a closely associated membrane pump or in themselves constitute the elements of pumping action is unknown. If the latter is the case, combination with ATP might impose one type of specificity on the binding sites for sodium and potassium, whereas splitting of ATP might impose the opposite type. How ions are translocated is, at present, a purely speculative matter. Skou (16) has persuasively reviewed the evidence that relates enzyme to pump. In all fairness, it must be emphasized that the evidence is circumstantial and that some believe that at least a part of ion transport across epithelial structures is independent of ATP and is powered more directly by the electron transport system.

POLARIZATION OF CELL MEMBRANES. — Cells are electrically polarized: negative inside, positive outside. Polarization is largely a function of the difference in potassium concentration on the two sides of the membrane, and the potential difference (PD) is described in a roughly quantitative manner by the simple Nernst equation

$$PD \ (in \ mV) = -61 \cdot \log \frac{(K^+_i)}{(K^+_e)}$$

in which (K^+_i) is the intracellular concentration of potassium and (K^+_e) is the extracellular concentration.

The potential difference is predominantly a potassium diffusion potential modified in variable degree by the restricted movements of less permeable ions. In Figure 2–7, curve 2 illustrates the effect of progressive substitution of potassium for sodium in the

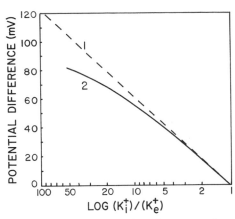

Fig. 2–7. — The relationship between the potential across the sarcolemma and the logarithm of the ratio of the concentration of potassium inside/outside skeletal muscle fibers. *Curve 1*, calculated from Nernst equation; *curve 2*, observed.

medium bathing a muscle fiber on the potential difference across the sarcolemma membrane. When the extracellular concentration of potassium is in the normal range of 3–4 mEq/L and the ratio $(K^+_i) / (K^+_e) = 40$ to 60, the potential difference is about 80–90 mV. As (K^+_e) is increased, thereby reducing the ratio, the potential difference decreases, reaching zero when $K^+_i / K^+_e = 1$; i.e., when the external potassium concentration equals the internal.

The origin of the potential difference is explained as follows: The cell membrane is absolutely impermeable to the large polyvalent protein and organic phosphate anions contained within the cell. The cell membrane is effectively, although not actually, impermeable to sodium as a result of the operation of the ion pumps, which continuously eject sodium. As a first approximation, one can consider the cell as permeable only to potassium and chloride ions. Positively charged potassium ions tend to diffuse out of the cell down a concentration gradient. They are restrained by the increasing negative charge left within the cell. A state is reached in which the outward diffusion of potassium, driven by concentration difference, is just balanced by increasing cell negativity, restraining further diffusion. This state is described by the Nernst equation and in Figure

2–7 by line 1. If the intracellular concentration of potassium were 10 times the extracellular concentration, the potential difference would be −61 mV (log 10 = 1). If the intracellular and extracellular concentrations were equal the potential difference would be 0 mV (log 1 = 0). Values of the potential difference for most mammalian cells are 60–90 mV when exposed to normal concentrations of potassium in extracellular fluid. From such potential difference values, one would predict intracellular potassium concentrations 10–30 times the extracellular concentrations. In a number of instances, the intracellular concentrations were observed to be higher—a fact which suggests that potassium is actively accumulated within cells; i.e., potassium is pumped into cells. Furthermore, it is evident from Figure 2–7 that the potential difference predicted by the Nernst equation (curve 1) exceeds the measured potential difference (curve 2). Other ions (e.g., sodium and chloride) no doubt diffuse into cells with sufficient ease to alter the relationship from that of a strict potassium diffusion potential. More complicated formulas have been devised to account for the shunting effects of other ions, but their consideration is beyond the scope of this discussion.

GIBBS-DONNAN DISTRIBUTION.—The concentration of nondiffusible ions in cells relative to interstitial fluid is far greater than that in plasma. The inequalities of distribution of diffusible cations and anions across cell membranes should therefore be more marked, and the osmotic forces correspondingly larger, than across the capillary endothelium if Donnan forces were to act unopposed. In fact, to prevent continuous diffusion of water into cells and progressive increase in cell volume, the osmolar concentration of cell contents must be maintained at a value less than that which would result from an unopposed Donnan distribution of diffusible ions. The active extrusion of sodium from cells accomplishes this end. Most investigators agree that the distribution of chloride between the interior of muscle fibers and the interstitial fluid is essentially that

predicted for a Donnan distribution and therefore is passive in nature.

If cells are permeable to bicarbonate, the intracellular concentration of this ion should be even lower than that of chloride. However, the partition of cellular carbon dioxide between bicarbonate ion and carbamino-bound carbon dioxide is unknown. It may be that the bicarbonate ion concentration is very low and that the intracellular carbon dioxide of muscle (8–10 mEq/L of water) is largely in carbamino combination. On the other hand, permeability to bicarbonate ion may be low, and the intracellular concentration may be determined by factors other than Gibbs-Donnan distribution. Cell contents are more acid (pH 6.8–7) than is interstitial fluid—a fact in line with that predicted from Donnan distribution.

OSMOTIC PRESSURE AND WATER DISTRIBUTION BETWEEN CELLS AND EXTRACELLULAR FLUID

Osmotic forces are of prime importance in determining the distribution of water among the several fluid compartments of the body. It is important, therefore, to have a clear appreciation of their operation. When a solution and pure solvent are separated by a membrane that is permeable to solvent but not to solute, the solvent passes into the solution by osmosis. The osmotic pressure (17) is the particular hydrostatic pressure that must be applied to the solution to prevent the entry of solvent (Fig. 2–8). Cell membranes are permeable to water but effectively impermeable to many crystalloidal solutes, such as sodium, chloride and bicarbonate. Cells thus behave as tiny osmometers.

ISOSMOTIC VS. ISOTONIC SOLUTIONS.—When red cells are placed in distilled water, they swell and hemolyze; i.e., they then discharge their hemoglobin. If they are placed in 0.93% (0.16 M) saline solution, they undergo no change in volume. The osmolar concentration of the saline solution (0.3 osmols per liter) is exactly equal to that of the cell contents; the two solutions have

SOLVENT   SOLUTION

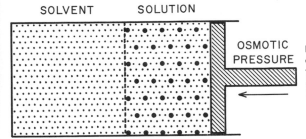

OSMOTIC
PRESSURE

Fig. 2—8. — Kinetic formulation of osmotic pressure based on diffusion of solvent but not of solute across a membrane. (From Pitts, R. F.: *The Physiological Basis of Diuretic Therapy* [Springfield, Ill.: Charles C Thomas, Publisher, 1959].)

the same osmotic pressure—they are isosmotic. Since no swelling or shrinking occurs, they are also isotonic. Basically, an isotonic solution is one that is physiologically isosmotic with cell fluid; i.e., when a solution is separated from cell contents by a semipermeable cell membrane, no transfer of water occurs.

A solution containing 1.8% urea has the same osmotic pressure as a solution containing 0.9% sodium chloride; i.e., the two solutions are isosmotic. However, the urea solution is not isotonic, for if red cells are added, they swell and hemolyze exactly as they do in distilled water. The reason for this is as follows: The membrane of erythrocytes, like that of most cells, is nearly as permeable to urea as to water. Therefore, urea exerts no osmotic effect when separated from cell contents by membranes permeable to it. A solution of urea is physiologically equivalent to distilled water.

The capillary endothelium is permeable to water and to all solutes of blood plasma other than proteins and lipids. Hence, only transient osmotic forces develop across capillary walls when solutions of crystalloids higher or lower in osmolar concentration than interstitial fluid are introduced into the circulation.

NATURE OF OSMOTIC FORCES.—To state that a concentrated solution has a higher osmotic pressure than a dilute solution is a bit ambiguous. In isolation, a solution, no matter how concentrated, has no osmotic pressure. An osmotic pressure develops only when a solution is separated from pure solvent or a more dilute solution by a semipermeable membrane. Furthermore, the force developed is dependent on the diffu-

sion of solvent and not necessarily on the presence of solute, except as it influences the concentration (or, better, the activity) of the solvent in a solution.

Figure 2–8 describes the origin of osmotic pressure in terms of the molecular motions of solvent on the two sides of a membrane. On the pure solvent side, molecules in their unordered agitation strike the membrane; and, because it is permeable, some pass through. The same thing happens on the side of the solution, except that the solvent is somewhat diluted by solute, so that its concentration (or, better, its activity, chemical potential or escaping tendency) is reduced. Accordingly, fewer solvent molecules pass from solution to pure solvent than in the reverse direction. Osmosis of solvent (i.e., net transfer of fluid) occurs from pure solvent to solution. The osmotic pressure is the pressure that must be applied to the solution to increase the activity, or escaping tendency, of solvent in the solution to equal that of the pure solvent.

MAGNITUDE OF OSMOTIC FORCES. — The osmotic forces that develop when blood plasma, interstitial fluid and cell fluid are separated from pure water by semipermeable membranes are surprisingly large. They are of the order of magnitude of 6.7 atmospheres (atm) or 5,100 mm Hg. The essential equality of the osmolar concentrations of extracellular, transcellular and intracellular fluids is a direct result of the rapid distribution of water through capillary walls and cell membranes, driven by forces of potentially great magnitude. Water diffuses so that its escaping tendency, or activity, in all body fluid compartments is the same.

UNITS OF OSMOTIC CONCENTRATION.— Osmotic pressure is one of the colligative properties of solutions: it depends on the numbers of particles per unit volume of solvent, not on their chemical characteristics. One gram-molecular weight of glucose, sucrose, urea or any nondissociating compound consisting of $6.023 \cdot 10^{23}$ molecules is termed 1 osmole (osmol). One osmole of any solute dissolved in 22.4 kg of water depresses the activity or escaping tendency of the water by 1 atm, or, dissolved in 1 kg of water, depresses activity by 22.4 atm. One milliosmole (mOsm) is 1/1,000th of an osmole. One milliosmole dissolved in 1 kg of water depresses the escaping tendency of water by 17 mm Hg.

One gram-molecular weight of sodium chloride, consisting of $6.023 \cdot 10^{23}$ molecules, dissociates into twice this number of ions in solution. Therefore, 1 mol of sodium chloride exerts an osmotic effect of nearly 2 osmol.* One gram-molecular weight of sodium sulfate dissociates into 3 times this number of ions and hence exerts an osmotic effect approaching 3 osmol.

The osmotic concentrations of solutions are customarily measured, not in terms of osmotic pressure but in terms of another colligative property: freezing-point depression. Pure water freezes at 0° C. A solution containing 1 osmol of an undissociated solute (such as glucose) per 1 kg of water freezes at −1.86° C. Such a solution is said to be 1 osmolal. If 1 osmol were dissolved in 1 L. of solution, the solution would be 1 osmolar. These terms are frequently confused; however, as it happens, differences are small in solutions of the concentration of body fluids. The blood plasma of man normally freezes at −0.553° C. Osmolal concentration is, therefore, $0.553 / 1.86 = 0.297$; i.e., 297 mOsm/kg H_2O. To find the concentration of a sodium chloride solution osmotically equivalent to plasma, one must divide the osmolality by the osmotic coefficient of sodium chloride at the appropriate concentration; i.e., $0.297 / 1.85 = 0.16$ molal.*

The osmotic concentrations of plasma, interstitial fluid, the transcellular fluids and intracellular fluid are all roughly equal and vary around 300 mOsm/kg H_2O. Because 1 mOsm/kg H_2O exerts an osmotic effect equivalent to 17 mm Hg, the osmotic pressure of the body fluids averages $300 \times 17 = 5,100$ mm Hg. The osmotically active solutes of the body fluids are, in large part, electrolytes. The univalent ions sodium, chloride and bicarbonate account for 90–95% of the osmotic activity of blood plasma and interstitial fluid. Other ions and organic compounds, such as glucose, amino acids and urea, account for the remainder.

WATER DISTRIBUTION BETWEEN INTRACELLULAR AND EXTRACELLULAR COMPARTMENTS

The distribution of water between intracellular and extracellular compartments corresponds to their contents of osmotically active substances, largely ions. Cell membranes permit the free movement of water in either direction, and water diffuses so that its escaping tendency is the same inside each cell as in the surrounding interstitial fluid. The interstitial compartment is kept well mixed, because of the rapid circulation of blood plasma and the free exchange of water between plasma and interstitial fluid across capillary membranes.

Figure 2–9 illustrates the changes in volume and osmolal concentration of extra- and intracellular compartments in a variety of circumstances in which ionic content or water content is altered (18). Volume is indicated by the width of a compartment; osmolal

---

*Actually, if 1 mol of sodium chloride were dissolved in an infinite volume of solution, the osmotic effect would be that of 2 osmol. In solutions having the same concentration as body fluids, the osmotic coefficient of sodium chloride is 1.85; i.e., each pair of sodium and chloride ions does not affect the activity of water as would two entirely independent particles but, rather, as would 1.85 particles.

---

*The osmotic coefficient of sodium chloride varies from 1.967 when concentration is 0.001 molal to 1.811 when concentration is 0.5 molal. The osmotic coefficient of 0.16 molal sodium chloride is 1.85.

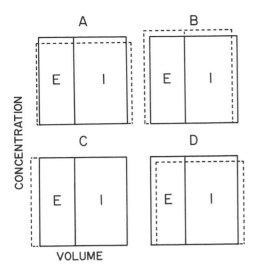

Fig. 2–9.—Changes in volume and osmolal concentration of intracellular (*I*) and extracellular (*E*) fluids on **A**, addition of water to the body; on **B**, addition of hypertonic salt solution; on **C**, addition of isotonic salt solution; and on **D**, loss of sodium chloride. Compartments enclosed by *solid lines* represent the initial normal state; those enclosed by *dashed lines* represent the final experimental state. Height of compartment represents osmolal concentration; width represents volume. (Adapted from Darrow, D. C., and Yannet, H.: Clin. Invest. 14:266, 1935.)

concentration, by the height. The normal condition is represented by the solid-line enclosures; the altered condition, by the dotted-line enclosures.

ADDITION OF WATER.—The effect of the oral ingestion of a large volume of water is shown in Figure 2–9, *A*. The water diffuses uniformly between extracellular and intracellular compartments, increasing volume and decreasing osmolal concentration. If the subject weighs 70 kg and is 60% water by weight (42 L), the intracellular volume might reasonably be 25 L and the extracellular volume (including transcellular volume) might be 17 L. If the subject were to ingest 3 L of water and to absorb it rapidly, and if he did not excrete any of this water, one would predict that extra- and intracellular concentrations would decrease from 300 mOsm to 280 mOsm/kg of water: 300 mOsm/kg · 42 kg/ (42 + 3) kg = 280 mOsm/kg. The water would diffuse in proportion to the initial volumes; thus, extracellular volume would increase by 17/42 · 3 L = 1.21 L, and intracellular volume would increase by 25/42 · 3 L = 1.79 L. Actually, increase in volume and decrease in concentration would be less in a normal person, for diuresis begins before absorption from the gut is complete.

ADDITION OF SOLUTE WITHOUT WATER. —If a strongly hypertonic solution of sodium chloride is infused intravenously, the volume of the extracellular compartment increases while that of the intracellular compartment decreases. Sodium chloride remains in the extracellular fluid, increasing osmolality. Water leaves the cells by osmosis until the osmolal concentration of the intracellular fluid rises to equal that of extracellular fluid. If one were to infuse 200 ml of 10% sodium chloride (20/58.5 ·1.85 = 633 mOsm) into a hypothetical normal subject, the increase in osmolal concentration of the body fluids would amount to 633 mOsm/42 kg = 15.1 mOsm/kg H_2O; i.e., to 315.1 mOsm/kg H_2O. It would appear that the sodium chloride had distributed between the extracellular and intracellular compartments in proportion to their water contents. Actually, the salt remains extracellular and water leaves the cells. The 25 L of cell water contain 7,500 mOsm of osmotically active materials (25 kg · 300 mOsm/kg). To increase concentration to 315.1 mOsm/kg requires reduction of intracellular water from 25 to 23.8 L (7,500 mOsm/315.1 mOsm/kg = 23.8 kg). Thus, the infusion of 200 ml of 10% sodium chloride causes the transfer of 1.2 L of cell water to the extracellular compartment. Thirst would induce the subject to ingest sufficient water to dilute the body fluids to 300 mOsm/ kg. Intracellular volume would return to normal, and extracellular volume would increase by a total of 2.11 L over the normal; i.e., enough to dilute 633 mOsm to 300 mOsm/L. The end result would be the same as the infusion of 2.11 L of isotonic saline solution (Fig. 2–9, *C*).

INFUSION OF ISOTONIC SALINE SOLUTION.—The infusion of isotonic saline solution expands the extracellular volume without producing any change in intracellular volume or in intra- or extracellular concentration (Fig. 2-9, *C*). This is because the osmolality of extracellular fluid is unchanged and the sodium chloride remains chiefly extracellular.

REMOVAL OF SODIUM CHLORIDE.—The removal of sodium chloride from the extracellular fluid without loss of water results in the transfer of water from the extracellular compartment to the intracellular compartment. If one introduces a large volume of 5% glucose into the peritoneum and allows it to remain for 3-4 hours, glucose is absorbed from, and sodium chloride diffuses into, the peritoneal dialysate. Because the solution is isotonic, little change in volume occurs; when the solution is withdrawn, sodium chloride is abstracted from the body with little or no change in total body water. However, as shown in Figure 2-9, *D*, extracellular water enters cells, and osmolal concentration of intracellular and extracellular phases decrease. Cell volume increases at the expense of extracellular volume.

TOTAL BODY STORES OF IONS

That the total body water is a function of the total body store of ions is evident. Furthermore, the distribution of water between cells and extracellular fluid is related to the distribution of ions. Finally, because sodium is largely an extracellular ion, whereas potassium is largely an intracellular ion, the distribution of water ultimately depends on the quantities of these ions contained within the body.

SODIUM.—The total body sodium of a normal adult male averages 60 mEq/kg of body weight. A 70-kg man contains some 4,200 mEq. Bone, which constitutes some 15-16% of body weight, contains between 40 and 45% of the total store of sodium; i.e., 1,800 mEq (19). Of the remaining 2,400 mEq, some 2,000-2,200 mEq is dissolved in extracellular fluid. Accordingly, about 50% of total body sodium is extracellular, 40% is associated with bone and 10% or less is intracellular. Such figures are derived from postmortem chemical analysis of the body.

The division of body sodium into exchangeable and nonexchangeable moieties is clinically useful. Exchangeable sodium, which can be readily measured in the living subject by the dilution of radioactive sodium (^{22}Na or ^{24}Na), amounts to 42 mEq/kg of body weight (20-22). This fraction includes all sodium of extracellular and intracellular fluids and somewhat less than half of bone sodium. The 18 mEq of nonexchangeable sodium is largely associated with the skeleton and is adsorbed on the surfaces of the hydroxyapatite crystals buried deep in the substance of the more dense long bones. Exchangeable sodium is of interest in that it is in diffusion equilibrium with plasma sodium. If sodium is lost in sweat, urine or diarrheal fluid, that present in the exchangeable reservoir, including the exchangeable sodium of cancellous bone, is available to mitigate the decrease in concentration that would otherwise occur when body water is restored. When sodium is retained, as it is when excesses are ingested by the potentially edematous patient, it is distributed into the subject's exchangeable reservoir.

POTASSIUM.—The total body potassium of a normal adult male averages 42 mEq/kg of body weight. A 70-kg man contains some 2,980 mEq, nearly all of which is intracellular, labile and readily exchangeable. Only about 2%, or 60 mEq, is distributed in extracellular fluid. The normal plasma concentration of potassium is 4 mEq/L. The shift of only a very small fraction of the intracellular store into extracellular fluid causes plasma concentration to rise to a dangerous, and perhaps lethal, level of 8-10 mEq/L if renal excretion is inadequate. Acidosis is associated with loss of cell potassium, hydrogen ions entering cells in exchange for potassium ions. In diabetic acidosis, the potassium lost from cells is rapidly excreted in the urine, and cell stores suffer progressive depletion. No increase in plasma potassium concentration occurs, and few, if any, symptoms and signs of potassium depletion are evident. On correction of the acidosis, potassium re-enters cells, and plasma concentration falls to levels of 1-2 mEq/L. Because the intracellular deficit may be large, weeks of normal intake may be required to replenish depleted stores. Potassium depletion manifests itself in the neuromuscular signs of diminished deep reflexes, muscular weakness progressing to flaccid paralysis, and mental confusion; in the gastrointestinal signs of anorexia, diarrhea, abdominal distention and paralytic ileus; in the renal signs of isosthenuria (loss of concentrating power of the kidneys); and in the cardiac signs of rapid rate and irregular rhythm.

In the acidosis of terminal renal disease, the ability of the kidney to excrete potassium is reduced and plasma potassium rises. More precipitous increases occur in acute renal failure, in which urine formation may be completely suppressed. The major manifestations of hyperkalemia are cardiovascular, although muscular weakness, areflexia and flaccid paralysis may develop much as they do in potassium depletion. When plasma concentration rises to 7 – 8 mEq/L, characteristic electrocardiographic changes occur: the T waves become high and peaked, the QRS complexes become broad and slurred, the P waves disappear and arrhythmias develop. Eventually the electrocardiogram shows complete disorganization, the heart becomes hypodynamic and death occurs, owing to circulatory collapse, which is often precipitated by ventricular fibrillation.

When potassium intake is reduced below rate of excretion, progressive loss of cellular potassium occurs. Plasma potassium decreases, but usually not to levels below 2 mEq/L. Unfortunately, the plasma potassium concentration is no measure of the extent of depletion of cellular stores. If one infuses 10% glucose into a normal person, plasma potassium may decrease to 2 mEq/L or less, because of enhanced uptake of potassium by cells; yet no intracellular deficit exists. On the other hand, a marked deficit may exist but plasma concentration may be as high as 3 mEq/L. The measurement of total body store by isotope dilution of radiopotassium (^{42}K) or the estimation of the deficit by therapeutic trial of increased intake is necessary if one is to establish the magnitude of the change in intracellular potassium.

CHLORIDE. – The total body chloride of a normal adult male averages 33 mEq/kg of body weight. A 70-kg man contains, in all, about 2,300 mEq. The major fraction, 70% or so, is contained in the plasma and interstitial fluid. Although primarily an extracellular ion, chloride is not exclusively so distributed. The remaining 30% of the body chloride is in part intracellular and in part localized in connective tissue, where it is perhaps bound to collagen. Of all cells, the erythrocytes contain the most chloride. Other tissues, such as gonads, gastric mucosa and skin, contain lesser amounts; muscle probably contains the least.

BICARBONATE. – Bicarbonate is a unique ion, in that it has no permanence. Its existence is fleeting – merely a step in the transfer of carbon dioxide between cells and lungs. In fact, one can best envision bicarbonate as an anion that represents the excess of cations, such as sodium, potassium, magnesium and calcium, over so-called fixed anions, such as chloride, sulfate, phosphate and protein. Any hydroxyl ion excess, imposed by the liberation of alkali within the body, is immediately corrected by the hydration of carbon dioxide to form bicarbonate ions and water. Conversely, any hydrogen ion excess, imposed by the liberation of acid in the body, is immediately corrected by conversion of bicarbonate ions to carbonic acid, which dehydrates to carbon dioxide and water.

The total body bicarbonate averages 10 – 12 mEq/kg of body weight. About half is distributed in the extracellular compartment, the remainder in cells. The carbon dioxide in bone is largely in the form of carbonate, bound in the crystal lattice, and is nonexchangeable. Presumably, all bicarbonate of cells is exchangeable. Cell concentrations are not known with any certainty, because the distribution of carbon dioxide between ionic and carbamino combination is unknown.

MAGNESIUM. – Knowledge of the body stores of magnesium has lagged behind that of other ions. However, in recent years, with the recognition of clinical deficiencies, interest has been kindled. Total body stores average 12–17 mEq/kg of body weight (23). A 70-kg man contains, in all, from 850 to 1,200 mEq, the major fraction of which is present in cells.

MEASUREMENT OF BODY STORES OF IONS

Studies of total ionic content of the human body are relatively few, in that they necessitate total dissolution of the body and meas-

equilibration period to determine the quantity of radiosodium excreted. The numerator of the above equation is the quantity of radiosodium retained in the body. The denominator is the specific activity of sodium in plasma; i.e., counts per minute per milliequivalent of total sodium.

If $45 \cdot 10^6$ counts per min. is administered and if $5 \cdot 10^6$ counts per min. is excreted, there remains in the body $40 \cdot 10^6$ counts per min. If the plasma contains $2 \cdot 10^3$ counts per minute per milliliter and 0.140 mEq of sodium per milliliter, then

$$\text{Exchangeable sodium} = \frac{40 \cdot 10^6 \text{ cpm}}{2 \cdot 10^3 \text{ cpm/ml and } 0.140 \text{ mEq Na/ml}} = \frac{40 \cdot 10^6 \text{ mEq}}{14.29 \cdot 10^3} = 2,800 \text{ mEq}$$

urement of the ionic composition of aliquots. Obviously, such a method cannot be used clinically. Measurements of total exchangeable ions, in contrast, are relatively easily performed and involve no hazard, even to the acutely ill patient. Exchangeable ion content approximates total body store except for sodium, a fair proportion of which is occluded in compact bone. An additional small moiety present in cerebrospinal fluid exchanges very slowly.

The procedure for measuring exchangeable ion content of the body may be illustrated as follows, using sodium as an example. Radioactive sodium (^{23}Na or ^{24}Na) diffuses throughout the body exactly as does nonradioactive sodium (^{28}Na), except for the bone and cerebrospinal fluid stores.

If one injects 20–40 microcuries (μCi) of radiosodium into a subject intravenously, allows 24 hours for equilibration, draws a sample of blood and analyzes the plasma for both radiosodium (in counts per minute) and nonradiosodium (in milliequivalents per milliliter), it is possible to calculate the total exchangeable sodium as follows:

If the subject weighs 70 kg, total exchangeable sodium amounts to 40 mEq/kg.

Total exchangeable chloride, potassium and bicarbonate have been determined by similar methods.

ONCOTIC PRESSURE AND FLUID DISTRIBUTION BETWEEN PLASMA AND TISSUE INTERSTICES

Since the molecular weights of the plasma proteins are high, varying from 69,000 for albumin to over 1,000,000 for certain globulins, the osmotic effects these proteins exert are small, even though their concentrations are relatively large (60–70 Gm/L). On average, the plasma proteins exert an osmotic pressure of 28 mm Hg. In comparison with the 5,100 mm Hg exerted by the crystalloidal solutes of plasma, this colloid osmotic pressure seems insignificant. However, it has a physiologic significance out of all proportion to its numerical value. As pointed out previously, the capillary walls are freely permeable to water and to crystalloidal solutes. Therefore, these solutes exert no osmotic

$$\text{Exchangeable sodium} = \frac{\text{Counts per min given} - \text{Counts per min excreted}}{\text{Counts per min per ml plasma/mEq Na per ml plasma}}$$

All urine is collected during the 24-hour

force across the endothelium, for they traverse it nearly as readily as does water. On the other hand, the capillaries are relatively impermeable to proteins, and the protein content of interstitial fluid of all organs except the liver is low. Therefore, nearly the full colloid osmotic effect of plasma proteins is exerted across the capillary endothelium, opposing the filtration of fluid from capillary lumen to tissue interstices and promoting its reabsorption into the vascular compartment. Because albumin is the most abundant of the plasma proteins and has the lowest molecular weight, it exerts the major fraction of the colloid osmotic effect.

STARLING HYPOTHESIS. — The forces that determine the distribution of fluid between the vascular and interstitial fluid compartments were first outlined by Starling (24) in 1896. The elements of his thesis are presented in Figure 2–10. The major pressure drop within the vascular system occurs within the terminal arterioles. Blood enters the true capillaries under a pressure head of 40–45 mm Hg. This pressure represents the force available to drive blood onward through capillaries, venules and veins to the heart. It also serves to filter fluid through the porous capillary walls into tissue interstices. Because the capillary wall largely restricts the passage of protein, a colloid osmotic force of 25–30 mm Hg opposes filtration. Tissue fluid is under a turgor pressure of some 2–5 mm Hg, which constitutes an additional small force opposing filtration. The sum of these forces at the arteriolar end of the capillary is equivalent to a net or effective filtration pressure of 10–15 mm Hg.

Energy is expended in driving blood along the capillary, for length is greater in relation to diameter than is shown in Figure 2–10. Hence, at the venular end of the capillary, hydrostatic pressure is reduced to 10–15 mm Hg. Oncotic pressure and turgor pressure remain essentially the same. Accordingly, the sum of the forces at the venular end of the capillary is equivalent to a net inward or absorbing pressure of 10–15 mm Hg. Starling postulated that fluid filters out at the arteriolar end of the capillary, circulates through the tissue interstices and is returned to the capillary at the venular end.

DIFFUSION VERSUS FILTRATION AND REABSORPTION IN TISSUE NUTRITION. — Bulk filtration and reabsorption of fluid at the ends of the capillary and circulation of fluid through tissue interstices are often misconstrued as the means of providing nutrients to and removing wastes from cells. Landis, Pappenheimer (25) and others have shown that the quantities of fluid that circulate in this manner are quite small. According to Pappenheimer, pressure gradients such as those shown in Figure 2-10 could cause the filtration and reabsorption of only 0.003 ml of fluid per minute across all of the capillaries contained in 100 Gm of tissue of the human forearm; i.e., a total volume of only 40 ml in 24 hours. Obviously, the transport of materials to and from tissues by such a mechanism would be entirely inadequate to supply their needs.

Diffusion of water and solutes across cap-

Fig. 2–10.—The Starling hypothesis of fluid distribution between blood plasma and interstitial compartments.

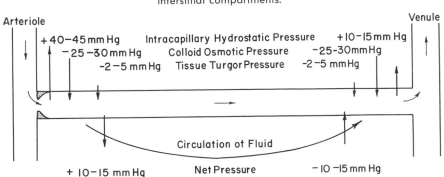

Arteriole   Venule

+40–45 mm Hg   Intracapillary Hydrostatic Pressure   +10–15 mm Hg
−25–30 mm Hg   Colloid Osmotic Pressure   −25–30 mm Hg
−2–5 mm Hg   Tissue Turgor Pressure   −2–5 mm Hg

Circulation of Fluid

+ 10–15 mm Hg   Net Pressure   − 10 −15 mm Hg

illary walls occurs at phenomenally high rates in comparison with rates of transport by bulk flow of fluid. Pappenheimer has calculated that the plasma contained in the capillaries of the forearm exchanges its water with that of interstitial fluid some 300 times per minute. The sodium chloride, urea and glucose of capillary plasma exchange 120, 100 and 40 times per minute, respectively, with like components of interstitial fluid. These rates, of course, relate to exchange, not to net transfer. However, if a tissue uses glucose and reduces concentration in interstitial fluid slightly, a net diffusion of glucose from plasma to tissue will occur. Similarly, any wastes produced by cells will appear in interstitial fluid in slightly higher concentration than in plasma and will be removed by diffusion down concentration gradients.

The capillaries behave as though perforated by aqueous pores 65 Å (10^{-7} mm) in diameter and having a population density of $10^9/cm^2$. However, pore orifices constitute only 0.1% of the endothelial surface of a capillary and, according to some, are restricted to the cement substance that joins adjacent endothelial cells. Oxygen and carbon dioxide, because of their lipid solubility, are free to diffuse across 100% of the capillary surface.

ROLE OF VASOMOTION IN TRANSCAPILLARY FLUID TRANSFER. — The Starling hypothesis of filtration of fluid at the arteriolar end of a capillary and reabsorption at the venular end is a gross oversimplification, as is the vascular arrangement diagramed in Figure 2–10. Zweifach (26, 27) has shown that the terminal vascular bed is better described in terms of the arrangement shown in Figure 2–11. Arterioles and metarterioles gradually lose their investment of smooth muscle and continue as endothelial tubes, known as preferential or thoroughfare channels, ultimately to become venules and veins. The true capillaries branch off at right angles from the preferential channel, anastomose freely with other capillaries and rejoin the thoroughfare. At the points of origin of the capillaries, smooth muscle fibers encircle the lumen, controlling the flow of blood through the loops. When the sphincters relax, flow is brisk; when they contract, flow ceases. Rhythmic contraction and relaxation of the precapillary sphincters and of the smooth muscle of the terminal arterioles and metarterioles is termed vasomotion. Frequency of vasomotion and relative duration of constrictor and dilator phases determine the minute volume of blood that perfuses the tissue and are themselves dependent on the vasomotor nerve outflow, the hormones carried in the blood stream and the local concentrations of metabolites in the tissues.

During the dilator phase, when blood perfusion is brisk, fluid filters out of the capillary loop along its entire length. During the constrictor phase, when flow ceases, fluid enters the capillary throughout its length.

Fig. 2–11. —Organization of the terminal vascular bed. (From Zweifach, B. W.: *Transactions of Third Josiah Macy, Jr., Conference on Factors Regulating Blood Pressure* [New York: Josiah Macy Foundation, 1949].)

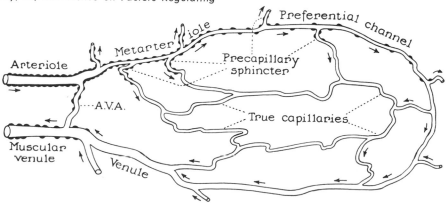

FACTORS AFFECTING INTERSTITIAL FLUID VOLUME.—It is apparent from Figure 2-10 that an increase in intracapillary hydrostatic pressure should increase filtration of fluid and expand interstitial volume, whereas a decrease in hydrostatic pressure should promote reabsorption and reduce interstitial volume. An increase in hydrostatic pressure can result either from dilation of arterioles and precapillary sphincters or from partial obstruction of venous outflow. In exercise, blood flow to active muscles increases markedly as a consequence of dilation of the terminal vascular bed; i.e., interstitial volume increases at the expense of plasma volume. In local inflammation, dilation of the terminal vascular bed results in increased warmth of the affected part, erythema and swelling; the latter is an expression of increased transudation of fluid, at least in part related to the hyperemia. An increase in interstitial volume occurs locally if veins draining the region are obstructed by thrombosis or, generally, if cardiac output is reduced and pressure increases throughout the venous system, as it does in congestive heart failure.

In a number of instances, the effects assigned to an increase in intracapillary pressure actually have their origin in prolongation of the dilator phase of vasomotion at the expense of the constrictor phase. The longer the phase of active blood perfusion during which filtration occurs and the shorter the phase of reduced perfusion during which absorption occurs, the greater will be the net transfer of fluid from plasma to interstitial compartment. Following a moderate hemorrhage, the circulating blood volume is restored promptly by the transfer of interstitial fluid to the vascular compartment. This is effected largely by prolongation of the constrictor phase of vasomotion and reduction of the dilator phase. In essence, what we are saying is that the product of intracapillary pressure and time of perfusion is of more significance in determining the distribution of fluid between plasma and interstitial compartments than is intracapillary pressure alone.

A reduction in the concentration of plasma protein reduces the oncotic pressure, which opposes transudation and promotes reabsorption of interstitial fluid. Hypoproteinemia is commonly associated with generalized expansion of interstitial volume. Albuminuria and hypoalbuminemia are characteristic features of the nephrotic syndrome in chronic glomerulonephritis and nephrosis. Massive edema occurs in both conditions; and, although low plasma protein concentration is not a complete explanation, it certainly contributes to expansion of interstitial volume. Hypoproteinemia, edema and ascites also occur in cirrhosis and in part are consequences of inadequate formation of albumin by the diseased liver.

The oncotic effect of plasma proteins is largely dependent on the concentration of albumin and suffers a larger decrement in both the nephrotic syndrome and chronic liver disease than might be anticipated from the reduction in total protein concentration. In both conditions, the concentration of albumin is much reduced, and the albumin/globulin ratio of $2+ : 1$ is often reversed.

Increase in capillary permeability with loss of protein into tissue interstices reduces the differential oncotic effects that ordinarily retain fluid in the vascular compartment. A number of factors account for the relative protein impermeability of normal capillaries. Protein (possibly fibrinogen), adsorbed on the inner surface of the capillary, leakproofs it. The endothelial cells are locked together in a lapjoint, and the chinks are sealed with a calcium-proteinate cement impermeable to colloids. The endothelial cells possess tone or turgescence, loss of which increases protein permeability. Physical damage to capillaries by heat or ultraviolet light, capillary poisons, increased acidity of blood, anoxia, lack of calcium and the liberation of histamine and proteolytic enzymes in damaged tissues all increase capillary permeability to protein and transudation of fluid.

Increased tissue distensibility, due to loss of subcutaneous adipose tissue or to previous episodes of edema, predisposes to expansion of interstitial fluid. Tissue turgor, although of minor proportions, resists outward filtration of fluid and favors reabsorption in capillaries that are minimally perfused.

Obstruction of lymphatic outflow results in edema of a peculiar brawny type, characterized by proliferation of connective tissue and by the collection of proteinaceous fluid in the tissue interstices. Lymphatic obstruction is almost always the result of long-standing chronic or repeated acute inflammatory processes. Lymphatics have a very great capacity for regeneration; only repeated insults result in permanent blockage and lymph edema. A major function of the lymphatic drainage of any tissue is the removal of proteins that leak through capillary walls. No mechanism exists for their direct return to the capillary lumen. Instead, they are absorbed into the lymphatic capillaries, which progressively coalesce to form the central lymphatic channels. These in turn form the thoracic duct and the right lymphatic duct, which empty into the venous system at the junction of the subclavian and jugular veins.

Summary

Water constitutes some 45–75% of body weight of normal man, varying inversely with the proportion of adipose tissue. This water can be considered as distributed among a plasma compartment (4.5%), an interstitial compartment (16–18%), a transcellular compartment (1–3%) and a cellular compartment (30–40%) of body weight.

In extracellular fluid, sodium is the major cation and chloride and bicarbonate are the major anions. These ions represent 90–95% of the osmotically active components of extracellular fluid. In intracellular fluid, potassium and magnesium are the major cations, and organic phosphate compounds and protein are the major anions. The marked differences in concentration of potassium and sodium inside and outside the cell are maintained by ion pumps, which are located in cell membranes, are metabolically activated and are concerned with the extrusion of sodium from, and the concentration of potassium within, cells. Cell membranes are impermeable to protein and to organic phosphate complexes, but they allow more or less free exchange of other ions between cell contents and extracellular fluid.

Water diffuses rapidly across cell membranes to establish essential equality of the osmolal concentrations in intra- and extracellular fluids. Relative volumes of cell contents and extracellular fluid depend on the quantities of ions contained within these compartments. Total body sodium averages 60 mEq/kg of body weight; potassium, 42 mEq/kg; chloride, 33 mEq/kg; bicarbonate, 10–12 mEq/kg; and magnesium, 12–17 mEq/kg. Only 60% of body sodium is readily exchangeable, whereas most of the potassium, chloride, bicarbonate and magnesium is exchangeable.

The distribution of fluid between the plasma and interstitial compartments is determined by the balance of the hydrostatic pressure, the colloid osmotic pressure and the tissue-turgor pressure operative across the capillary endothelium. The relative durations of the dilator versus the constrictor phases of vasomotion, the permeability of the capillaries, the distensibility of the tissues and the adequacy of lymphatic drainage all play ancillary roles.

REFERENCES

1. Elkinton, J. R., and Danowsky, T. S.: *The Body Fluids: Basic Physiology and Practical Therapeutics* (Baltimore: Williams & Wilkins Company, 1955).
2. Peters, J. P.: *Body Water: The Exchange of Fluids in Man* (Springfield, Ill.: Charles C Thomas, Publisher, 1935).
3. Strauss, M. B.: *Body Water in Man* (Boston: Little, Brown & Company, 1957).
4. Welt, L. G.: *Clinical Disorders of Hydration and Acid Base Balance* (Boston: Little, Brown & Company, 1955).
5. Manery, J.: Water and electrolyte metabolism, Physiol. Rev. 34:334, 1954.
6. Robinson, J. R.: Metabolism of intracellular water, Physiol. Rev. 40:112, 1960.
7. Schloerb, P. R.; Friis-Hansen, B. J.; Edelman, I. S.; Solomon, A. K., and Moore, F.

D.: The measurement of total body water in the human subject by deuterium oxide dilution with consideration of the dynamics of deuterium distribution, J. Clin. Invest. 29: 1296, 1950.

8. Skelton, H.: The storage of water by various tissues of the body, Arch. Int. Med. 40:140, 1927.

9. Bernard, C.: *Leçons sur les phénomènes de la vie communs aux animaux et aux végétaux* (Paris: Baillière, 1885).

10. Schultz, A. L.; Hammersten, J. F.; Heller, B. I., and Ebert, R. V.: A critical comparison of the T-1824 dye and iodinated albumin methods for plasma volume measurement, J. Clin. Invest. 32:107, 1953.

11. Swan, R. C.; Madisso, H., and Pitts, R. F.: Measurement of extracellular fluid volume in nephrectomized dogs, J. Clin. Invest. 33: 1447, 1954.

12. Gaudino, M.; Schwartz, I. L., and Levitt, M.: Inulin volume of distribution as measure of extracellular fluid in dog and man, Proc. Soc. Exper. Biol. & Med. 68:507, 1948.

13. Behnke, A. R., Jr.: Physiological studies pertaining to deep sea diving and aviation, especially in relation to the fat content and composition of the body, Harvey Lect. 37:198, 1941–42.

14. Pace, N., and Rathbun, E. N.: Studies of body composition: III. The body water and chemically combined nitrogen content in relation to fat content, J. Biol. Chem. 158:685, 1945.

15. Glynn, I. M.: Sodium and potassium movements in human red cells, J. Physiol. 134:278, 1956.

16. Skou, J. C.: Enzymatic basis for active transport of Na^+ and K^+ across cell membrane, Physiol. Rev. 45:596, 1965.

17. Pitts, R. F.: *The Physiological Basis of Diuretic Therapy* (Springfield, Ill.: Charles C Thomas, Publisher, 1959).

18. Darrow, D. C., and Yannet, H.: The changes in the distribution of body water accompanying increase and decrease in extracellular electrolyte, J. Clin. Invest. 14:266, 1935.

19. Bergstrom, W. H., and Wallace, W. M.: Bone as a sodium and potassium reservoir, J. Clin. Invest. 33:867, 1954.

20. Edelman, I. S.; Liebman, J.; O'Meara, M. P., and Berkenfeld, L. W.: Interrelations between serum sodium concentration, serum osmolality and total exchangeable sodium, total exchangeable potassium and total body water, J. Clin. Invest. 37:1236, 1958.

21. James, A. H.; Brooks, L.; Edelman, I. S.; Olney, J. M., and Moore, F. D.: Body sodium and potassium: I. The simultaneous measurement of exchangeable sodium and potassium in man by isotope dilution, Metabolism 3: 313, 1954.

22. Warner, G. F.; Sweet, N. J., and Dobson, E. L.: Sodium space and body sodium content, exchangable with sodium-24 in normal individuals and in patients with ascites. Circulation Res. 1:486, 1953.

23. Widdowson, E. M.; McCance, R. A., and Spray, C. M.: Chemical composition of human body, Clin. Sc. 10:113, 1951.

24. Starling, E. H.: Physiological factors involved in the causation of dropsy, Lancet 1: 1405, 1896.

25. Pappenheimer, J. R.: Passage of molecules through capillary walls, Physiol. Rev. 33:387, 1953.

26. Zweifach, B. W.: Basic mechanisms in peripheral vascular homeostasis, in *Transactions of Third Josiah Macy, Jr., Conference on Factors Regulating Blood Pressure* (New York: Josiah Macy Foundation, 1949).

27. Zweifach, B. W.: *Functional Behavior of the Microcirculation* (Springfield, Ill.: Charles C Thomas, Publisher, 1961).

3

Elements of Renal Function

FOR MORE than 100 years, glomerular ultra-filtration, tubular reabsorption and tubular secretion have been considered as contributing in varying degree to urine formation. However, rigorous proof of the contributions of each of these discrete renal processes is of relatively recent origin, the major evidence having accumulated over the past 40 years. This chapter considers briefly the historical development of concepts* concerning the role these processes play and the basis for the present view that all processes are involved in the elaboration of urine.

Historical Development of Concepts

According to Aristotle, the kidneys are not vital organs; rather, they provide a "greater finish and perfection to the body." His concept that urine is formed in the bladder was corrected by Galen, who rightly inferred that the kidneys form urine, the ureters are conduits and the bladder is an organ of storage.

The tubular structure of the kidney was first recognized (in 1662) by Bellini, who described the large papillary ducts that bear his name. However, a true appreciation of the complexity of the renal tubular system awaited the microscopic studies of Malpighi, published in 1666. Malpighi discovered that the cortex, which other anatomists had believed to be coagulated blood, is in reality a

compact mass of minute, tortuously coiled tubules, connected ultimately with the papillary ducts of Bellini. Furthermore, he observed, for the first time, many tiny spherical bodies (malpighian corpuscles) scattered throughout the cortex, and he saw that each is connected with a renal tubule. Although he noted that the corpuscles are attached to arteries and veins, he failed to recognize that their contents are tufts of capillaries. Rather, he thought that they were glands for the secretion of urine, which drains via the tubular system into the renal pelvis, ureter and bladder.

The precise morphologic studies of Bowman (3) in 1842 provided a basis for subsequent advances in knowledge of function. Working without benefit of microtome or stains and with a microscope that magnified only 300 times, he described accurately the glomerular capillary tuft, the afferent and efferent arterioles and the continuity of the capsule of the renal corpuscle (Bowman's capsule) and the tubular basement membrane. He observed that the capsule opens into the tubule and that it is tightly fused to afferent and efferent arterioles at its vascular pole. Thus, any fluid extruded by the capillaries drains from the capsular space into the tubular lumen. He described the tubule as formed of a single layer of epithelial cells resting on a basement membrane. Each tubule, he found, is connected with a single glomerulus, and each drains into a branched collecting duct. By injecting the renal artery

---

*Essays by Dr. Homer W. Smith (1, 2) are recommended to those having a special interest in the history of renal physiology.

and vein with water-insoluble colored materials and by teasing apart bits of tissue, he discovered the portal character of the peritubular capillary circulation and correctly inferred that all of the peritubular blood passes through the glomerular capillaries.

Bowman's functional speculations were somewhat less astute. He believed that the glomerular capillaries secrete water, which serves to dissolve and to flush out of the tubular lumen the excretory solutes secreted by the tubular cells. In keeping with the then current belief, he considered that secretion involves rupture of the luminal membranes of tubular cells and discharge of their contents into the tubular urine.

At the same time and quite independently, Ludwig (4) studied the microscopic anatomy of the kidney, and on all essential points his findings were in agreement with those of Bowman. From his studies on the relationship between renal arterial blood pressure and urine flow, Ludwig developed a physical theory of urine formation, remarkable for its prescience.

According to Ludwig, urine formation begins with the separation of a protein-free ultrafiltrate of blood plasma in the glomerular capillary tuft. The responsible force is the hydrostatic pressure imparted to the blood by the beat of the heart. The filtrate is formed in volume sufficient to account for the rate of excretion of all urinary solutes; volume is reduced and excretory products are concentrated by the reabsorption of the bulk of the filtrate as it flows along the renal tubules. Ludwig maintained that the glomerular capillaries are semipermeable, permitting free passage of water and solutes of small dimensions while restraining colloids and formed elements. His thesis of glomerular ultrafiltration is, thus, completely acceptable today.

Tubular secretion, which played so prominent a role in Bowman's hypothesis, was denied by Ludwig, who maintained that the volume of filtrate was sufficiently large to account for all solutes present in the urine without invoking secretion. He presumed that tubular reabsorption, like filtration, depends on pure physical forces. He recognized that the hydrostatic pressure of the blood in the peritubular capillaries must be lower than that in the glomerular capillaries and therefore unfavorable for filtration. He also recognized that the proteins and formed elements of postglomerular blood are concentrated by the formation of glomerular filtrate, and he postulated that, by a process of "endosmosis," tubular fluid is reabsorbed into the peritubular capillaries.

One might read into Ludwig's hypothesis a belief that the colloid osmotic force exerted by the plasma protein could cause the endosmosis of fluid across the tubular epithelium. However, it was not until 1896 that colloid osmotic pressure was first described, by Starling; hence, such an extrapolation is unjustified. Although Ludwig's generalization that tubular reabsorption, like glomerular filtration, is dependent on physical rather than "vital" forces* was brilliantly conceived, it is unacceptable in the light of present knowledge. Most solutes are now known to be reabsorbed by active mechanisms, which require the expenditure of metabolic energy by the cells effecting transport. Water is reabsorbed by diffusion along an osmotic gradient generated by the reabsorption of solutes, mainly ions.

Some 30 years after its proposal by Bowman, Heidenhain (5) revived the theory that urine is formed by the combined secretory activities of the glomerular capillary tufts and the renal tubules. Heidenhain injected indigo carmine into rabbits that had been made hypotensive by spinal transection or

---

*The term "vital" as applied to biologic processes had a different connotation in the 19th century than it has today. Then, it alluded to mysterious characteristics peculiar to living systems — neither physical nor chemical in nature, not subject to experimental elucidation and beyond the ken of mortal man. Now the term is used more generally to indicate only that the process is carried out in a living system. Although many living processes are beyond our understanding today, there is no reason to believe that they will not eventually be explained in terms of physics and chemistry. The "vitalists" of the 19th century opposed such a view; the "mechanists," including Ludwig, were its strong proponents.

by hemorrhage. These animals produced no urine, owing, according to Ludwig's hypothesis, to failure of glomerular filtration. However, when the kidneys were removed after 15 minutes, the tubular cells were stained a deep blue. An hour or more later, the dye was present in the tubular lumens in high concentration. No dye was seen at any time in the glomerular capillaries or in Bowman's capsule. Heidenhain concluded that tubular cells take up dye from the peritubular capillaries and secrete it into the lumen.

Heidenhain calculated that some 70 L of glomerular filtrate would have to be formed each day to account for the observed rate of excretion of urea. This value he considered preposterous,* especially in view of the fact that some 68 L of fluid would have to be reabsorbed to form 2 L of urine. He further pointed out that the glomerular capillaries are not naked vessels, as Bowman had claimed, but arc covered with a layer of epithelial cells. He inferred that this epithelial covering would prevent filtration but would contribute to urine formation by secretion. Heidenhain's thesis thus resembled Bowman's, in that it postulated that the glomeruli secrete mainly water, whereas the tubules secrete other urinary constituents.

The relationship between urine flow and blood pressure, which formed the basis of the filtration-reabsorption theory of Ludwig, was explained by Heidenhain as being due to the dependence of glomerular and tubular secretion on renal blood flow. He thought pressure to be significant only in that it determines flow. Furthermore, he observed that the infusion of saline or urea solutions has no effect on blood pressure but markedly augments urine flow, whereas partial occlusion of the renal vein, which might be expected to raise glomerular capillary pressure and filtration rate, actually reduces urine flow. He concluded that the kidneys, like other glands,

are influenced in their rate of secretion of urine by the composition of the blood and by the rate of blood flow.

Heidenhain's views of tubular secretion must have been similar to ours today, for his illustrations show that indigo carmine is transported across intact tubular cells without rupture of the luminal membrane. Today, renal tubular secretion is believed to depend on carrier molecules located in intact cellular membranes. No rupture of the apical membrane with discharge of cell contents occurs in the kidney. Heidenhain created the term "active force" to account for transcellular movement of solutes. Today we use the term "metabolic energy." Whereas Ludwig's kidney was a physical machine, Heidenhain's was a chemical one. Both investigators were mechanists in the true sense of the word, and both were partly correct in their interpretations of renal function.

However, neither Ludwig nor Heidenhain had proved either glomerular ultrafiltration or tubular secretion. Variations in rate of urine flow and solute excretion, such as those observed by Ludwig, might, as Heidenhain claimed, be determined by a relationship between renal blood flow and rate of glomerular and tubular secretion and not by changes in rate of glomerular filtration. Similarly, the dye that Heidenhain observed in tubular cells might have been taken up from the tubular lumen, not from the peritubular blood. Furthermore, dye might be concentrated in the tubular lumen by the filtration of a highly dilute solution, invisible in the capsular space, followed by the reabsorption of a large proportion of the filtered water. No critical experimental test of either thesis had been made, nor was it to be made for the next 50 years.

In 1917, Cushny published the first monograph to be devoted entirely to the physiology of the kidney, *The Secretion of Urine* (6). Cushny introduced no new experimental evidence; in fact, he contributed nothing to an already extensive, if not critical, experimental literature. Rather, he read widely,

---

*It is now known that the rate of glomerular filtration of plasma averages 180 L/day in man and that water equivalent to that contained in 178 L of plasma is reabsorbed.

discarded that which smacked of vitalism, which by his definition included tubular secretion, and developed a mechanistic thesis he termed "the modern theory." The best parts of "the modern theory" were Cushny's reiteration of Ludwig's concept that the glomeruli are ultrafilters and of Claude Bernard's concept that the kidneys regulate the composition of the internal fluid environment. His views on tubular reabsorption and his rejection of tubular secretion were founded more on prejudice than on fact, and are both incorrect. Nevertheless, his monograph constituted a milestone in renal physiology: the time was ripe; "the modern theory" was lucidly, if not consistently, expounded; and it provided a clear-cut target at which an imaginative new group of experimentalists could shoot.

"The modern theory" included Ludwig's view that the hydrostatic pressure imparted to the blood by the beat of the heart forces a protein-free ultrafiltrate of plasma through the glomerular capillaries. The volume of filtrate is adequate to account for all excretory products; the tubules do not secrete. Because all solutes of small molecular dimensions must enter the glomerular filtrate in concentrations essentially equal to their concentrations in the aqueous phase of plasma, those of value must, obviously, be reabsorbed. Those completely reabsorbed (e.g., glucose and amino acids) and those partially reabsorbed (e.g., sulfate, urea and chloride) he designated "threshold solutes," presuming that all have more or less biologic value and that for each some threshold plasma concentration exists, below which reabsorption is complete. He designated creatinine and certain other wastes "no-threshold solutes," for he believed that all of these substances that enter the filtrate are excreted in the urine.

Cushny properly rejected Ludwig's physical endosmosis as the mechanism of tubular reabsorption, for he recognized that it could explain neither the formation of urine more concentrated than plasma nor the complete reabsorption of certain threshold solutes from the tubular fluid. Having rejected Heidenhain's thesis of tubular secretion as involving "vitalistic" discriminatory capacities on the part of tubular cells, he faced the problem of devising a "nonvitalistic" mechanism of reabsorptive transport in the reverse direction. He maintained that the tubules blindly and unvaryingly reabsorb a fluid of constant composition, a sort of idealized Ringer-Locke solution. Nonideal plasma is filtered through the glomeruli; ideal fluid is reabsorbed; and whatever is left over is excreted as urine. Active forces, chemical rather than physical in nature, power the reabsorptive machinery.

Cushny's thesis of "reabsorption of an idealized fluid of constant composition" is a simplification, in a semantic but not in a mechanistic sense, of current concepts. The capacity of tubular cells to reabsorb a fluid of constant and ideal composition, independent of the composition of the fluid presented in the filtrate, is no less demanding of discriminatory powers than is the secretion of an "idealized urine" in the reverse direction. In fact, both theses are wrong. Many solutes present in the filtrate are reabsorbed independently by specific cellular transport mechanisms. Other solutes, in addition to being filtered, are secreted into the urine by one or another of several independent secretory mechanisms. A few solutes are known to be filtered and both reabsorbed and secreted.

Proof of Glomerular Ultrafiltration

A simple filter removes only gross particulate matter from solution. With a fine-enough filter (Millipore filter), red cells can be separated from blood plasma, but the process is still one of simple filtration. Ultrafiltration goes a step further: not only particulate matter but also colloidal materials, such as proteins and lipids, are removed from solution. However, an ultrafilter does not sieve out solutes of small molecular dimensions, i.e., the so-called crystalloidal, as opposed to colloidal,* solutes.

CRITERIA OF ULTRAFILTRATION

If we are to accept ultrafiltration of plasma through the glomerular capillary tuft as the initial process in urine formation, three criteria must be met: (1) The ultrafiltrate must be protein-free. (2) The ultrafiltrate must contain all crystalloids (solutes of small molecular dimensions) in the same concentrations as in the aqueous phase of the plasma from which it is formed. The glomerular capillary membrane must not alter the proportions of these constituents of plasma with respect to each other or with respect to water.† (3) The hydrostatic pressure of the blood within the glomerular capillaries must constitute a force adequate to separate this protein-free fluid from the plasma in the amounts known to be formed.

MICROPUNCTURE TECHNICS. — Micropuncture technics in the hands of A. N. Richards and his colleagues have provided incontrovertible proof that the above criteria of glomerular ultrafiltration are met in the amphibian, reptilian and mammalian kidney. A micromanipulator carrying needles for microdissection was first suggested by Purkinje about 1844, and a working model was first built by Schmidt in 1859. A micropipet was first constructed in 1907 by McClendon. The technics of microdissection and microinjection were developed to a high degree of perfection over the period 1912–24 by Robert Chambers. Using these tech-

nics, Chambers contributed immensely to our knowledge of the physical and chemical properties of the cytoplasm and plasma membrane of living cells.

FIRST CRITERION. — In the spring of 1921, Richards observed a demonstration of Chambers' micromanipulator at a meeting of the American Association of Anatomists, in Philadelphia. Richards had had a long-sustained interest in renal physiology, had recently studied the glomerular circulation in the transilluminated kidney of the living frog and was well acquainted with the accessibility of the glomeruli on the ventral surface of the amphibian kidney. With Wearn, Richards (7) began the arduous task of puncturing Bowman's capsule in the kidney of the living frog and of analyzing the minute quantities of fluid that could be collected in a micropipet (Fig. 3–1). Their initial studies were relatively simple: the fluid obtained was free of protein within the limits of their analytic methods, although it contained glucose and chloride. At least the first criterion of glomerular ultrafiltration was met: the fluid was protein-free.

SECOND CRITERION. — Proving that representative crystalloidal solutes are present in the glomerular filtrate in the same concentrations as in the aqueous phase of plasma was far more demanding, for it required the

Fig. 3–1. — Collection of glomerular filtrate by micropuncture.

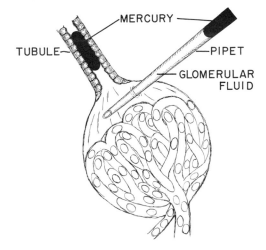

---

*Colloids exhibit a Tyndall effect; i.e., the path of a light beam through a solution of a colloid is visible. This means that particle size is great enough to scatter visible light. Solutions of crystalloids do not exhibit a Tyndall effect; the particles are so small that they do not scatter light.

†Charged particles have slightly different concentrations in glomerular ultrafiltrate and in plasma water: diffusible cations are slightly less concentrated, and diffusible anions are slightly more concentrated. This inequality of concentration results from the presence of negatively charged protein only in the plasma and is an expression of a Gibbs-Donnan distribution of diffusible ions (see Chapter 2).

perfection of a system of microchemical analysis of samples a fraction of a microliter in volume. In studies carried out over a period of years, Richards (8) and his colleagues observed equality of composition of filtrate and plasma with respect to osmotic pressure, electrical conductivity, glucose, pH, chloride, potassium, phosphate, urea, creatinine and uric acid. Most of their experiments were performed on the frog and *Necturus*, for in these animals the glomeruli are large and easily visible through the thin peritoneal layer that covers the kidney. However, data obtained on the rat, guinea pig and opossum are in complete agreement with those obtained on the frog and *Necturus*. Thus, the second criterion of glomerular ultrafiltration was met: the composition of glomerular fluid with respect to crystalloidal solutes is identical with that of the aqueous phase of plasma.

THIRD CRITERION. — The minimal force required to filter fluid through a porous membrane is set by (1) the force required to overcome frictional resistance to fluid flow through minute channels in the membrane and (2) the force required to separate fluid from dissolved constituents. Because the glomeruli separate only proteins from an aqueous medium containing all other solutes, the force required is small: 25 – 30 mm Hg in the mammalian kidney and 5 – 15 mm Hg in the amphibian kidney. This force is equal to the oncotic pressure of the plasma proteins; and, because the protein concentration of amphibian plasma is low, the force required is small. If the glomeruli separated pure water from the dissolved salts and organic constituents of mammalian plasma, the force needed would be incredibly great — some 5,100 mm Hg, i.e., equal to the osmotic pressure of blood plasma.*

Table 3 – 1 summarizes the balance of forces involved in glomerular ultrafiltration in the amphibian and mammalian kidney. The mean arterial pressure of *Necturus* is 25 mm Hg; that of man is 100 mm Hg. Because

---

*The total molecular concentration of mammalian blood plasma is 300 mOsm/L; therefore the osmotic pressure is 5,100 mm Hg (see Chapter 2).

TABLE 3–1. — BALANCE OF FORCES INVOLVED IN GLOMERULAR ULTRAFILTRATION

	NECTURUS*	MAN†
Mean arterial pressure (mm Hg)	25.0	100
Glomerular capillary pressure (mm Hg)	17.7	50
Intracapsular pressure (mm Hg)	1.5	10
Net filtration pressure (mm Hg)	16.2	40
Colloid osmotic pressure (mm Hg)	10.4	30
Pressure to overcome frictional resistance in membrane (mm Hg)	5.8	10

*From White, H. L.: Am. J. Physiol. 90:689, 1929.
†Estimated by author.

the vessels connecting the aorta and afferent arterioles are short and direct, pressure at the beginning of the afferent arterioles approaches the arterial pressure. In *Necturus*, the glomerular capillary pressure is 70% of mean arterial pressure. Obviously, in man, one can only make a reasonable guess of capillary pressure; but, on the basis of recent work on the rat, the author's estimate is 45 – 50% of mean arterial pressure — a value that may well vary in the diseased kidney. The intracapsular pressure opposes filtration; hence, the net or effective filtration pressure is equal to the intracapillary pressure minus the intracapsular pressure. The colloid osmotic pressure also opposes filtration. Accordingly, the pressures available to overcome frictional resistance to flow through the porous glomerular membranes of *Necturus* (9) and man are 5.8 and 10 mm Hg, respectively. Such pressures are presumably adequate to account for the observed rates of glomerular filtration set forth in Chapter 4. Accordingly, the third and final criterion of glomerular ultrafiltration has been satisfied: the force is adequate.

A major stumbling block to an exact measurement of glomerular capillary pressure in mammals is that glomeruli, for the most part, are not visible on the surface of the kidney. Even the most superficial ones lie deep in the cortex and therefore are unavailable to micropuncture measurement of pressure. This seemingly insurmountable difficulty has been overcome by Gertz *et al.* (10) in an ingenious way. As shown in Figure 3 – 2, *A*, surface loops of proximal tubules of the rat kidney were identified by the intravenous injection of lissamine green, a dye which is in part bound to plasma proteins and in part filterable through glomeruli. A loop immediately distal to a glomerulus is blocked with viscous oil, and a pressure-measuring micropipet is introduced just proximal to the block. Pressure in this segment rises due to continued filtration without egress of tubular urine until back pressure stops filtration. This intratubular stop-flow pressure (P_{SF}) is presumably equal to glomerular capillary pressure (P_{GC}) minus colloid osmotic pressure (P_{CO}) of plasma proteins; or, rewriting

$$P_{GC} = P_{SF} + P_{CO}$$

As shown in Figure 3–2, B, intratubular stop-flow pressures were measured over a range of arterial pressure: lowered, by partial clamping of the aorta above the renal arteries, and raised, by carotid ligation. The dotted line, designated glomerular capillary pressure, is the sum of the stop-flow pressure and colloid osmotic pressure. An interesting feature illustrated by this graph is that, at arterial pressures below 90 mm Hg, the capillary pressure is essentially equal to the arterial pressure; the pressure drop in lobar and interlobular arteries and across the afferent arteriole is nil. At pressures above 90 mm Hg, capillary pressure becomes constant and independent of arterial pressure. The pressure drop, presumably across the afferent arteriole, exactly equals the increase in arte-

rial pressure. This fact is illustrated in Figure 3–2, C. These observations correlate well with certain characteristics of the renal circulation, loosely grouped as autoregulation of glomerular filtration rate and renal blood flow and described in more detail on p. 168. Both parameters—filtration rate and renal blood flow—vary directly with arterial pressure over the range of 50–90 mm Hg. From 90 to 180 mm Hg, both become constant and relatively independent of pressure. Increasing afferent arteriolar constriction over this latter range of pressures could maintain both variables constant.

Recently, Brenner *et al.* (11) and Deen *et al.* (12) have made direct measurements of glomerular capillary pressures in the rat that give a different picture of glomerular dynamics than the indirect measurements of Gertz. Such direct measurements have been made possible by discovery of a mutant strain of Wistar rats, which is characterized by having a number of surface glomeruli available for micropuncture. Lacking evidence to the contrary, the estimates of glomerular dynamics in man have been taken from this experimental work of Brenner on the rat (with adjustments for differences between rat and man). Glomerular capillary pressures (P_{GC}), which were measured in single glomerular capillary loops of this mutant strain of rats, were 49–78 cm H_2O (on average, equal to 44.3 mm Hg; note that, in Table 3–1, all pressures have been converted from centimeters of

Fig. 3–2.—Estimation of glomerular capillary pressure in the rat and of the pressure drop across the afferent arteriole. *A*, method of measurement of intratubular stop-flow pressure; *B*, relationship between intratubular stop-flow, glomerular capillary and mean arterial pressures; *C*, pressure drop across the afferent arteriole. (Modified from Gertz, K. H.; Mangos, J. A.; Braun, G., and Pagel, H. D.: Pflügers Arch. 288: 369, 1966.)

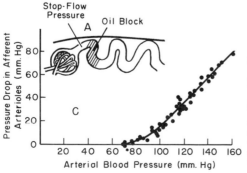

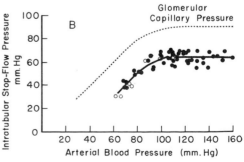

water to millimeters of mercury, a more familiar hemodynamic unit). The mean arterial pressure of these anesthetized rats was 132 mm Hg; that of normal man is about 100 mm Hg.

Pressure in Bowman's capsule, measured simultaneously, averaged 11.3 cm H_2O (8.3 mm Hg). The hydrostatic pressure difference (effective hydrostatic pressure), therefore, was 36 mm Hg (44.3 mm Hg − 8.3 mm Hg). Also opposing glomerular filtration was the colloid osmotic pressure (P_{CO}) of the plasma proteins: 5.5 Gm/100 ml of arterial plasma entering the glomerulus and 8.4 Gm/100 ml of efferent arteriolar plasma leaving the glomerulus. The colloid osmotic pressure exerted at the middle of the effective glomerular capillary filtration length was calculated as half the sum of the colloid osmotic pressures at the beginning and end of the capillary. The average colloid osmotic pressure was 26.1 mm Hg. The net effective filtration pressure, therefore, was about 10 mm Hg (36.0 mm Hg − 26.1 mm Hg). The increase in protein concentration as plasma flows along the capillary loop was obviously due to the expression of protein-free filtrate through the capillary wall. An increase from 5.5 to 8.4 Gm% indicates that about 35% of the plasma flowing through the capillary loops was filtered through the capillary walls (filtration fraction). Because the net hydrostatic pressure in the latter reaches of glomerular capillaries is essentially the same as the colloid osmotic pressure of efferent arteriolar plasma, filtration equilibrium had been achieved somewhere along the glomerular capillary filtration length. By filtration equilibrium is meant equality of the outwardly directed forces (hydrostatic pressure) and inwardly directed forces (colloid osmotic pressure and Bowman's capsule pressure).

The filtration rates of single glomeruli were measured, in these studies, by free-flow collection methods (see Chapter 7). Knowing the net filtration pressures (much lower than previously estimated) and single nephron glomerular filtration rates permitted the calculation of the filtration coefficient (K_f), which is a measure of glomerular capillary fluid permeability. This value $-0.32 \cdot 10^{-8}$ ml/sec per millimeter of mercury for one glomerulus — was, therefore, much higher than previously estimated; i.e., the glomerular capillaries were shown to be at least 10 times more permeable than estimated in Chapter 4. Thus, it is possible that filtration equilibrium is achieved early in the glomerular capillaries and that a large fraction of capillary length is essentially nonfunctional as a filter. A consequence would be that glomerular filtration is flow-dependent; i.e., the greater the volume flow of plasma, the greater the capillary length involved in filtration and the greater the filtration rate.

In more recent studies, Deen *et al.* (12) have confirmed the above-mentioned view. Expansion of extracellular fluid volume increases glomerular filtration rate and glomerular plasma flow proportionally, with no significant change in net ultrafiltration pressure at the afferent-most reaches of the glomerular capillary loop.

Whether or not these findings of Brenner and his colleagues are applicable to man is unknown, although estimates have been made (see Table 3 − 1). Thus, the filtration fractions (glomerular filtration rate/renal plasma flow) in man, dog and rat are 0.20, 0.25 and 0.35, respectively. Even more controversial is whether or not they apply to the diseased kidney in man. However, it seems better to equate human renal functions to directly measured rat renal functions than to estimate from indirectly derived data. One line of evidence, adduced from calculations of indirect measurements in the dog, shows that glomerular capillary pressures are essentially as low as in the rat (13).

Proof of Tubular Reabsorption

Once glomerular ultrafiltration is proved, tubular reabsorption follows directly, for many of the filterable constituents of blood plasma are absent from the urine. However, the technics of micropuncture of the renal tubules and analysis of the fluid withdrawn at various sites have, in the hands of Richards (14) and his associates, provided experimen-

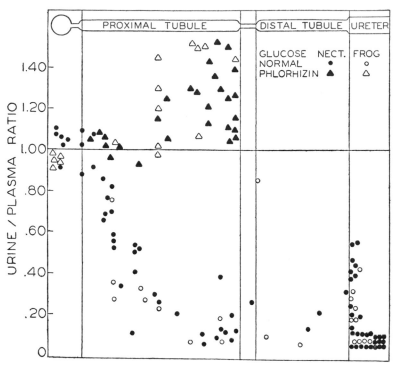

Fig. 3—3.—Reabsorption of glucose from proximal tubular fluid of the normal frog and *Necturus* and progressive concentration of unreabsorbed glucose following administration of phlorhizin as a consequence of continued reabsorption of fluid. (Data from Walker, A. M., and Hudson, C. L: Am. J. Physiol. 118:130, 1937; figure from Smith, H. W.: *The Kidney: Structure and Function in Health and Disease* [New York: Oxford University Press, 1951].)

tal confirmation of tubular reabsorption and—more important—evidence as to the location within the nephron of certain reabsorptive mechanisms. In recent years, these technics have contributed immensely to our knowledge of mechanisms of reabsorption of ions and of concentration of the urine.

Figure 3–3 illustrates the site of reabsorption of glucose in the renal tubules of the frog and *Necturus* (15). A schematic nephron, consisting of glomerulus and proximal and distal tubules, is shown at the top of the figure. The site of puncture is indicated by the placement of each datum at the appropriate locus along the nephron. On the ordinate is plotted the ratio of the concentration of glucose in the tubular fluid to that in the plasma.* The values obtained by glomerular

puncture cluster around a ratio of 1:1, for the concentration of glucose in the filtrate is the same as that in the plasma. The ratio decreases rapidly as the fluid flows along the proximal segment, indicating that glucose is reabsorbed much more rapidly than water. Although glucose† is completely reabsorbed by the time the filtrate has traversed the first half of the proximal segment, the more distal portion of the proximal tubule also has latent reabsorptive capacity, for, when perfused with glucose solution, reabsorption can be demonstrated. However, perfusion of the distal tubule has shown that this segment is incapable of reabsorbing glucose. Rather, any glucose that enters the distal tubule is concentrated by the reabsorption of water.

Phlorhizin has long been known to cause

---

*During the collection of fluid from Bowman's capsule and from any given point along the tubule, the tubular lumen distal to the site of puncture is blocked with a globule of oil or mercury to prevent reflux.

†The total reducing substance was measured. That which remains at the midpoint of the proximal segment is largely, if not entirely, non-glucose-reducing materials. Glucose is completely reabsorbed.

glucosuria. In frogs and *Necturus* given phlorhizin, the ratio of the concentration of glucose in the tubular fluid to that in the plasma increases, rather than decreases, as the filtrate flows along the proximal tubule. This does not indicate that glucose is secreted; rather, it shows that reabsorption is blocked and that the filtered glucose is concentrated by the reabsorption of water.

Figure 3–4 illustrates certain characteristics of the reabsorption of ions and water (16). Total molecular concentration, largely of sodium, chloride and bicarbonate ions, was measured by a micro-vapor-pressure method. Chloride was measured nephelometrically. The total molecular concentration (osmolar concentration) of the glomerular filtrate is the same as that of the plasma from which it is formed. Total molecular concentration does not change as the filtrate flows along the proximal segment. Because fluid is reabsorbed, ions and water must be reabsorbed proportionally. The present view is that sodium is actively, and chloride is

passively, reabsorbed in the proximal tubule. The tubule is freely permeable to water. The osmotic force created by the transport of ions causes the reabsorption of an osmotically equivalent fraction of the water.

In the distal tubule, both total osmolar concentration and chloride concentration decrease relative to plasma, indicating that ions are reabsorbed more rapidly than is water in this segment. The urine is thus diluted; i.e., osmotic pressure is reduced relative to plasma. Water is eliminated without proportional loss of ions.

Proof of Tubular Secretion

Of the three discrete renal processes involved in urine formation, tubular secretion was the last to be generally accepted. In fact, Richards and his colleagues long argued against its existence, accepting it only when their own observations on urea excretion in the frog could be explained in no other way. The reason is fairly evident. Any substance

Fig. 3—4.—Isosmotic reabsorption of ions and water in the proximal tubule and dilution of the urine in the distal tubule of the amphibian kidney. (Data from Walker, A. M., Hudson, C. L., Findley, T., Jr., and Richards, A. N.: Am. J. Physiol. 118:121, 1937; figure from Smith, H. W.: *The Kidney: Structure and Function in Health and Disease* [New York: Oxford University Press, 1951].)

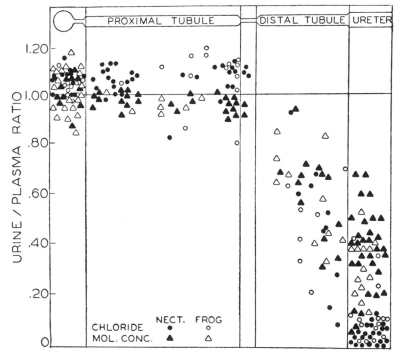

that is secreted will also be filtered. Only if that which is excreted in the urine exceeds that which could be accounted for by filtration alone, can tubular secretion be demonstrated. Micropuncture methods did not contribute significantly to proof of tubular secretion; the fact that the concentration of a substance progressively increases as the tubular fluid flows along a given segment may indicate only that water is reabsorbed, not necessarily that the substance is secreted. Now it is possible to assess the degree of water reabsorption by the infusion of inulin, a substance that is freely filterable through glomerular capillaries but not reabsorbed by the renal tubules. If a substance increases in concentration to a greater degree than does inulin, it must be added to the tubular fluid by secretion. Such methods were unavailable to the early micropuncture workers.

EVIDENCE FROM RATE OF EXCRETION

Evidence for secretion from the rate of excretion was first adduced for the indicator dye phenol red by Marshall and Vickers (17). The rate of excretion of phenol red (phenolsulfonphthalein) was introduced in 1910 by Rowntree and Geraghty as an empirical renal function test and has been widely used in the diagnosis of renal disease over the succeeding years. When administered parenterally, phenol red is rapidly and quantitatively excreted in the urine. Marshall and Vickers observed that some 60% of the dye is bound to plasma albumin and therefore is nonfilterable through glomerular capillaries. They calculated that, if the dye were excreted solely by glomerular filtration, the rate of filtration would have to be impossibly high to account for the observed rates of excretion. Marshall and Crane (18) noted further that, as the plasma concentration of phenol red is gradually increased, the rate of excretion at first increases and then tends to level off. If excretion were solely a function of rate of filtration, the quantity of phenol red eliminated each minute should increase in exact proportion to plasma concentration.

These investigators interpreted their findings as indicating that the tubular secretory mechanism is saturated at moderate plasma concentrations and so can transport no more at high concentrations. They also observed that, at low plasma concentrations, as much as 70% of the dye could be extracted from the renal blood. Because only 40% of the dye is filterable and only a fraction of the total blood plasma perfusing the kidney is filtered, the conclusion was inescapable that the tubular cells must secrete it. More recent evidence concerning tubular secretion will be considered later (Chapter 8).

EVIDENCE FROM COMPARATIVE PHYSIOLOGY

From comparative physiologic studies of renal function, the evidence for secretion is impressive. Certain marine teleost fish, including the goosefish, pipefish, sea horse and toadfish, have aglomerular nephrons. The kidneys of these fish receive only a portal blood supply, the arterial supply having disappeared with the glomeruli. Blood pressure in the peritubular capillaries is less than the colloid osmotic pressure of the plasma proteins; hence, filtration cannot, in any way, contribute to urine formation. Nevertheless, these fish excrete all the constituents typical of the urine of marine glomerular fish. They also secrete various foreign substances, such as phenol red, indigo carmine and tetraethylammonium ion. Of special import is the fact that they cannot secrete glucose even when hyperglycemia is induced or when phlorhizin is administered. Neither can they secrete sucrose, xylose, inulin or ferrocyanide. Although such observations by no means constitute evidence for tubular secretion in mammals, they at least suggest the possibility that certain urinary constituents may be secreted in the higher forms.

EVIDENCE FROM IN VITRO PREPARATIONS

Chambers and Cameron (19) and Chambers and Kempton (20) found that the mesonephros of 8 – 10-day chick embryos can be cultured in vitro. Isolated fragments of proximal tubules become closed cysts and secrete fluid into their lumina. When placed in dilute solutions of phenol red, the cells making up these cysts become stained and secrete the dyes in high concentration. At 38° C, secretion is active; at 3 – 6° C, no dye is secreted, and any that had accumulated in the lumen diffuses out. Secretion is blocked by cyanide, hydrogen sulfide, phenylurethane and iodoacetate. These inhibitors apparently block the uptake of dye into the cell at the basal membrane, for extrusion of dye already in cells into the lumen is not affected. Distal tubules do not take up the dye nor secrete it; hence, the phenol-red secretory mechanism is restricted to the proximal tubule. Essentially similar results were obtained on isolated tubules cultured from the metanephros of a human embryo.

Tubules teased from the kidneys of the flounder and immersed in a balanced salt medium were observed by Taggart and Forster (21) to take up phenol red from dilute solution and secrete it in high concentration into the lumens. Slices of mammalian kidneys likewise concentrate a number of substances, including phenol red, *p*-aminohippurate (22) and tetraethylammonium ion (23). These latter in vitro preparations have been extremely useful in assessing metabolic requirements of secretory processes.

Summary

Three discrete renal processes are now known to be involved in the elaboration of urine: glomerular ultrafiltration, tubular reabsorption and tubular secretion. Among the early workers, Ludwig and Cushny were proponents of glomerular filtration and tubular reabsorption as the processes of major import, whereas Bowman and Heidenhain championed glomerular and tubular secretion. Definitive proof of the contribution of glomerular ultrafiltration awaited the precise micropuncture studies of Richards and his colleagues, who demonstrated that the following three criteria of ultrafiltration are met in amphibian and mammalian glomeruli: (1) the ultrafiltrate is protein-free; (2) the ultrafiltrate contains all crystalloidal solutes in essentially the same concentrations as the aqueous phase of plasma; and (3) the hydrostatic pressure within the glomerular capillaries is adequate to produce filtrate in the volume known to be formed. Although demonstration of glomerular ultrafiltration necessitates acceptance of tubular reabsorption, the micropuncture studies of Richards' group provided direct confirmation of reabsorption and an indication of the sites at which reabsorptive processes are located.

Tubular secretion, although more difficult to establish, is no less significantly involved in urine formation. Comparative physiologic studies on urine formation in aglomerular fish, the observation of secretion of phenol red in vitro by isolated renal tubules in a variety of animals, and data on the rates of excretion of dyes and certain other substances by the kidneys of the dog and man all demand acceptance of tubular secretion.

REFERENCES

1. Smith, H. W.: Highlights in the history of renal physiology, Bull. Georgetown Univ. M. Center 13:4, 1959.
2. Smith, H. W.: *Lectures on the Kidney* (Lawrence: University of Kansas Press, 1943).
3. Bowman, W.: On the structure and use of the malpighian bodies of the kidney with observations on the circulation through that gland, Phil. Trans. Roy. Soc., London 132:57, 1842.
4. Ludwig, K.: Nieren und Harnbereitung, in Wagner, R.: *Handwörterbuch der Physiologie* (Brunswick: F. Vieweg, 1844).
5. Heidenhain, R.: Mikroskopische Beiträge zur Anatomie und Physiologie der Nieren, Arch. f. mikr. Anat. 10:1, 1874.
6. Cushny, A. R.: *The Secretion of Urine* (London: Longmans, Green & Co., Ltd., 1917).
7. Wearn, J. T., and Richards, A. N.: Observations on the composition of glomerular urine with particular reference to the problem of reabsorption in the renal tubules, Am. J. Physiol. 71:209, 1924.
8. Richards, A. N.: Kidney function, Harvey Lect. 16:163, 1920 – 21.
9. White, H. L.: Observations on the nature of

glomerular activity, Am. J. Physiol. 90:689, 1929.

10. Gertz, K. H., Mangos, J. A., Braun, G., and Pagel, H. D.: Pressure in the glomerular capillaries of the rat kidney and its relation to arterial blood pressure, Pflügers Arch. 288: 369, 1966.

11. Brenner, B. M., Troy, J. L., and Daugarty, T. M.: The dynamics of glomerular ultrafiltration in the rat, J. Clin. Invest. 50:1776, 1971.

12. Deen, W. M., Roberts, C. R., Brenner, B. M.: A model of glomerular ultrafiltration in the rat, Am. J. Physiol. 223:1178, 1972.

13. Lambert, P. P., Gassee, J. P., Verniory, A., and Fichourille, P. F.: Measurement of the glomerular filtration pressure from sieving data for macromolecules, Pflügers Arch. 329:34, 1971.

14. Richards, A. N.: Urine formation in the amphibian kidney, Harvey Lect. 30:93, 1934–35.

15. Walker, A. M., and Hudson, C. L.: The reabsorption of glucose from the renal tubule in Amphibia and the action of phlorhizin upon it, Am. J. Physiol. 118:130, 1937.

16. Walker, A. M., Hudson, C. L., Finley, T., Jr., and Richards, A. N.: The total molecular concentration and the chloride concentration of fluid from different segments of the renal tubule of Amphibia: The site of chloride reabsorption, Am. J. Physiol. 118: 121, 1937.

17. Marshall, E. K., Jr., and Vickers, J. L.: The mechanism of the elimination of phenolsulfonphthalein by the kidney, a proof of secretion by the convoluted tubules, Bull. Johns Hopkins Hosp. 34:1, 1923.

18. Marshall, E. K., Jr., and Crane, M. R.: The secretory function of the renal tubules, Am. J. Physiol. 70:465, 1924.

19. Chambers, R., and Cameron, G.: Intracellular hydrion concentration studies: VII. The secreting cells of the mesonephros in the chick, J. Cell. & Comp. Physiol. 2:99, 1932.

20. Chambers, R., and Kempton, R. T.: Indications of function of the chick mesonephros in tissue culture with phenol red, J. Cell. & Comp. Physiol. 3:131, 1933.

21. Taggart, J. V., and Forster, R. P.: Renal tubular transport: Effect of 2,4-dinitrophenol and related compounds on phenol red transport by the isolated tubules of the flounder, Am. J. Physiol. 161:167, 1950.

22. Cross, R. J., and Taggart, J. V.: Renal tubular transport: Accumulation of p-aminohippurate by rabbit kidney slices, Am. J. Physiol. 161: 181, 1950.

23. Farah, A., Rennick, B., and Frazer, M.: The influence of some basic substances on the transport of tetraethylammonium ion, J. Pharmacol. & Exper. Therap. 119:122, 1957.

4

The Nature of Glomerular Filtration

THE FILTRATION OF FLUID through glomerular capillary membranes does not involve the local expenditure of metabolic energy. Rather, filtration depends on the hydrostatic pressure, imparted to the blood by the beat of the heart (1). As pointed out in the preceding chapter, the minimum force needed to filter fluid through a porous membrane is determined by the force required to overcome frictional resistance to flow of fluid through channels in the membrane and by the force required to separate fluid from its dissolved constituents. Because the glomerular capillaries separate only the proteins from the blood plasma, the latter force is small and is equal to the colloid osmotic pressure. The filtration characteristics of glomerular capillary membranes are strikingly similar to those of artificial porous membranes, such as collodion, Cellophane and unglazed porcelain.

Accordingly, the pore concept of glomerular filtration is generally accepted today. However, there is no agreement concerning the structural basis for the porelike properties of glomerular capillaries.

The architecture of the glomerular capillary membranes may be described in two ways: visually, in terms of appearance in electron micrographs, and functionally, in terms of filtration characteristics.

The seemingly direct microscopic approach is complicated by problems of artifacts that may develop in protein and lipoprotein ultrastructures made electron-dense with heavy metals and dehydrated with organic solvents. The functional description, based on filtration characteristics, is complicated by the necessity for making many simplifying assumptions.

Functional Description of Glomerular Capillaries

The functional approach has been most ingeniously employed by Pappenheimer *et al.* (2–5). They assumed that the pores of glomerular capillaries are straight-bore cylindrical channels, all having identical radii (r) and all leading directly from capillary lumen to glomerular capsule, and so of equal length (ΔX). Length has been taken as 400–600 Å (0.04–0.06 μ), which is the thickness of the basement membrane. The total number of pores in all glomerular capillaries of both kidneys has been assigned the value N. Pappenheimer further assumed that flow of fluid along these channels is streamline in nature and describable by Poiseuille's equation.* If the rate of glomerular filtration of fluid in milliliters per minute is $\dot{Q}_f$, if the pressure drop across the capillary membrane is ΔP and if the viscosity of the filtrate is η, then Poiseuille's equation for N pores states that the rate of glomerular filtration is

---

*Poiseuille's equation adequately describes hydrodynamic flow in small-bore rigid tubes and approximates flow in minute blood vessels. That it does so in channels of the diameter of membrane pores is not accepted by all.

49

$$\dot{Q}_f = \frac{N\pi r^4}{8\eta} \cdot \frac{\Delta P}{\Delta X} \tag{1}$$

The cross-sectional area of a single pore is πr^2; therefore, the total pore area, A_p, is $N\pi r^2$.

Substituting A_p in Poiseuille's equation 1 yields

$$\dot{Q}_f = \frac{A_p r^2}{8\eta} \cdot \frac{\Delta P}{\Delta X} \tag{2}$$

The filtration coefficient, K_f, is an expression of fluid permeability of the membrane and has the dimensions of milliliters per minute per 1 mm Hg of effective filtration pressure:

$$K_f = \frac{\dot{Q}_f}{\Delta P} \tag{3}$$

Substituting K_f in equation 2 yields

$$K_f = \frac{A_p \cdot r^2}{8\eta \cdot \Delta X} \tag{4}$$

Solving equation 4 for r, the radius of a pore, yields

$$r = \sqrt{\frac{8\eta \cdot K_f}{Ap/\Delta X}} \tag{5}$$

Because η, the viscosity of the filtrate, and K_f, the filtration coefficient, and ΔX, the membrane thickness, can all be measured more or less directly for artificial membranes, it is necessary only to measure total pore area to obtain an estimate of pore radius.

For artificial membranes such as collodion, Cellophane and unglazed porcelain, total pore area can be measured simply by weighing the membrane dry, soaking it in water and reweighing it. The increase in weight is equal to $Ap \cdot \Delta X$, the product of pore area and membrane thickness; i.e., total pore volume. However, artificial membranes have some pores that do not completely penetrate the membrane; so the method of wet-weight increase gives a total pore area that is too large and, consequently, a pore radius that is too small.

The molecular diameter of tritiated water (HTO) is minute in comparison with the diameter of the pores. The rate of diffusion of HTO through an artificial membrane in comparison with its rate of free diffusion through water is proportional to pore area. If D_{HTO} is the coefficient of free diffusion of HTO in water, if ΔC is the difference in concentration of HTO on the two sides of the membrane and if dn (HTO)$/dt$ is the rate of passage of HTO across the membrane, then, according to the Fick diffusion equation

$$\frac{A_p}{\Delta X} = \frac{dn \text{ (HTO)}/dt}{D_{HTO} \cdot \Delta_c} \tag{6}$$

Substituting

$$\frac{dn \text{ (HTO)}/dt}{D_{HTO} \cdot \Delta c} \text{ for } \frac{A_p}{\Delta X}$$

in equation 4 permits solution for r, the pore radius. Radii, so defined, correspond closely to those predicted in other ways.

Unfortunately, such simple methods cannot be applied directly to the measurement of pore size in the glomerular membranes of the normally functioning kidney. However, an adaptation of these methods can be so applied. It has long been known that certain proteins of small molecular dimensions are excreted in the urine when administered intravenously. Bott and Richards (6) studied protein excretion by the perfused kidney of *Necturus* and by the kidney of the intact frog. They observed that horse serum albumin (mol. wt. 70,000) is not excreted in significant amounts by either preparation, whereas hen and duck albumin, lactoglobulin and crystalline zinc insulin (mol. wt. ± 35,000) are excreted, although less readily than are substances of lower molecular weight, such as purified protein derivative (PPD) tuberculin (mol. wt. 14,500) and inulin (mol. wt. 5,000). Bott and Richards concluded that the pores of glomerular capillaries are all large enough to permit filtration of particles 40 Å in diameter but that only half of them permit passage of particles 50 Å in diameter and none permit passage of 70 Å particles.

Differences in rates of penetration of glomerular capillaries by various proteins relative to water cannot be ascribed a priori

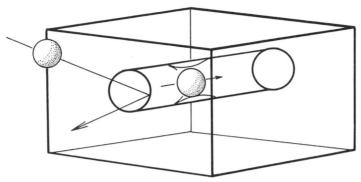

Fig. 4—1.—Mechanics of steric hindrance and viscous drag. (See text.)

to a spectrum of pore sizes. Steric hindrance and viscous drag restrict filtration of proteins, even though maximum particle size is less than minimum pore size. A molecule whose diameter is a significant fraction of pore diameter is far more likely to strike the edge of a pore and bounce off than to enter the pore (Fig. 4 – 1). The greater the diameter of the molecule relative to that of the pore, the less frequently will it strike sufficiently head-on to enter (steric hindrance). Viscous drag of the stationary layer of fluid lining the pore slows the movement of a particle along the pore. Again, the greater the diameter of the molecule relative to that of the pore, the greater is the viscous drag (Fig. 4 – 1).

The molecular sieving equation, given below (equation 7), was initially developed to measure numbers and dimensions of pores in muscle capillaries of the isolated hind leg of the cat (2, 3). It has since been used to characterize the glomerular capillaries of intact animals and man (5, 7). If a protein, such as myoglobin or egg albumin, is infused intravenously, it is excreted in the urine. By the use of clearance methods to be described later, C_2, the concentration of protein in the glomerular filtrate, can be calculated from C_1, the plasma concentration of the protein, the renal plasma threshold for the protein, the rate of excretion of the protein and the rate of glomerular filtration. The molecular sieving equation corrects for both steric hindrance and viscous drag. Its derivation is beyond the scope of this text, but it takes the following form:

$$\frac{C_2}{C_1} = \frac{1 + \dfrac{D}{\dot{Q}_f} \cdot \dfrac{8\eta K_f}{r^2}}{\dfrac{1 + 2.4a/r}{2(1 - a/r)^2 - (1 - a/r)^4}} + \frac{D}{\dot{Q}_f} \cdot \frac{8\eta K_f}{r^2} \quad (7)$$

The radius of the protein particle (a) is its Einstein-Stokes radius; i.e., the radius of a sphere that would diffuse at the same rate as the particle. The molecules of neither myoglobin nor egg albumin are spherical; the former are lozenge-shaped, the latter ellipsoid (Fig. 4 – 2). The coefficients of free diffusion (D) and the Einstein-Stokes radii (a) are known for both myoglobin and egg albumin. Restriction of filtration of these two proteins (C_2/C_1) has been measured by Yuile and Clark (8) and by Marshall and Deutsch (9), respectively, and amounts to 0.75 for myoglobin and 0.22 for egg albumin.* The rate of glomerular filtration, $\dot{Q}_f$, is also readily measurable. Substituting known constants and variables measured in experiments with myoglobin and egg albumin in simultaneous glomerular sieving equations permits solution for r (pore radius) and K_f (filtration coefficient).

According to Pappenheimer, the glomerular pores of the dog have a diameter of 75 Å, and K_f amounts to 1.9 – 4.5 ml/min per 1 mm Hg of effective filtration pressure per 100

*The glomerular clearance of myoglobin is 75%, and that of egg albumin is 22%, of the clearance of inulin in the dog. The latter clearance measures the rate of glomerular filtration. Clearance methods and interpretations are described in Chapter 5, and the specific method used in calculating glomerular clearance of proteins is described in the section on protein reabsorption in Chapter 6.

SUBSTANCE	MOL.WT. Grams	Radius from Diffusion Coefficient	Dimensions from X-Ray Diffraction	(FILTRATE) (FILTRAND)
WATER	18	1.0		1.0
UREA	60	1.6		1.0
GLUCOSE	180	3.6		1.0
SUCROSE	342	4.4		1.0
INULIN	5,500	14.8		0.98
MYOGLOBIN	17,000	19.5	⊢8, 54	0.75
EGG ALBUMIN	43,500	28.5	88, 22	0.22
HEMOGLOBIN	68,000	32.5	54, 32	0.03
SERUM ALBUMIN	69,000	35.5	150, 36	<0.01

Fig. 4–2.—Relationship between molecular weight, molecular dimensions and glomerular sieving of solutes.

Gm of kidney. Presumably, these values are essentially the same for man. Pores 75 Å in diameter should permit the filtration of a minute fraction of the normally circulating plasma albumin molecules. Experiments of Bieter (10), Rigas and Heller (11), Oliver *et al.* (12), Smetana (13) and Terry *et al.* (14) support the view that plasma albumin is filtered in very low concentration by the glomeruli of the normal kidney and is largely reabsorbed in the proximal convoluted tubules. Free hemoglobin, when present in the plasma in significant amounts, should and does enter the glomerular filtrate and appear in the urine (hemoglobinuria). The degree of sieving of hemoglobin is roughly in accord with a pore diameter of 75 Å.

The total pore area of the glomerular capillaries of both kidneys of a 10–15-kg dog has been calculated to be 430 cm², whereas the total glomerular capillary area from anatomic measurements (15) amounts to 8,000 cm². Thus, aqueous pores occupy about 5.5% of the glomerular capillary surface; the remainder of the surface is water-impervious and, presumably, lipid in nature. In comparison, pores occupy only 0.1% of the surface of muscle capillaries. Furthermore, the pores of muscle capillaries are smaller: about 60 Å in diameter. The hydrostatic pressure within the arteriolar portions of muscle capillaries is much lower than that within glomerular capillaries. These three facts account for the low rate of formation of interstitial fluid in muscle in comparison with the high rate of glomerular filtration in the kidney.

By means of the following equation:

$$\dot{Q}_f = K_f \, (\Delta P - \pi)$$

where π is the colloid osmotic pressure exerted by plasma proteins in glomerular capillaries,* the pressure drop across the capillary membrane, ΔP, can be calculated to be roughly 60 mm Hg in the dog. This pressure minus the colloid osmotic pressure gives the pressure required to overcome viscous resistance to flow of fluid through the glomerular pores.

The functional characteristics of the glomerular capillary membranes are summarized

---

*Because fluid is filtered, plasma proteins are concentrated, and the mean colloid osmotic pressure is greater than that in capillaries in which no net loss of fluid occurs.

TABLE 4–1.— OPERATIONAL CHARACTERISTICS OF
GLOMERULAR CAPILLARIES*

Total glomerular capillary area	5,000–15,000 cm²/100 Gm kidney
Total capillary pore area	500–1,000 cm²/100 Gm kidney
Fractional pore area	1/10–1/20
Pore diameter	70–100 Å
Pore length	400–600 Å
Filtration coefficient	1.9–4.5 ml/min./mm Hg/100 Gm
Pressure drop across capillary wall	45–75 mm Hg
Colloid osmotic pressure	25–30 mm Hg
Pressure to overcome viscous resistance to flow	20–45 mm Hg

*From Pappenheimer, J. R.: Über die Permeabilität der Glomerulummembranen in der Niere, Klin. Wchnschr. 33:362, 1955.

in Table 4–1. They are operational characteristics; i.e., the glomeruli behave as though these were, indeed, the characteristics. However, one must accept absolute values with reservation, for the many simplifying assumptions necessary for their derivation are certainly not all valid; the pores may well be larger than 75 Å. Wallenius (16) has shown that, if their dimensions are calculated from data on the sieving of dextrans of graded molecular sizes, their diameters approach 100 Å. Dextrans are uncharged molecules, whereas myoglobin, hemoglobin and egg albumin are charged at the pH of the plasma and glomerular filtrate. Hence, the proteins may suffer some electrical, as well as steric and viscous, hindrance to filtration—the more so, the greater the charge on the membrane. No correction for electrical hindrance is included in the sieving equation.

The ingenuity and completeness of Pappenheimer's description of the operational characteristics of glomerular capillaries in the dog must be balanced against the more precise and limited measurements of Brenner *et al.* in the rat outlined in Chapter 3 on page 42. Brenner's direct measurements of pressure drop across glomerular capillaries are much lower and the permeability of capillary walls to the aqueous phase of plasma is much higher than those calculated by Pappenheimer. While placing my faith on the direct measurements of Brenner, I admire intellectually the indirect approach of Pappenheimer.

Even the presence of pores is not accepted by all. Chinard (17, 18) maintained that the colloid restrictive barrier of the glomerular capillary membrane is a hydrated gel. He has proposed that the glomerular fluid is formed by a process of diffusion, not by bulk filtration. Water and small molecules have essentially the same diffusivities in this gel; the diffusivities of larger molecules diminish progressively with increasing particle size. According to this view, the entire glomerular capillary surface is involved in the production of glomerular fluid; pores, as such, do not exist. An increase in hydrostatic pressure increases the electrochemical potential of water and solutes, and so increases their diffusivities in the membrane.

In the author's opinion, the pore concept is useful if certain reservations are kept firmly in mind. The glomerular capillaries behave as though they were penetrated by uniform pores 75–100 Å in diameter, occupying 5% or so of the capillary surface. The pores probably do not have these postulated uniform dimensions. Indeed, true pores, as stable anatomic structures, may not exist at all. The filtering membrane may well be a hydrated gel, the protein and lipid components of which are loosely bonded. Water and dissolved molecules may migrate along devious aqueous channels that have no permanence; i.e., channels that are continually collapsing and reforming. Whether water and solutes are driven through the membrane by gradients of electrochemical potential (diffusion) or by a gradient of hydrostatic pressure (bulk filtration) becomes an academic question when one attempts to visualize a restrictive barrier at the molecular level.

Electron-Microscopic Description of Glomerular Capillaries

If glomerular capillaries are perforated by anatomically stable cylindrical pores 75–100 Å in diameter, that fact should be readily demonstrable in electron micrographs. Although, in his early studies, Hall observed such pores penetrating the basement membrane, he and others have subsequently shown them to be artifacts. Hall (19, 20) and Rhodin (21) believe that the slit pores between adjacent foot processes of epithelial cells restrict the filtration of protein but permit the relatively free passage of water and solutes. In contrast, Pease (22), Yamada (23) and others (24–26) consider the basement membrane to be the semipermeable barrier. They consider it to be a gel that permits free passage of small molecules through its aqueous phase but restricts the movement of colloids. Although the electron microscope has not resolved, to the satisfaction of all, either the site or the nature of the colloid-restrictive element of glomerular capillaries, it has demonstrated an amazing complexity of structure only vaguely suggested by the most precise observations with the light microscope.

The glomerular capillary wall is composed of three layers: an endothelial cell layer, a noncellular basement membrane and an epithelial cell layer (Figs. 4–3 and 4–4). The endothelial cells that line the capillary have large, oblate nuclei, which bulge into the lumen and balloon the wall. Peripheral to the nucleus, the cytoplasm of the endothelial cells spreads out into a thin sheet, 250–500 Å in thickness, which is fused into a continuous tube in intimate contact with the blood (Fig. 4–3, layer 5). According to some investigators, this tube is perforated by myriad tiny holes, roughly 1,000 Å (0.1 μ) in diameter. Others maintain that the wall is highly attenuated but not perforated at these points. Accordingly, the innermost lining of the capillary has been named either the "lamina fenestra" or "lamina attenuata," depending on the investigator's bias. In any event, these fenestrations or attenuations, while small enough to restrict the passage of cellular elements, are far too large to restrict the

Fig. 4–3. — Schematic representation of the structure of a glomerular capillary as revealed by electron microscopy. (See text.) (From Pease, D. C.: J. Histochem. 3:259, 1955.)

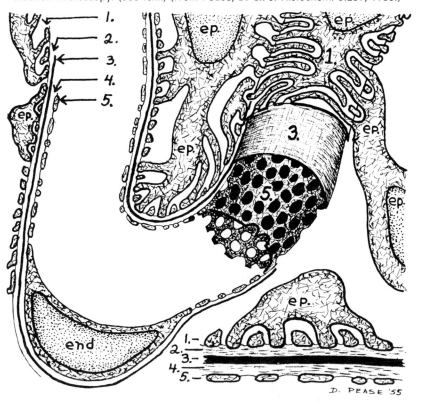

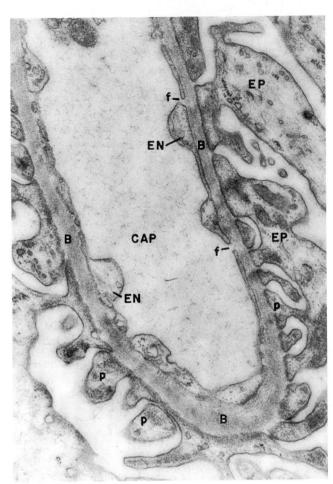

Fig. 4—4. — Electron micrograph of a glomerular capillary loop of the rat, illustrating endothelium (*EN*) with fenestrae (*f*), basement membrane (*B*), epithelium (*EP*) with podocytes (*p*) and capillary lumen (*CAP*). (From Farquhar, M. G., Wissig, S. L., and Palade, G. E.: J. Exper. Med. 113:47, 1961.)

passage of proteins. This lining is, therefore, not the semipermeable barrier of the glomerular capillary.

The middle layer of the capillary wall is the basement membrane. It forms a continuous tube immediately surrounding and closely applied to the endothelial cylinder. The basement membrane is a laminated structure, composed of a central osmophilic layer termed the lamina densa (Fig. 4–3, layer 3) sandwiched between two osmophobic cement layers (layers 2 and 4). Most investigators now agree that the basement membrane is a gel without demonstrable porous structure. This gel in its hydrated form in life could well be the semipermeable barrier that restricts the passage of plasma colloids.

The outermost layer of the capillary wall is by far the most complex. It is composed of epithelial cells, also called podocytes, which are suspended in the fluid of Bowman's capsule and make contact with the capillary wall only by myriad tiny terminal foot processes, or pedicels. The somata of epithelial cells give rise to numerous arms, or trabeculae, which encircle the capillary tube. Trabeculae of epithelial cells located on the same capillary or adjacent capillaries interdigitate (Fig. 4–4, *EP*, and Fig. 4–3, layer 1). The trabeculae in turn give rise to pedicels that are embedded in the outer cement layer of the basement membrane. The pedicels of adjacent trabeculae interdigitate in a complex fashion. According to Hall (19, 20), the spacing of adjacent pedicels in well-fixed tissue specimens is remarkably uniform and amounts to about 100 Å. He expressed the belief that the slits represent filtration pores that restrict the passage of colloids but allow the free passage of water and small molecules. The aggregate length of these slit pores has been calculated to be 2,000–4,000 miles. Hall maintained that the following factors account for the high filtration capacity of the glomerular capillaries in comparison with capillaries of other tissues: (1) a triangular profile of the pedicels, such that the slit pore is restricted to molecular dimensions only near the lamina densa; (2) an aggregate slit-pore area that is large; (3) wide gutters and channels beneath trabeculae, which connect the slit pores with Bowman's capsule; (4) fenestrations in the endothelial layer, which permit free egress of plasma fluid; and (5) high effective filtration pressure.

Observations on the structure of the glomerular capillaries in biopsy specimens from patients with the nephrotic syndrome cast some doubt on Hall's thesis. The nephrotic syndrome is characterized, among other things, by massive proteinuria. In the childhood disease known as "genuine lipoid nephrosis," glomerular filtration may be higher than normal, although in adults in the nephrotic stage of chronic glomerulonephritis, filtration rate is commonly reduced. However, independent of the nature of the disease, the epithelial layer of the glomerular membranes of patients with the nephrotic syndrome exhibits striking alterations (25, 26). Pedicels are lost, and the cytoplasm of the epithelial cells flattens out into an undifferentiated sheet closely applied to the basement membrane. Slit pores disappear.

These findings are difficult to reconcile with the view that the relative protein impermeability of glomerular capillaries depends on critical dimensions of slit pores. Indeed, they introduce the added difficulty of explaining the transfer of filtrate across the flattened and confluent sheets of epithelial cells. In contrast, the massive proteinuria of the nephrotic syndrome has been explained by Farquhar *et al.* (25) and Spiro (26) as due to

degenerative changes in the basement membrane, including loss of homogeneity and a punched-out or moth-eaten appearance. They maintained that the changes in the epithelial cells are a reaction to injury of the basement membrane. They suggested that the epithelium initially lays down, maintains and repairs the basement membrane. These changes in the epithelial cell layer and basement membrane in nephrosis are reversible in patients who respond favorably to steroid therapy (27).

Rinehart (24) believed that the basement membrane is the semipermeable barrier of the capillary wall but that fluid is transported across both the endothelial and epithelial cell layers by the formation of vesicles at the inner surface, their migration across the cell and their rupture at the outer surface. In the nephrotic syndrome, vesicles are especially prominent. This concept is in accord with the views of Palade (28), who suggested that fluid traverses the capillary walls of most tissues by the formation and rupture of vesicles. It is, of course, opposed to the views of Zweifach (29) and Pappenheimer *et al.* (2), as well as others, who proposed that the filtration of fluid in capillaries other than those of the glomeruli occurs through the intercellular cement that fills the crevices between adjacent endothelial cells.

More recent observations of Graham and Karnovsky (30) seem to have demonstrated finally that the slit pores of Hall (19, 20), or the membranes covering them, constitute the semipermeable portions of the glomerular capillary walls. Glomerular filtration of two peroxidases was studied in the mouse by electron-microscopic cytochemical methods following intravenous administration. One, horseradish peroxidase (HRPO), with a molecular weight of 40,000, rapidly traverses the endothelial fenestrations, basement membrane and slit pores to enter the urinary space of Bowman's capsule. The other, myeloperoxidase (MPO), with a molecular weight of 160,000–180,000, also readily traverses the endothelial fenestrations and crosses the basement membrane. As shown in Figure 4–5, it piles up beneath the surfaces of overlying pedicels and at the slit junctions of adjacent pedicels. This suggests that the primary filtration barrier to molecules of the size of albumin and certain globulins is the slit pore, or, as stated above, the membrane covering the slit pore.

Farquhar *et al.* (31) had, earlier, developed the thesis that the basement membrane constitutes the protein-impermeable layer, on the basis of studies on filterability of ferritin. This iron-containing protein has a molecular weight of 462,000. It is largely excluded from the basement membrane; i.e., it passes no farther than the lamina fenestra. Thus, the filtration of high-molecular-weight plasma proteins, such as lipoproteins, fibrinogen and α_2-macroglobulins, may be restricted by the basement membrane. Because both HRPO and MPO are taken up by mesangial cells, Graham and Karnovsky (30) suggested that an important function of these cells is incorporation and disposal of glomerular filtration residues.

Summary

The hydrostatic pressure, imparted to the blood by the beat of the heart, forces a "protein-free" filtrate of plasma through the walls of the glomerular capillaries. These capillaries function as ultrafilters: as though they were perforated by cylindrical pores some 75–100 Å in diameter and 400–600 Å in length, occupying about 5% of their surface area. Albumin molecules, which have a diameter slightly less than that of the pores, are largely sieved (restrained) by the combined effects of steric hindrance, viscous drag and electrical hindrance. The albumin, which normally enters the filtrate in very low concentration, is reabsorbed in the proximal convoluted tubules. The characteristics of the glomerular membranes cited above are operational, not structural, characteristics. Cylindrical pores of the dimensions indicated cannot be demonstrated by electron microscopy. Rather, the structural basis for the relative impermeability of glomerular capil-

Fig. 4–5. — Electron micrograph of a portion of a glomerular capillary of a mouse given myeloperoxidase (MPO) intravenously. L, lumen of capillary, extending along left border and bottom of figure; next, lamina fenestra; then, basement membrane; and, finally, the foot processes of epithelial cells (*Ep*). Note the black deposit of MPO concentrated along the outer border of the basement membrane immediately under the foot processes and slit pores of epithelial cells. (From Graham, R. C., and Karnovsky, M. J.: J. Exper. Med. 124:1123, 1966.)

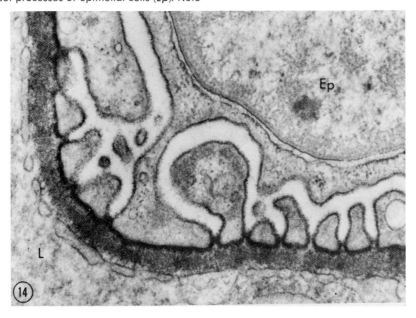

laries to colloids may be the slit pores, which lie between adjacent pedicels of the epithelial cells, or the gelatinous basement membrane, which allows free passage of small molecules through its aqueous phase but restrains the larger proteins. The massive proteinuria of the nephrotic syndrome is more readily explained in terms of the latter concept, for the basement membrane undergoes degenerative changes that probably render it more permeable to large molecules.

REFERENCES

1. Ludwig, K.: *Beiträge zur Lehre vom Mechanismus der Harnsekretion* (Marburg: N. G. Elwert, 1843).
2. Pappenheimer, J. R., Renkin, E. M., and Borrero, L. M.: Filtration, diffusion and molecular sieving through peripheral capillary membranes: A contribution to the pore theory of capillary permeability, Am. J. Physiol. 167: 13, 1951.
3. Pappenheimer, J. R.: Passage of molecules through capillary walls, Physiol. Rev. 33:387, 1953.
4. Pappenheimer, J. R.: The Passage of Substances across Capillary Walls, in *Transactions of the Third Josiah Macy, Jr., Conference on Renal Function* (New York: Josiah Macy Foundation, 1952).
5. Pappenheimer, J. R.: Über die Permeabilität der Glomerulummembrane in der Niere, Klin. Wchnschr. 33:362, 1955.
6. Bott, P. A., and Richards, A. N.: Passage of protein molecules through glomerular membranes, J. Biol. Chem. 141:291, 1941.
7. Lambert, P. P., Grégoire, F., and Malmendier. C.: La perméabilité glomérulaire aux substances protidiques, Rev. franç. clin. et biol. 2:15, 1957.
8. Yuile, C. L., and Clark, W. F.: Myohemoglobinuria: A study of the renal clearance of myohemoglobin in the dog, J. Exper. Med. 74:187, 1941.
9. Marshall, M. E., and Deutsch, H. F.: Clearances of some proteins by the dog kidney, Am. J. Physiol. 163:461, 1950.
10. Bieter, R. N.: Albuminuria in glomerular and aglomerular fish, J. Pharmacol. & Exper. Therap. 43:407, 1931.
11. Rigas, D. A., and Heller, G. G.: The amount and nature of urinary proteins in normal human subjects, J. Clin. Invest. 30:853, 1951.
12. Oliver, J., MacDowell, M., and Lee, Y. C.: Cellular mechanisms of protein metabolism in the nephron: I. The structural aspects of proteinuria; tubular absorption, droplet formation, and the disposal of proteins, J. Exper. Med. 99:589, 1954.
13. Smetana, H.: Permeability of renal glomeruli of several mammalian species to labeled proteins, Am. J. Path. 23:255, 1947.
14. Terry, R., Hawkins, D. R., Church, E. H., and Whipple, G. H.: Proteinuria related to hyperproteinemia in dogs following plasma given parenterally: A renal threshold for plasma proteins, J. Exper. Med. 87:561, 1948.
15. Vimtrup, B. J.: On number, shape, structure and surface area of glomeruli in kidneys of man and mammals, Am. J. Anat. 41:123, 1928.
16. Wallenius, G.: Renal clearance of dextran as a measure of glomerular permeability, Acta Soc. med. upsal., suppl. 4, 1954.
17. Chinard, F. P.: Derivation of an expression for the rate of formation of glomerular fluid (GFR): Applicability of certain physical and physicochemical concepts, Am. J. Physiol. 171:578, 1952.
18. Chinard, F. P.: Possible Mechanisms of Formation of Glomerular Fluid, in *Transactions of the Third Josiah Macy, Jr., Conference on Renal Function* (New York: Josiah Macy Foundation, 1952).
19. Hall, B. V.: Further Studies of the Normal Structure of the Renal Glomerulus, in *Proceedings of the Sixth Annual Conference on the Nephrotic Syndrome* (New York: National Nephrosis Foundation, 1955).
20. Hall, B. V.: The protoplasmic basis of glomerular ultrafiltration, Am. Heart J. 54:1, 1957.
21. Rhodin, J.: Electron microscopy of the kidney, Am. J. Med. 24:661, 1958.
22. Pease, D. C.: Fine structure of the kidney seen by electron microscopy, J. Histochem. 3:295, 1955.
23. Yamada, E.: The fine structure of the renal glomerulus of the mouse, J. Biophys. & Biochem. Cytol. 1:551, 1955.
24. Rinehart, J. F.: Fine structure of renal glomerulus as revealed by electron microscopy, A.M.A. Arch. Path. 59:439, 1955.
25. Farquhar, M. G., Vernier, R. L., and Good, R. A.: Studies on familial nephrosis: II. Glomerular changes observed with the electron microscope, Am. J. Path. 33:791, 1957.
26. Spiro, D.: The structural basis of proteinuria in man: Electron microscopic studies of renal biopsy specimens from patients with lipoid nephrosis, amyloidosis and subacute and chronic glomerulonephritis, Am. J. Path. 35: 47, 1959.
27. Folli, G., Pollack, V. E., Reid, R. T. W., Pir-

ani, C. L., and Kark, R. M.: Electron microscopic studies of reversible glomerular lesions
in the adult nephrotic syndrome, Ann. Int.
Med. 49:775, 1958.

28. Palade, G. E.: Fine structure of blood capillaries, J. Appl. Physics 24:1424, 1953.

29. Zweifach, B. W.: *Functional Behavior of the
Microcirculation* (Springfield, Ill.: Charles C
Thomas, Publisher, 1961).

30. Graham, R. C., and Karnovsky, M. J.:
Glomerular permeability: Ultrastructural,
cytochemical studies using peroxidases as
protein tracers, J. Exper. Med. 124:1123,
1966.

31. Farquhar, M. G., Wissig, S. L., and Palade,
G. E.: Glomerular permeability: I. Ferritin
transfer across the normal glomerular capillary wall, J. Exper. Med. 113:47, 1961.

5

Clearance and Rate
of Glomerular Filtration

MICROPUNCTURE METHODS, developed and exploited by Richards and his colleagues, provided the first definitive evidence that glomerular filtration is the initial step in urine formation. However, these methods cannot be used to measure the glomerular filtration rate (GFR) in intact animals and man. This datum, which is highly significant for an understanding of the pathophysiology of the kidney and for the quantitative assessment of tubular reabsorption and tubular secretion, must be obtained by clearance methods.

In intrinsic renal disease, congestive heart failure, acute peripheral circulatory failure (shock), cirrhosis with ascites, eclampsia and states associated with dehydration, the rate of glomerular filtration is modestly to markedly reduced. All excretory products are filtered; in addition, some are secreted. However, basically, the elimination of most of these products depends on the adequacy of the filtering process. When the filtration rate falls, the plasma levels of the excretory products rise. Uremia, with its associated increases in plasma urea nitrogen, creatinine, uric acid, sulfate, phosphate, potassium, etc., is severe in proportion to the reduction in glomerular filtration rate.

In studying reabsorption or secretion of any substance, it is necessary to know the rate at which it is filtered and excreted. The rate of reabsorption of any substance equals its rate of filtration minus its rate of excretion. The rate of secretion of any substance is equal to its rate of excretion minus its rate of filtration. In each instance, it is necessary to have a measure of both the rate of filtration and the rate of excretion of the substance in question. Precise clearance methods are available for measuring these variables.

The basis of the methods for measuring the rate of glomerular filtration and the application of these methods in intact animals and man are subjects of this chapter.

Clearance

In the early 1920s, Austin *et al.* (1) compared the ability of the normal kidney of man to excrete urea with that of the diseased kidney. Strangely, the rate of excretion per minute, per hour or per day is no measure of intrinsic excretory capacity, for the rate of excretion is determined ultimately by the rate of production of urea. Neither is the plasma concentration of urea a satisfactory index, for it is determined by rate of production and by body hydration as well as by intrinsic excretory capacity.

The function of the kidney, in one very limited sense, is to clear urea from the blood. A measure of this function is the volume of blood completely cleared of urea in 1 minute.

Obviously, this is a *virtual volume*, not a *real volume*. No single milliliter of blood has all of its urea removed in one transit through the kidney; rather, a little urea is removed from each of the many milliters of blood perfusing the kidneys. One may add up this urea and express it as though it were derived by completely clearing a much smaller volume of blood of all of its contained urea. This datum, the blood urea clearance,* is an empiric measure of one renal function: the ability of the kidney to remove urea from the blood and to deliver it into the urine. It tells us nothing about the mechanism of removal.

If U_u represents the quantity of urea in 1 ml of urine (concentration) and V is the milliliters of urine formed per minute (volume), then $U_u \cdot V$ equals the quantity of urea excreted in 1 minute. If P_u represents the quantity of urea in 1 ml of plasma, then

centration and rate of excretion of urea. If urine flow is maintained above 2 ml/min, the urea clearance is a measure of urea excretory ability and varies more or less proportionally with filtration rate.

In renal disease, the urea clearance is reduced and the extent of the reduction can, within limits, be used as a measure of the extent of the disease process. In severe congestive failure, dehydration, shock and cirrhosis with ascites, the urea clearance is also reduced, not owing to intrinsic renal disease but to unfavorable hemodynamic relationships and to oliguria (low urine flow). When these conditions improve, the urea clearance returns to its normal value. There is little doubt that the clearance concept was initially developed to obtain a clinically useful standard of reference, and not as a functionally useful concept.

$$\frac{U_u \cdot V}{P_u} = \frac{\text{Quantity of urea excreted in 1 min}}{\text{Quantity of urea in 1 ml of plasma}} = \text{Number of ml of plasma completely cleared of urea in 1 min}$$

In normal adults with moderately high rates of urine flow, the urea clearance, calculated as above, is relatively constant and averages 75 ± 15 ml/min. Note that the urea clearance is a *volume of plasma* completely cleared of urea, not a quantity of urea removed from plasma. In a person on a high-protein diet, or in one who has ingested urea, the plasma concentration of urea (P_u) increases. Because the rate of excretion of urea $(U_u \cdot V)$ increases in direct proportion, the ratio $\frac{U_u \cdot V}{P_u}$, the urea clearance, remains unchanged. The urea clearance is, therefore, independent of plasma urea con-

---

*The urea clearance was initially described as a whole-blood clearance. However, the kidney operates on blood plasma and treats the red cells as mere floating inert bodies. It is, therefore, more meaningful to study plasma clearance than whole-blood clearance. In the measurement of glomerular filtration rate, one must use plasma clearance, for only plasma is filtered. Plasma urea clearances are now more commonly measured than blood urea clearances. The clearance formula was devised in 1917 by Thomas Addis; the term "clearance" was first used by Möller *et al.* (2) in 1929.

Measurement of Glomerular Filtration Rate

In 1926, Poule Rehberg (3) of Copenhagen saw what the clearance formula really meant, or rather, what it could mean under specific circumstances. Let us suppose that there exists a substance with the following properties: (1) It is freely filterable through glomerular capillary membranes; i.e., it is not bound to plasma proteins or sieved in the process of ultrafiltration. (2) It is biologically inert and is neither reabsorbed nor secreted by the renal tubules. (3) It is nontoxic and does not alter renal function when infused in quantities that permit adequate quantification in plasma and urine. (4) It can be quantified in plasma and urine with a high degree of accuracy.

The clearance of such a substance is equal to the rate of glomerular filtration; i.e., it measures the volume of plasma filtered through the glomeruli in 1 minute. This fact is illustrated in Figure 5–1, which represents

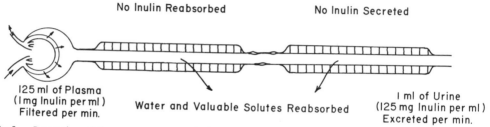

Fig. 5–1.—Principles of the measurement of glomerular filtration rate by the inulin clearance method.

the kidney as though it were a single large nephron rather than a multitude of minute ones operating in parallel. On average, 1,300 ml of whole blood or 700 ml of plasma perfuse the kidney each minute; and 125 ml of plasma per minute are filtered through the glomeruli.

If each milliliter of plasma contains 1 mg of our hypothetical ideal measuring substance, X (in Fig. 5 – 1, the substance is inulin), and if 125 ml of plasma is filtered through the glomeruli each minute, 125 mg of X will be delivered into the tubules each minute. If no X is reabsorbed and none is secreted, and if steady-state conditions prevail, 125 mg of X will appear in the urine each minute. If the bulk of the water is reabsorbed and only 1 ml of urine is excreted each minute, the urinary concentration of X will be 125 mg/ml, as follows:

Because inulin is hydrolyzed to fructose in the gastrointestinal tract and is poorly absorbed from subcutaneous tissue or muscle, it must be administered intravenously. To avoid pyrogenic reactions, the inulin must be specially processed. It must be administered in a concentrated priming dose adequate to raise the plasma concentration to 10–20 mg/100 ml and then infused at such a rate as to maintain the plasma level constant; i.e., at the same rate at which it is excreted. Frequent blood samples must be drawn, preferably without stasis at the midpoint of short urine collection periods. Urine collections must be accurate; and, if urine flow is low or if the subject cannot void in sufficient quantity, the bladder must be catheterized and washed with sterile water. Finally, the chemical analysis of plasma and urine for inulin must be carried out precisely. Clearly, the

$$\text{Clearance of } X = C_X = \frac{U_X \cdot V}{P_X} = \frac{125 \text{ mg/ml} \cdot 1 \text{ ml/min}}{1 \text{ mg/ml}} = 125 \text{ ml/min}$$

It is apparent that the clearance of X is equal to the originally postulated rate of glomerular filtration.

METHOD OF MEASURING GLOMERULAR FILTRATION RATE IN MAN

We can now state that the fructose polysaccharide, inulin, is a substance that appears to have all of the properties outlined above. Its clearance, when determined with suitable care, is an accurate measure of the rate of glomerular filtration in all animals from fish to man.

determination of glomerular filtration rate is not a bedside procedure. The urea clearance will give about as much clinically useful information for assessing renal function and making a prognosis as will the inulin clearance. However, if one wishes to study secretion or reabsorption, only an exactly performed inulin clearance test will suffice.

HISTORICAL ASPECTS

The historical aspects of the problem of finding a substance whose clearance is an adequate measure of filtration rate are both interesting and informative. Rehberg, in

1926, approached the problem with the following question: What normal urinary constituent of man is most concentrated with respect to the plasma? The answer is creatinine, if one disregards hippuric acid, ammonia and hydrogen ions; Rehberg knew nothing about them. Thus, U/P is greatest for creatinine; hence, the clearance of creatinine, $U/P \cdot V$, will exceed that of all other constituents. Because Rehberg chose the creatinine clearance as his measure of filtration rate, he ended up with the idea of a filtration-reabsorption type of kidney. This kidney need not secrete any normal urinary constituent, for the rate of the glomerular filtration was so high that all urinary solutes known at that time could be accounted for in terms of quantities filtered. Many investigators still use the creatinine clearance in man as a measure of the rate of glomerular filtration. Although acceptable in the dog, it is not acceptable in man, because it yields variable results that, on average, are too high, for creatinine is not only filtered but is also secreted by the renal tubules.

Marshall had clearly demonstrated tubular secretion of phenol red in the dog. Because the aglomerular kidneys of the goosefish and toadfish secrete not only phenol red but also creatinine, the use of the creatinine clearance in man as a measure of glomerular filtration rate was suspect until proved otherwise.

Smith began his epic work on renal function at about this time, namely, 1930. He argued that carbohydrates are valuable substances throughout the animal kingdom. Hence, it would be unlikely that any animal would develop a tubular secretory mechanism to eliminate them; rather, because they are valuable, all useful carbohydrates would likely be reabsorbed. However, it was known that certain pentoses, such as xylose,* and polysaccharides, such as sucrose and raffinose, when given intravenously, are

not metabolized, are rapidly excreted and can be quantitatively recovered in the urine.

One of the first experiments was to inject large quantities of these sugars into the aglomerular goosefish. None of these sugars was excreted. Glucose in amounts sufficient to cause a marked hyperglycemia was also not excreted. The administration of phlorhizin, which causes glycosuria in glomerular animals by blocking tubular reabsorption, did not alter these results. Thus, the aglomerular kidney does not secrete carbohydrates — whether useful or not — under any circumstance.

The logical experiment was then performed in the dog: xylose was administered and its clearance measured; phlorhizin was given parenterally; and both xylose and glucose clearances were measured simultaneously. The results are shown in schematic form in Figure 5–2. For the moment, the inulin clearance should be disregarded, for at the time this experiment was first performed, inulin clearances had not been measured.

The xylose clearance of the dog is unchanged by phlorhizin; the glucose clearance rises promptly to equal the xylose clearance (4). In normal dogs, the xylose, sucrose and raffinose clearances are equal within limits of experimental error. The conclusion was drawn, therefore, that the clearances of these three sugars in normal animals and also that of glucose, when reabsorption is blocked by

Fig. 5–2.—Clearances of inulin, xylose and glucose in the normal and phlorhizinized dog.

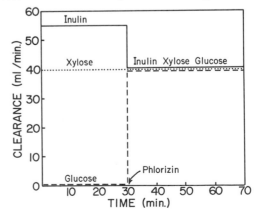

---

*Xylose can be administered orally. Sucrose and raffinose are hydrolyzed when administered by mouth, and the resulting monosaccharides are metabolized; therefore, sucrose and raffinose must be given parenterally.

phlorhizin, are adequate measures of rate of glomerular filtration.

The argument would have been a good one had it not been that xylose is reabsorbed from the filtrate to the extent of 20–30%. Furthermore, the reabsorptive mechanism for xylose is the same as that for glucose. Phlorhizin blocks the reabsorption of both sugars. As an additional complicating factor, phlorhizin causes a generalized autonomic disturbance, reducing filtration rate and renal blood flow. The true clearance relationships are shown in Figure 5–2, if one now considers the inulin clearance. Some 20–30% of xylose is reabsorbed in the normal animal; i.e., its clearance is 20–30% below glomerular filtration rate, measured by the inulin clearance. Phlorhizin blocks the reabsorption of both xylose and glucose. The drug also reduces filtration rate some 20–30%. In the animal given phlorhizin, the clearances of xylose, glucose and inulin are all adequate measures of glomerular filtration rate; in the normal animal, only the clearance of inulin is an adequate measure.

Clearance of Inulin

The clearance of inulin, a fructose polysaccharide derived from dahlia roots and Jerusalem artichokes, was proposed as a measure of glomerular filtration rate more or less simultaneously by Richards *et al.* (5) and by Shannon and Smith (6) about 1935. The inulin molecule has an Einstein-Stokes rad-

ius of 15Å; i.e., it diffuses as would a spherical body of such radius. Inulin is, therefore, not likely to be reabsorbed passively by back diffusion through the tubular epithelium. It is inert, is not metabolized and can be recovered quantitatively in the urine following parenteral administration. For these reasons, it seemed probable that inulin would neither be secreted nor reabsorbed.

INULIN CLEARANCE AS MEASURE OF RATE OF GLOMERULAR FILTRATION. — The following lines of evidence suggest that the inulin clearance is a valid measure of glomerular filtration rate:

1. The rate of excretion of inulin ($U \cdot V$) is directly proportional to, and a linear function of, the plasma concentration of inulin (P) over a wide range (Fig. 5–3, *left*). Accordingly, the clearance of inulin, $U \cdot V/P$, is constant and is independent of plasma inulin concentration (Fig. 5–3, *right*). Although such relationships must hold if inulin is freely filterable through the glomeruli and neither secreted nor reabsorbed, they are by no means proof, per se, that inulin behaves in this manner.

2. Identity of simultaneously measured clearances of two or more substances differing widely in physical and chemical properties constitutes more convincing evidence. In the normal dog, the inulin clearance agrees (within ±5%) with the simultaneously determined creatinine (6), ferrocyanide (7), or allantoin clearance (8). In the dog given phlorhizin, the inulin clearance additionally

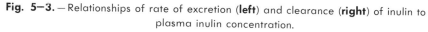

Fig. 5–3. —Relationships of rate of excretion (**left**) and clearance (**right**) of inulin to plasma inulin concentration.

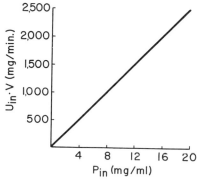

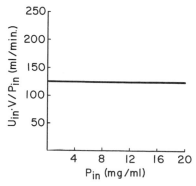

agrees, within the same limits, with the glucose or xylose clearances. The above clearance identities hold over wide ranges of plasma concentrations of the measured substances. One may reasonably argue that it is highly unlikely that inulin, a fructose polysaccharide, would be restricted in filtration or be secreted or reabsorbed to the same extent as creatinine, a nitrogenous waste product, or as ferrocyanide, a polyvalent anion, when the plasma levels of all are varied over wide ranges.

3. The clearance of most substances known to be secreted decreases as plasma concentration increases. This results from saturation of the secretory system at a relatively low plasma level. As the plasma concentration increases further, secretion contributes in diminishing proportion, and filtration contributes in increasing proportion, to excretion. As shown in Figure 5–4, the clearance of the secreted substance, p-aminohippurate (PAH), asymptotically approaches the inulin clearance at high plasma PAH concentrations. At infinitely high plasma PAH levels, the clearance of PAH would be determined solely by the rate of glomerular filtration; the contribution of secretion would be negligible.

Fig. 5–4. — Relation of clearances to plasma concentrations of p-aminohippurate, inulin and glucose in man.

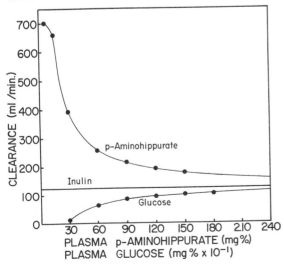

4. The clearance of many substances known to be reabsorbed increases as plasma concentration increases. This results from saturation of the reabsorptive mechanism at a moderate plasma level. As the plasma concentration increases further, the substance is excreted at a rate that increases in direct proportion to plasma level. Reabsorption reduces excretion in diminishing proportion, and filtration contributes in increasing proportion, with increasing plasma concentration. As shown in Figure 5–4, the clearance of the reabsorbed substance, glucose, asymptotically approaches the inulin clearance at high plasma glucose levels. At infinitely high plasma glucose concentrations, the clearance of glucose would be determined solely by its rate of filtration; the reduction in clearance due to reabsorption would be negligible.

The considerations presented above illustrate clearly the distinction between evidence for and proof of a thesis. Until recently, there has been no absolute proof that the inulin clearance measures filtration rate; rather, there has been much evidence that it does. If a substance were found whose clearance is higher than that of inulin and whose rate of excretion is proportional to and a linear function of plasma concentration over a wide range, one would be forced to accept its clearance and discard that of inulin as a measure of filtration rate. In nearly 40 years of investigation, no such substance has been found. Because there is no evidence to the contrary, and much in favor, the inulin clearance has been widely accepted as a measure of glomerular filtration rate in all vertebrates.

Within the past few years, several groups have provided direct proof of the adequacy of the inulin clearance as a measure of rate of glomerular filtration in the rat and *Necturus* (9–12). What they have shown is that inulin is neither reabsorbed nor secreted, its complete filterability from plasma having been demonstrated earlier by Richards *et al.* (5). The procedures used were the following:[14]C-carboxyl-labeled or ^{3}H-methoxy-labeled inulin of high specific activity was infused into a single proximal nephron through a micropipet inserted into the lumen. Urine was collected separately through catheters inserted into the two ureters. If any inulin was reabsorbed from the perfused nephron, it would enter the general circulation and return equally to both kidneys, whence it would be excreted equally by both. Actually, less than 1% of the inulin perfused into one nephron of the experimental kidney appeared in urine collected from the control kidney. Accordingly, less than 2% was reabsorbed—an amount of debatable significance, in view of the fact that a tiny quantity of labeled inulin, deposited beneath the capsule, was rapidly excreted by the two kidneys. If a proximal tubule was blocked close to the glomerulus and was perfused immediately below the block with inulin and the perfusate was collected from a distal loop of the same nephron, recovery averaged 99.3%. If, in addition, inulin was infused systemically, recovery of inulin from the perfused nephron was unchanged. Such a direct demonstration that inulin is neither secreted nor reabsorbed by the tubules of the rat and *Necturus* not only proves the adequacy of its clearance as a measure of filtration rate in these forms; it also strengthens the view that it is an adequate measure in all forms.

CREATININE CLEARANCE

The creatinine clearance has been shown to be a valid measure of glomerular filtration rate in *Necturus* and in the rabbit, sheep, seal and dog. The major evidence in each instance is agreement of simultaneously measured inulin and creatinine clearances over wide ranges of plasma concentrations of both. For precise work, creatinine must be infused in amounts sufficient to raise plasma concentration to 15 mg/100 ml or more. The clearance of endogenous creatinine (± 1 mg/100 ml) is not a valid measure of filtration rate, because the Jaffé chromogen in plasma is not all true creatinine, whereas most of that in urine is. The clearance of apparent endogenous creatinine is, therefore, lower

than the filtration rate in the forms mentioned above.

In contrast, the clearance of exogenous (i.e., infused) creatinine exceeds the rate of glomerular filtration in the fish, frog, reptile, bird, guinea pig, rat, monkey, ape, and man. In these forms, creatinine is not only filtered but is also secreted by the tubules. In certain instances in man, the clearance of endogenous creatinine agrees reasonably well with the clearance of inulin. Agreement results from the balance of two errors: (1) the apparent clearance of creatinine is lower than the true clearance, because the apparent creatinine concentration of plasma is higher than the true concentration; and (2) the true clearance of creatinine is higher than filtration rate, because of tubular secretion. The difference between animal species that apparently do not secrete creatinine and those that do may be a quantitative rather than a qualitative difference. Thus, a creatinine secretory mechanism may exist in the dog, and possibly in other species as well, yet possess an activity so low that no statistically significant difference exists between the creatinine clearance and the inulin clearance under the usual conditions of clearance measurement. However, under the highly abnormal conditions of the stop-flow technic (see Chapter 6), even this very minor secretory capacity is unmasked (13, 14). Under such conditions, secretion is more apparent in male than in female dogs. Secretion can be enhanced in the female dog by pretreatment with testosterone. The mechanism for secretion of creatinine may be identical with that for PAH, inasmuch as both are blocked by dinitrophenol and probenecid. Furthermore, the administration of large amounts of PAH depresses creatinine secretion. These latter two observations have also been made in man. However, no differences in secretion of creatinine have been described in relation to sex in the human.

In the squirrel monkey, creatinine is secreted to an even greater extent than in the chimpanzee and man. According to Selkurt *et al.* (15), the creatinine secretory mechanism is identical with the strong base secretory mechanism (see Chapter 8), rather than with the mechanism for the secretion of PAH, as noted above. Thus quinine sulfate, a known inhibitor of the strong base system, blocks creatinine secretion, whereas PAH, probenecid and EDTA do not.

NORMAL VALUES OF INULIN CLEARANCE

The glomerular filtration rate of normal young men averages 125 ± 15 ml/min per 1.73 m² of surface area; that of normal young women averages 110 ± 15 ml/min per 1.73 m² of surface area (16). Filtration rate varies not only with body size—more specifically with surface area—but also with age. It is quite low in the newborn,* even in comparison with the obviously low surface area; but it increases rapidly, reaching the adult relationship to surface area by the age of 2 years (17). Filtration rate is also moderately reduced in the aged (18), even in the absence of renal disease.

The glomerular filtration rate in normal man is found to be remarkably constant on repeated measurement from day to day and from month to month over years. In the dog, filtration rate is less stable. A change from a high-carbohydrate to a high-protein diet may double the filtration rate in the dog (19). The infusion of isotonic or hypertonic saline solution at a high rate also increases the filtration rate in the dog. Neither circumstance appreciably affects the filtration rate in man.

AMBIGUITY IN TERMINOLOGY

Glomerular filtration rate is expressed in terms of milliliters of plasma filtered through glomerular capillaries per minute. This introduced an ambiguity in terminology, for plasma is 93–94% water and some 6–7% protein, and only the aqueous phase is filtered. All of the true crystalloids of plasma are dissolved in the aqueous phase; yet their concentrations are commonly expressed in terms of milligrams per 100 ml, or mEq/L, of plasma, not of plasma water. Thus, all of the crystalloids in 125 ml of plasma are filtered each minute when the rate of glomerular filtration is 125 ml/min. However, only 0.93×125 ml $= 116$ ml of water are filtered. The student should keep in mind that glomerular filtration rate is defined as volume of plasma filtered per minute, not as volume of plasma water, although obviously only the water and its dissolved crystalloids are actually filtered.

GLOMERULAR FILTRATION IN OLIGURIA AND DIURESIS

Normal variations in urine flow are effected by changes in water reabsorption, not by changes in filtration rate. In moderate hydropenia (water-withholding to the point of thirst):

Volume of plasma filtered	=	125 ml/min
Volume of water filtered	=	116 ml/min
Volume of water reabsorbed	=	115.5 ml/min
Volume of urine excreted	=	0.5 ml/min

In a well-hydrated person who additionally ingests a liter or so of water:

Volume of plasma filtered	=	125 ml/min
Volume of water filtered	=	116 ml/min
Volume of water reabsorbed	=	100 ml/min
Volume of urine excreted	=	16 ml/min

In extreme dehydration, in which urine flow may drop to 0.2–0.3 ml/min, filtration rate is significantly reduced, in association with reduced circulating blood volume and signs of peripheral circulatory insufficiency. The oliguria of the patient with congestive heart failure accumulating edematous fluid or of the patient with cirrhosis accumulating ascitic fluid is also frequently associated with a low rate of glomerular filtration. However, the fact remains that normal physiologic variations in urine flow are brought about by variations in the rate of water reabsorption, not by variations in the rate of glomerular filtration.

---

*Low filtration rate is associated in the newborn, and especially in the premature infant, with a prominent cuboidal or columnar visceral epithelial layer enfolding the loops of glomerular capillaries.

GLOMERULAR FILTRATION IN RENAL DISEASE

The measurement of glomerular filtration rate in renal disease provides an estimate of the degree of impairment of one discrete renal function. Repeated measurements at intervals enable one to study the course of renal disease and to sharpen one's prognosis. However, it is true that nearly as much clinically useful information can be obtained from properly performed tests of urea clearance, for, although the urea clearance is no measure of filtration rate, it varies roughly in proportion to filtration rate in renal disease.

As was mentioned earlier, many excretory products find their way into the urine mainly in consequence of their being filtered through the glomeruli. In renal disease, reduction in filtration rate results in elevated plasma concentrations of excretory products. Thus, the plasma concentrations of urea, creatinine, phosphate, sulfate and uric acid increase as filtration rate declines. The elevated plasma levels balance reduced filtration rate; the total quantities excreted remain the same.

It is commonly stated that renal function (either inulin or urea clearance) must be reduced to one half to one third of normal before plasma concentrations of excretory products increase. While practically so, this hypothesis is untrue. It arises from the rather broad range of normal. For example, halving the filtration rate doubles the plasma concentration of urea, but the value may still be within the upper range of normal. If filtration rate is reduced to 25% of normal, plasma urea increases fourfold—definitely out of the range of normal. If filtration rate is reduced to 10% of normal, plasma urea increases roughly 10-fold. The patient is now in a precarious state—not so much from elevated blood urea, for this compound is remarkable benign, but from other deficiencies in regulatory capacity that are more significant. High fluid intake and generous salt intake can compensate, to a remarkable degree, for renal damage by supporting filtration rate at the maximum possible level and by reducing

the reabsorption of certain excretory products (most notably urea) that occurs when the urine is highly concentrated. Frank uremia is frequently precipitated by excessive sweating, purgation, ill-considered use of diuretics or restriction of intake of salt and water, all of which result in dehydration and oliguria. A patient with chronic renal disease with any significant elevation of plasma urea should never be placed on a low-salt diet in the absence of gross edema.* All too frequently, such ill-advised therapy precipitates uremia.

INULIN SUBSTITUTES FOR ASSESSMENT OF RENAL FUNCTION

A major deterrent to the widespread use of the inulin clearance as a measure of filtration rate in the assessment of renal function in disease has been the technical problem of accurate analysis of inulin in plasma and urine. Although not especially difficult, the analytic technics are sufficiently demanding to render them unsuitable for occasional use in a routine clinical laboratory. Accordingly, interest has centered on a search for equivalent compounds labeled with gamma-emitting isotopes, such as ^{125}I, ^{131}I and ^{60}Co. Inulin can be labeled by substituting allyl ether groups for some of the hydroxyl groups of the fructofuranose units of inulin, followed by iodination at the double bonds [20]. Difficulties of preparation, lability of some of the substituent iodines and radiosensitivity of the compound have militated against its use. Radioactive cyanocobalamin (vitamin B_{12}) has also been proposed as an inulin substitute [21]. Major deterrents to its use have been high cost and plasma binding. When given in tracer amounts, ^{60}Co-vitamin B_{12} is

---

*The azotemic end-stage of chronic renal disease is characterized more by salt and water loss than by retention as edema. However, if the patient is also in severe congestive failure or has cirrhosis with massive ascites, treatment creates a dilemma. Shall the physician restrict salt intake, use diuretics and run the risk of precipitating uremia? Or shall he ignore fluid accumulation, with its attendant disability? Here caution is the better part of wisdom.

quantitatively bound to a specific plasma globulin and therefore is not filterable. If the binding sites are saturated with relatively large amounts of carrier vitamin B_{12}, some 10% of the radioactivity is still bound nonspecifically to plasma albumin. When specific binding sites are saturated and correction is made for nonspecific binding, clearance of radiocyanocobalamin compares favorably with clearance of inulin. Certain urologic contrast agents—Hypaque, Renografin and Conray—are excreted primarily by glomerular filtration. All are iodinated benzoic acid derivatives. Of these, radioiodinated Conray (sodium iothalamate) shows the most promise as a possible inulin substitute. In a series of 100 simultaneous clearance comparisons in 16 patients, the mean iothalamate/inulin clearance ratio was 1.005; i.e., the clearances of these two substances are apparently identical (22). However, more penetrating physiologic studies and more extensive clearance comparisons in patients in different stages of renal disease are indicated before true identity of iothalamate and inulin clearances can be considered firmly established. The virtue of the iothalamate clearance, if indeed it is equivalent to the inulin clearance, is simplicity of analysis of iothalamate in plasma and urine. One need only pipet accurately 1 ml of plasma and 1 ml of diluted urine into separate test tubes and count them for a statistically significant period of time in a well-type scintillation spectrometer to obtain valid radioconcentration measurements. From these, a clearance may be calculated.

Summary

The renal clearance of a substance is defined as the number of milliliters of plasma completely cleared of that substance in 1 minute's time. If the substance is freely filterable through glomerular capillaries, if it is neither actively nor passively reabsorbed or secreted, if it is inert and, per se, exerts no effect on renal function and if it can be accurately quantified in plasma and urine, then its clearance will be a valid measure of the rate of glomerular filtration. Good evidence exists that inulin exhibits these properties; thus the clearance of inulin is a measure of the volume of plasma filtered through the glomeruli.

In man, the inulin clearance is the only satisfactory measure of filtration rate. In the dog, both the creatinine clearance and the inulin clearance are adequate measures. The rate of glomerular filtration in normal men averages 125 ml/min and in normal women 110 ml/min, both expressed per 1.73 m^2 of surface area. In normal man, filtration rate is remarkably stable from day to day over a period of years. In patients with renal disease, filtration rate is reduced. The degree of disturbance in regulation of composition of the body fluids is in rough proportion to the reduction in filtration rate. When filtration rate declines to 10–15% of normal, the patient is in a precarious state and exhibits signs of frank uremia.

REFERENCES

1. Austin, J. H., Stillman, E., and Van Slyke, D. D.: Factors governing the excretion rate of urea, J. Biol. Chem. 46:91, 1921.
2. Möller, E., MacIntosh, J. R., and Van Slyke, D. D.: Studies of urea excretion: II. Relationship between urine volume and rate of urea excretion by normal adults, J. Clin. Invest. 6: 427, 1929.
3. Rehberg, P. B.: Studies on kidney function: I. The rate of filtration and reabsorption in the human kidney, Biochem. J. 20:447, 1926.
4. Joliffe, N., Shannon, J. A., and Smith, H. W.: The excretion of urine in the dog: III. The use of nonmetabolized sugars in the measurement of the glomerular filtrate, Am. J. Physiol. 100:301, 1932.
5. Richards, A. N., Westfall, B. B., and Bott, P. A.: Renal excretion of inulin, creatinine and xylose in normal dogs, Proc. Soc. Exper. Biol. & Med. 32:73, 1934.
6. Shannon, J. A., and Smith, H. W.: The excretion of inulin, xylose and urea by normal and phlorizinized man, J. Clin. Invest. 14:393, 1935.
7. Van Slyke, D. D., Hiller, A., and Miller, B. F.: The clearance, extraction percentage and estimated filtration of sodium ferrocyanide in the mammalian kidney: Comparison with inulin, creatinine and urea, Am. J. Physiol. 113: 611, 1935.

8. Friedman, M., and Byers, S. O.: Clearance of allantoin in the rat and dog as a measure of glomerular filtration rates, Am. J. Physiol. 151:192, 1947.

9. Baumann, K., Oelert, G., Rumrich, G., and Ullrich, K. J.: Ist Inulin zur Messung des Glomerulumfiltrates beim Warmblüter geeignet? Arch. ges. Physiol. 282:238, 1965.

10. Gutman, Y., Gottschalk, C. W., and Lassiter, W. E.: Micropuncture study of inulin absorption in the rat, Science 147:753, 1965.

11. Marsh, D., and Frasier, C.: Reliability of inulin for measuring volume flow in rat renal cortical tubules, Am. J. Physiol. 209:283, 1965.

12. Tanner, G. A., and Klose, R. M.: Micropuncture study of inulin reabsorption in Necturus kidney, Am. J. Physiol. 211:1036, 1966.

13. Swanson, R. E., and Hakim, A. A.: Stop-flow analysis of creatinine excretion in the dog, Am. J. Physiol. 203:980, 1962.

14. O'Connell, J. M. B., Romeo, J. A., and Mudge, G. H.: Renal tubular secretion of creatinine in the dog, Am. J. Physiol. 203:985, 1962.

15. Selkurt, E. E., Wathen, R. L., and Santos-Martinez, J.: Creatinine excretion in the squirrel monkey (*Saimiri sciureus*), Federation Proc. 26:266, 1967.

16. Smith, H. W.: *Principles of Renal Physiology* (New York: Oxford University Press, 1956).

17. Barnett, H. L.: Kidney function in young infants, Pediatrics 5:171, 1950.

18. Shock, N. W.: Renal function tests in aged males, Geriatrics 1:232,1946.

19. Pitts, R. F.: The effect of protein and amino acid metabolism on the urea and xylose clearance, J. Nutrition 9:657, 1935.

20. Concannon, J. P., Summers, R. E., Brewer, R., Weil, C., and Foster, W. D.: I^{125} allyl inulin for the determination of glomerular filtration rate, Am. J. Roentgenol. 92:302, 1964.

21. Nelp, W. B., Wagner, H. N., Jr., and Reba, R. C.: Renal excretion of vitamin B_{12} and its use in the measurement of glomerular filtration rate in man, J. Lab & Clin. Med. 63:480, 1964.

22. Sigman, E. M., Elwood, C. M., and Knox, F.: The measurement of glomerular filtration rate in man with sodium iothalamate ^{131}I (Conray), J. Nuclear Med. 7:60, 1965.

6

Tubular Reabsorption

THE ACCEPTANCE of glomerular ultrafiltration as the initial step in urine formation necessitates the acceptance of tubular reabsorption, for many filterable solutes of plasma are absent from the urine.

General Considerations

MAGNITUDE OF THE PROBLEM

The magnitude of the reabsorptive problem is illustrated by the following considerations. At a filtration rate of 125 ml of plasma per minute, 160 L of water enters the renal tubules each day. A 70-kg man contains, in all, about 40 L of water. His extracellular fluid volume amounts to 14 L, and his circulating plasma volume to 3.5 L. Obviously, the filtration of 160 L of water per day from a volume of only 3.5 L demands the cyclical return and refiltration of water. It likewise demands the cyclical return and refiltration of the many valuable constituents dissolved in the plasma water. One hundred and sixty liters of filtrate contain more than 1 kg of sodium chloride, 500 Gm of sodium bicarbonate, 250 Gm of glucose, 100 Gm of free amino acids, 4 Gm of vitamin C and significant quantities of many other valuable constituents. In most instances, the quantities filtered each day far exceed body stores and,

even more so, the quantities present in the circulating plasma volume. The quantities excreted are negligible fractions of the quantities filtered.

QUANTIFICATION

The rate of filtration of any substance, F_x (milligrams per minute), is equal to the product of the glomerular filtration rate, C_{in} (milliliters per minute), and the plasma concentration of the substance in question, P_x (milligrams per milliliter). The rate of excretion of that substance, E_x (milligrams per minute), is equal to the product of its urine concentration, U_x (milligrams per milliliter), and the urine flow, V (milliliters per minute). The rate of reabsorption, T_x (milligrams per minute), is the difference between the rate of filtration and the rate of excretion. All variables must be measured simultaneously:

$$T_x = F_x - E_x = C_{in} \cdot P_x - U_x \cdot V$$

As an example, let us consider the reabsorption of glucose under conditions of hyperglycemia induced by the infusion of glucose:

Clearance of inulin = 100 ml/min
Plasma glucose (arterial) = 300 mg % (3 mg/ml)
Urine glucose = 1,000 mg % (10 mg/ml)
Urine flow = 5 ml/min

Glucose filtered	= 100 ml/min · 3 mg/ml	= 300 mg/min
Glucose excreted	= 5 ml/min · 10 mg/ml	= 50 mg/min
Glucose reabsorbed		= 250 mg/min

71

Corrections must be made in the calculated rate of filtration of a substance if it is bound in part to plasma protein (thus, not freely filterable through the glomerular membranes) or if it is an ion. In the example cited above, no correction is needed, because glucose is not bound to protein, nor does it carry a charge.

Types of Reabsorptive Transport

Many more or less discrete mechanisms are involved in the reabsorption of the various components of the glomerular filtrate. Certain of these mechanisms reabsorb more than one component. For example, a single mechanism reabsorbs glucose, fructose, galactose and xylose; another reabsorbs sulfate and thiosulfate; and a third reabsorbs arginine, lysine, ornithine and cystine. Other mechanisms—namely, those that reabsorb glucose, phosphate, sulfate, acetoacetate and certain amino acids—although basically discrete seem to share and compete for some common step in transport. A few mechanisms (e.g., that for malate and possibly that for urate) are capable of transporting in both directions; i.e., they secrete or reabsorb, depending on the condition of the moment. Two exchange mechanisms have been described: one reabsorbs sodium ions and secretes hydrogen ions; the other reabsorbs chloride ions and secretes organic acid anions. Still other reabsorptive mechanisms appear to be completely independent of one another.

ACTIVE VERSUS PASSIVE REABSORPTION

Reabsorptive mechanisms can be grossly categorized as active or passive. A mechanism is active if it transports a substance from tubular lumen to peritubular fluid against an electrochemical gradient; i.e., against a gradient of electrical potential, of chemical concentration, or both. Work is performed directly on the substance reabsorbed by the cells effecting transport, and energy is expended in the process. A mechanism is passive if the substance reabsorbed migrates from tubular lumen to peritubular fluid down an electrochemical gradient. No energy is expended directly in moving the substance in question. However, energy is expended indirectly in establishing the concentration or potential gradient down which the substance diffuses.

ACTIVE REABSORPTION.—*Mechanisms exhibiting transport maxima* (Tm).—Glucose, phosphate, sulfate, malate, lactate, β-hydroxybutyrate, acetoacetate, vitamin C, certain amino acids and a number of other constituents of the glomerular filtrate are reabsorbed by mechanisms that are capable of transporting more or less fixed and limited quantities of solute per minute. When more than saturation quantities are presented to the tubules in the filtrate, the excess is excreted in the urine. This does not imply that transport capacity is invariable if conditions are changed. For example, phosphate reabsorption is depressed by parathyroid hormone, and malate reabsorption is markedly enhanced by the infusion of catalytic amounts of fumarate. Nevertheless, under given experimental conditions, only a limited number of milligrams or millimoles of glucose, phosphate, malate, etc., can be reabsorbed per minute; any excess delivered into the tubules is excreted. All of these substances can be more or less completely reabsorbed from the urine when plasma concentrations are low, and reabsorption of each is therefore active; i.e., it occurs against a concentration gradient.

Mechanisms exhibiting gradient-time limitation of transport capacity.—Sodium is reabsorbed against both a potential and a concentration gradient; therefore, the transport mechanism is active. However, in contrast to the mechanisms described above, that for sodium is not limited to some fixed number of milliequivalents that can be transported per minute; rather, it appears to be limited by the gradient that can be established across the tubular wall within the interval of time that the fluid is in contact with the epithelium.

Although the bulk of the filtered chloride is reabsorbed passively, the fact that it is the major anion accompanying sodium accounts for the observation that its reabsorption is also gradient-time limited. Thus, the sodium reabsorptive mechanism imposes its characteristics on the reabsorption of chloride. The reabsorption of bicarbonate, which is accomplished indirectly by sodium-hydrogen exchange, is likewise gradient-time limited. Accordingly, the three major ions of extracellular fluid exhibit similar over-all reabsorption characteristics. The gradient-time-limited mechanisms will not be further considered in this chapter; instead, they will be dealt with in the chapters on sodium reabsorption (Chapter 7) and regulation of acid-base balance (Chapter 11).

PASSIVE REABSORPTION. — Passive reabsorption occurs by diffusion of substances down gradients either of chemical activity or of electrical potential. Throughout all segments of the renal tubule, water diffuses passively from lumen to peritubular fluid down an osmotic gradient established and maintained largely by the reabsorption of sodium. Expressed in a different way, the transport of sodium creates an osmotic force that causes the movement of water. Chloride diffuses passively across the proximal tubular epithelium down a potential gradient likewise established and maintained by the active transport of sodium. Urea migrates passively from lumen to peritubular fluid down a concentration gradient established by the reabsorption of water. In each instance, no work is performed directly on the substance in question (water, chloride or urea) to move it from a region of higher to one of lower electrochemical potential. However, work is performed in establishing and maintaining the gradients down which water, chloride and urea diffuse. The passive reabsorption of all substances depends predominantly on the work performed and the gradients established by the active reabsorption of sodium.

Characteristics of Tm-Limited Reabsorptive Mechanisms

GLUCOSE

The reabsorptive mechanism for glucose illustrates in classic fashion the characteristics of an active system of limited transport capacity and was the first such mechanism to be clearly delineated (1, 2). Under normal conditions, no glucose is excreted in the urine; all that is filtered is reabsorbed. As the plasma concentration of glucose is increased above some critical level, termed the renal plasma threshold, glucose appears in the urine. The higher the plasma concentration of glucose, the greater is the quantity excreted in the urine.

In any given person, the quantity of glucose filtered per minute is a linear function of plasma concentration when measurements are made under such conditions that filtration rate remains stable. Glucose filtered = $C_{in} \cdot P_G$. Thus, filtered glucose, F_G, varies directly and proportionally with P_G when C_{in} is constant: $F_G = K \cdot P_G$ (Fig. 6–1). The quantity of glucose excreted per minute, E_G, is also a linear function of plasma concentration once the plasma threshold concentration is exceeded: $E_G = K \cdot (P_G - \text{threshold})$. The difference between the quantity filtered per minute and the quantity excreted per minute is the quantity reabsorbed per minute. Over a range of 350–2,200 mg/100 ml of plasma glucose, a constant amount of glucose is reabsorbed per minute. This amount, expressed in milligrams per minute, represents the tubular maximal reabsorptive capacity for glucose and is abbreviated Tm_G. For any one person, Tm_G has a remarkably constant value. The average value for man is 375 mg/min per 1.73 m² of surface area and for women is 303 mg/min per 1.73 m² of surface area.

In Figure 6–1, the curves for reabsorption and excretion are drawn in two ways: (1) as idealized, sharply breaking curves and (2) as rounded curves, more descriptive of the true relationships. The experimental determination of such curves by the gradual elevation

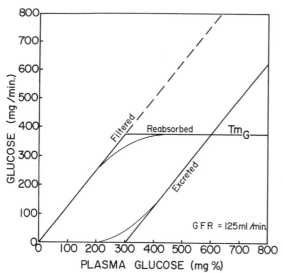

Fig. 6–1. — Titration of the renal tubules of man with glucose.

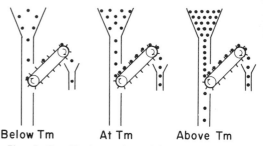

Fig. 6–2. — Mechanical model of a reabsorptive mechanism which exhibits limitation of transport capacity.

of plasma glucose concentration, measuring simultaneously the inulin clearance and both plasma concentration and rate of excretion of glucose, is termed a glucose titration of the renal tubules. The rounding of the curve of reabsorption is termed the splay of the titration curve. If the titration curve were to break sharply, the renal plasma threshold for glucose would be 300 mg/100 ml (3.0 mg/ml). This follows from the consideration: $Tm_G = P_G \cdot C_{in} - U_G \cdot V$. At the plasma concentration just equal to the renal threshold and just capable of saturating the reabsorptive mechanisms, $U_G \cdot V = 0$. Therefore,

$$P_G = \frac{Tm_G}{C_{in}} = \frac{375 \text{ mg/min}}{125 \text{ ml/min}} = 3 \text{ mg/ml} = 300 \text{ mg/100 ml}$$

The true renal plasma threshold is more nearly 180–200 mg/100 ml, indicating that the titration curve exhibits splay and glucose appears in the urine prior to complete saturation of tubular reabsorptive capacity.

MEANING OF Tm_G. — The limitation of the capacity of tubular cells to reabsorb glucose is illustrated in Figure 6–2, a model adapted from a toy once possessed by the author. An endless-belt conveyor, running at constant speed, delivers glucose from tubular lumen into peritubular fluid. If the glucose concen-

tration of the filtrate is low, all is reabsorbed; none appears in the urine. When the filtrate concentration is just sufficient to saturate the reabsorptive mechanism, all carrier sites are occupied. Further increase in filtrate concentration results in the appearance of glucose in the urine. Since, by definition, the conveyor operates at constant speed and has a fixed and limited number of carrier sites, transport of glucose attains a maximum value independent of the amount of glucose presented in the filtrate.

A more acceptable description is the following kinetic description based on the views of Shannon (3).* A carrier substance, B, is present in the luminal membrane of proximal tubular cells in fixed and limited amount. At the luminal surface, this carrier combines reversibly with glucose, G, present in the tubular fluid, to form a complex, $G \cdot B$, within the membrane. The complex $G \cdot B$ then migrates to the cytoplasmic surface of the luminal membrane, where it is split; the glucose is delivered into the cytoplasm of the tubular cell, and the membrane carrier, B, returns to the luminal surface to accept another glucose molecule.

| Glucose | | Membrane | | Cytoplasm |

$$G \quad + \quad B \rightleftarrows G \cdot B \rightarrow B \quad + \quad G$$

*Shannon originally described substance B as a cytoplasmic component of tubular cells. Since the rate-limiting step in glucose reabsorption probably resides in the luminal membrane, I have taken certain liberties with Shannon's views. The entire process of glucose reabsorption may be quite complex and involve a series of subsequent steps, none of which, however, is rate limiting.

If the affinity of B for G present in the tubular fluid is high, and if the rate of combination at the luminal surface is inherently rapid in comparison with the rate of breakdown of the complex at the cytoplasmic surface, two predictions can be made: (1) When sufficient glucose is present in the filtrate, all of the membrane carrier, B, will exist in the form $G \cdot B$. Transport will then be limited by the rate of breakdown of $G \cdot B$ at the cytoplasmic surface. (2) When less than saturation quantities of glucose are present in the filtrate, all of the glucose will be reabsorbed; none will be excreted. If the two assumptions made at the beginning of this paragraph were absolutely true, the titration curve would exhibit no splay. In the dog, little splay is evident; in man, splay is significant.

ORIGIN OF SPLAY.—The origin of splay in the glucose titration curve has two explanations, both of which no doubt contain an element of truth; one is kinetic, the other morphologic. The combination of glucose with the membrane carrier at the luminal surface, $G + B \leftrightharpoons G \cdot B$, is reversible and can be described by the following mass law expression: $K = \dfrac{[G] \cdot [B]}{[G \cdot B]}$. The symbol K represents the dissociation constant for the glucose carrier complex, and the symbols enclosed in brackets are concentrations. The smaller the value of K, the greater is the affinity of the carrier for glucose and the more completely will glucose be removed from the tubular fluid up to the point of complete saturation of the carrier. However, K probably has a finite value, and an appreciable concentration of glucose in the tubular fluid may be needed to saturate the carrier. Glucose will therefore be spilled in the urine before the carrier is completely saturated.

The morphologic explanation of splay introduces the concept of glomerulotubular balance. All nephrons are not equipotent in all respects. As illustrated in Figure 6–3, the glomeruli of some nephrons with normal tubular reabsorptive capacities produce less than average volumes of filtrate. These neph-

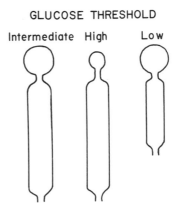

GLUCOSE THRESHOLD

Fig. 6–3.—Glomerulotubular imbalance as a cause of splay in the glucose titration curve.

rons saturate and spill glucose only at high plasma glucose levels. Other nephrons, with average filtration characteristics, have subnormal tubular reabsorptive capacities. These nephrons saturate and spill glucose at low plasma levels.

Figure 6–4 illustrates the analysis of an

Fig. 6–4.—Analysis of splay of the glucose titration curve in terms of numbers of nephrons exhibiting varying degrees of glomerulotubular imbalance. (Adapted from Smith, H. W.: *Lectures on the Kidney* [Lawrence: University of Kansas Press, 1943].)

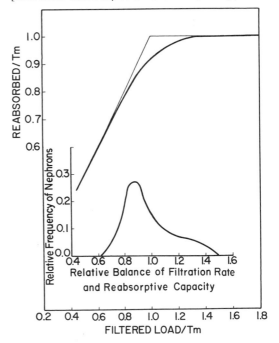

experimentally determined titration curve on a normal man, based on the assumption that each nephron individually exhibits ideal saturation characteristics (K, infinitely low) and that splay results solely from heterogeneity of nephron population (glomerulotubular imbalance). This analysis indicates that individual nephrons of the normal kidney may deviate in their filtration reabsorption characteristics by as much as $\pm 50\%$ from the norm, but that, on the whole, the population is relatively uniform (4).

GLUCOSE THRESHOLD. — From these facts, it can be seen that the renal plasma threshold, far from being a simple constant, is actually the resultant of three variables: (1) glomerular filtration rate, (2) tubular reabsorptive capacity (Tm_G) and (3) the degree of splay of the glucose titration curve. The renal plasma threshold varies inversely with filtration rate and directly with Tm_G. The greater the splay to the lower side of the inflection of the titration curve, the lower is the threshold.

In the young diabetic patient who is otherwise healthy, the renal threshold for glucose is normal, because filtration rate, Tm_G and splay are all within accepted normal limits. Glucosuria results solely from the high plasma concentration of glucose: more glucose is filtered than can be reabsorbed. In the elderly diabetic whose disease is of long standing, the plasma threshold is often high. Glucosuria may not occur, even though plasma glucose increases to levels well above the commonly accepted renal threshold. Such patients have glomerular filtration rates be-

tion may account for absence of glucosuria in some patients in diabetic coma: filtration rate is reduced because of extreme dehydration (6). Some nephrons are nonfunctional; and those that are functional are supplied with minimal volumes of filtrate. Because the filtered load is small, even though plasma concentration is high, all glucose may be reabsorbed.

RENAL GLUCOSURIA. — Renal glucosuria illustrates the operation of the other two variables (7, 8). The condition is congenital, often demonstrably familial, and benign. It is characterized by the excretion of moderate amounts of glucose in the urine; but the polyuria, polydipsia and polyphagia that characterize diabetes mellitus are absent. Renal glucosuria is compatible with continued good health and is a matter of concern only until established as renal in origin. In one type of renal glucosuria, Tm_G is reduced and the threshold is reduced in proportion. The splay of the titration curve is within normal limits. In the other type, Tm_G is normal but splay is markedly increased. Whether increased splay is due to excessive glomerulotubular imbalance or to altered kinetics of the carrier system is unknown. In neither type of benign renal glucosuria are other tubular functions altered.

GLUCOSE TRANSPORT MECHANISM. — The nature of the glucose transport mechanism is poorly understood. At one time, it was thought that glucose is phosphorylated in the process of reabsorption and that the following equations describe the basic aspects of transport:

$$\text{Glucose} + \text{ATP} + \text{Hexokinase} \rightleftharpoons \text{Glucose} - 6 - \text{PO}_4$$
$$\text{Glucose} - 6 - \text{PO}_4 + \text{Alkaline phosphatase} \rightarrow \text{Glucose} + \text{PO}_4$$

low normal. The filtering surface is reduced in consequence of the deposition of a mucopolysaccharide-protein complex in the glomerular capillary tufts (intercapillary glomerulosclerosis). The tubules retain their ability to reabsorb glucose, but the filtered load is less than expected because of reduced filtration (5). A somewhat similar explana-

Cold, azide, cyanide and anoxia, which interfere with oxidative processes supplying adenosine triphosphate (ATP), block glucose reabsorption. Phlorhizin was also thought to interfere with the phosphorylation of glucose. However, dinitrophenol, which uncouples oxidation and phosphorylation, does not block the reabsorption of glucose in any dose tolerated by an intact animal (9). It is therefore probable that glucose is not phosphorylated in the course of transport. Phlorhizin is now thought to bind strongly to the membrane carrier, preventing the attachment of glucose and its entry into the cell. It apparently does not exert its effects by interfering with the metabolic reactions that supply energy to the system—a view which was once held.

The term "membrane carrier" is a popular one today; it covers thinly our profound ignorance. A carrier is thought to be a macromolecule with a prosthetic group specific for the transported substance. The carrier is presumed to shuttle back and forth between the two surfaces of the membrane, combining solute at one surface and freeing it at the opposite. Energy must be supplied either to effect combination of the solute with the carrier or to split the carrier-solute complex. The distance involved in transport is small and is equal to the thickness of the cell membrane (50 Å or less). According to Chinard (9a), the glucose molecule traverses the tubular epithelium from lumen to peritubular capillary in 5 seconds without undergoing any fundamental structural change; i.e., without any splitting of the carbon chain.

CLEARANCE OF GLUCOSE.—The clearance of glucose is normally zero. As the plasma concentration increases and the threshold is exceeded, glucose appears in the urine, and the clearance becomes finite. The higher the plasma glucose concentration, the greater is the clearance; and at very high concentrations the glucose clearance, C_G, approaches the inulin clearance asymptotically (Fig. 6–5). The reason for these relationships is evident from the following equation:

$$C_G = U_G \cdot V/P_G \qquad (1)$$

The excreted glucose at high plasma concentrations is equal to the filtered glucose minus Tm_G:

$$U_G \cdot V = C_{in} \cdot P_G - Tm_G \qquad (2)$$

Substituting $C_{in} \cdot P_G - Tm_G$ for excreted glucose in equation 1 gives

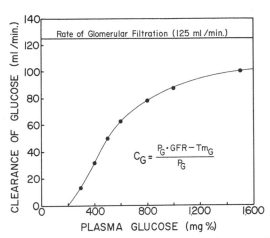

Fig. 6–5.—Clearance of glucose as a function of plasma concentration of glucose.

$$C_G = \frac{C_{in} \cdot P_G - Tm_G}{P_G} \qquad (3)$$

and, by rearranging, yields the following expression:

$$C_G = C_{in} - \frac{Tm_G}{P_G} \qquad (4)$$

As P_G increases, the ratio Tm_G/P_G becomes progressively smaller and smaller. At infinitely high values of P_G, the clearance of glucose becomes equal to the clearance of inulin. These general relationships are evident in Figure 6–5.

COMPETITIVE INHIBITION OF REABSORPTION.—Certain Tm-limited reabsorptive mechanisms transport two or more substances. Xylose, fructose, galactose and glucose are reabsorbed by a single mechanism; phlorhizin blocks the reabsorption of all four sugars. Shannon (10) observed that raising the plasma glucose concentration to 300 mg/100 ml or more—i.e., to a level sufficient to saturate the glucose reabsorptive mechanism—completely blocks all reabsorption of xylose. The clearance of xylose becomes equal to glomerular filtration rate. Because the membrane carrier is the same, occupation of transport sites by glucose excludes xylose. Elevation of plasma xylose concentration neither increases the rate of xylose reabsorption appreciably nor reduces the reabsorption of glucose. Accordingly, the affinity of glucose for the carrier far exceeds the affinity of xylose. The dissociation constant of the carrier-xylose complex, K_X, must therefore be much larger than that of the glucose complex, K_G. Phlorhizin itself may be reabsorbed by the same carrier. If so, its dissociation constant must be several orders of magnitude smaller than that of glucose, because its affinity for the carrier is much higher.

PHOSPHATE

Phosphate plays a variety of roles in the body. Calcium phosphate is a prominent constituent of skeletal structures; organic phosphate complexes are key substances in energy transformations within cells; and, as the major buffer component of the urine, inorganic phosphate contributes to the balancing of the acid-base requirements of the body. The plasma concentration of phosphate is maintained at a level of about 1 mM/L; the person who is in balance excretes each day, largely in the urine, the amount of phosphate ingested.

The tubular mechanism that reabsorbs inorganic phosphate resembles in many respects that which reabsorbs glucose, but it differs in at least two important respects: (1) The reabsorptive capacity for glucose is set so high that, under normal conditions, it is never exceeded; accordingly, the kidney does not regulate plasma glucose concentration. In contrast, the reabsorptive capacity for phosphate is poised at such a value that a slight increase or decrease in plasma concentration results in a change in rate of excretion; accordingly, the kidney participates in the regulation of plasma phosphate concentration. (2) The reabsorptive capacity for glucose is remarkably stable from day to day; it is relatively insensitive to changes in the ionic composition and hormone levels of the plasma. The reabsorptive capacity for phosphate is much more variable and is influenced significantly by body stores of ions and by the circulating levels of parathyroid and adrenal cortical hormones.

Figure 6-6 illustrates the relationship between the filtered load of phosphate* $(GFR \cdot P_{PO_4})$ and the phosphate reabsorbed and excreted in the normal dog (11). During the initial periods of this experiment, the filtered load of phosphate was extremely low, owing to low plasma concentration, and excretion was negligible. As a result of the infusion of phosphate at progressively increasing rates, filtered load rose and excretion increased rapidly. Tm_{PO_4} was attained at a filtered load of 0.125 mM/min and remained constant to the highest value reached, namely, 0.775 mM/min. In this experiment, Tm_{PO_4} averaged 0.100 mM/min. Comparable results have been obtained in man, differing only in greater splay of the titration curves and, of course, higher Tm_{PO_4} values. The Tm_{PO_4} values in man are also less stable from day to day than in the dog.

In the dog, it is possible to vary the rate of glomerular filtration from −30% to +50% of the mean normal value by altering the protein content of the diet. Tm_{PO_4} remains constant under these conditions; hence, it

Fig. 6–6. — Reabsorption and excretion of phosphate as functions of filtered load. (Adapted from Pitts, R. F., and Alexander, R. S.: Am. J. Physiol. 142: 648, 1944.)

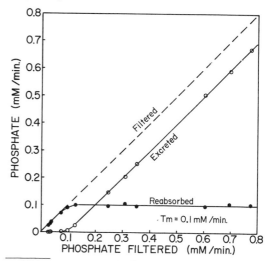

---

*It is customary to plot filtered load, rather than plasma concentration, on the abscissa. When so represented, the glomerular clearance (i.e., filtered load of the substance in question), plotted against itself, forms the 45° line passing through zero on both axes. This becomes a handy reference line with which to compare rate of excretion.

is independent of glomerular filtration rate. Because phosphate can be almost completely reabsorbed from the urine, it is evident that the reabsorptive mechanism is both an active one and one that is truly Tm-limited.

FACTORS AFFECTING PHOSPHATE REABSORPTION. — Metabolic acidosis does not alter Tm_{PO_4} in either dog or man, although it increases the splay of the titration curves. However, acidosis mobilizes soft-tissue and skeletal stores of phosphate, accounting for the phosphaturia observed early in metabolic acidosis. Tm_{PO_4} is reduced, and phosphate excretion is increased, by excessive amounts of cortisone — effects that no doubt underlie the phosphaturia and osteomalacia of hyperadrenocorticism.

The infusion of glucose in amounts sufficient to saturate the glucose reabsorptive mechanism reduces Tm_{PO_4}. The administration of phlorhizin increases Tm_{PO_4}. Apparently, some step in the reabsorptive mechanism for glucose is common to that for phosphate. However, the mechanisms must be largely independent, for phlorhizin inhibits glucose transport but increases phosphate transport. When glucose reabsorption is blocked by phlorhizin, the step common to the two mechanisms is freed to transport more phosphate, and Tm_{PO_4} increases (11). The nature of this interaction of phosphate and glucose reabsorption has not been clearly defined. It is possible that it is an expression of limitation of the supply of energy to tubular cells, which reabsorb both substances. Blockade of glucose reabsorption by phlorhizin would free the energy normally directed into glucose reabsorption and make it available for phosphate reabsorption. Phosphate reabsorption is also depressed significantly by the infusion of the amino acid alanine and the keto acid acetoacetate.

Prolonged infusion of phosphate reduces Tm_{PO_4}, an effect that is abolished by the simultaneous infusion of potassium salts. High dietary intake of phosphate in the newborn infant is also associated with reduction in Tm_{PO_4}. The infusion of calcium gluconate and the administration of large amounts of vitamin D also depress Tm_{PO_4}. All of these effects except that induced by vitamin D may well be mediated by increased secretion of parathyroid hormone in response to altered ionic composition of the body fluids.

EFFECTS OF PARATHYROID HORMONE. — Albright (12) first proposed the thesis that parathyroid hormone, by increasing the urinary excretion of phosphate, induces hypophosphatemia. Because of reduced phosphate concentration, the serum becomes unsaturated with respect to calcium phosphate and, as a consequence, calcium enters the serum in increased quantities from the gastrointestinal tract and from bone. Hypercalcemia develops. However, parathyroid transplants adjacent to osseous structures cause the local solution of bone. Furthermore, parathyroid hormone mobilizes skeletal stores of calcium and phosphate in nephrectomized animals, much as in normal animals. The hypercalcemia induced by parathyroid hormone is not, therefore, obligatorily dependent on its renal actions. However, the administration of parathyroid hormone does cause phosphaturia; in fact, the assay procedure is based on this action. The mechanism of the renal action of the hormone has now been somewhat clarified (13 – 15).

When large doses of parathyroid hormone are given intravenously to normal men, phosphate excretion increases promptly. This phosphate diuresis results from an increase in filtered load of phosphate secondary to an increase in glomerular filtration rate. When parathyroid hormone is given intravenously to a hypoparathyroid patient, an even more marked phosphaturia results, secondary both to an increase in filtration rate and to a decrease in Tm_{PO_4}. Prolonged administration of hormone depresses phosphate reabsorption in the normal person, as well as in the hypoparathyroid patient. In both normal and hypoparathyroid individuals, the depression of Tm_{PO_4} observed on the long-term administration of hormone is independent of changes in filtration rate. The increased sensitivity of the hypoparathyroid patient to parathyroid hormone is unexplained; however, a similar sensitivity to thyroid hormone in patients with myxedema and to cortisone in patients with adrenal insufficiency is well known. It is probable that much of the variability of Tm_{PO_4} in man is due to fluctuations in the rate of secretion of parathyroid hormone.

Parathyroid hormone causes hypercalciuria largely, if not entirely, because it mobilizes osseous stores and increases the plasma concentration of filterable calcium. Tubular reabsorption of calcium is increased in hyperparathyroidism because of the marked increase in filtered load; a portion of the excess is reabsorbed, and a portion is excreted.

SULFATE

Inorganic sulfate is formed in the body in the metabolism of sulfur-containing amino acids. It is incorporated into cartilage as chondroitin sulfate, can apparently serve as a source of sulfur in the synthesis of cystine and methionine, and enters into a variety of detoxification reactions. The plasma concentration of sulfate is maintained within limits of $1-1.5$ mM/L under normal conditions. At low plasma concentrations, reabsorption is essentially complete; hence, the reabsorptive mechanism is active. As is evident in Figure

$6-7$, the reabsorptive mechanism for sulfate in the dog resembles that for phosphate (16). Tm_{SO_4} is of the same order of magnitude as Tm_{PO_4}; titration curves for sulfate, as well as for phosphate, exhibit little splay. Saturation of the phosphate reabsorptive mechanism depresses sulfate Tm; and, conversely, saturation of the sulfate reabsorptive mechanism depresses phosphate Tm. However, the extent of depression of Tm in either instance is small and may indicate competition for energy rather than for a common carrier. Sulfate Tm, like phosphate Tm, is depressed by saturation of the glucose reabsorptive mechanism and is elevated above normal by inhibition of glucose reabsorption with phlorhizin. Sulfate Tm, again like phosphate Tm, is depressed by saturation of the reabsorptive mechanisms for alanine and for acetoacetate.

The sulfate reabsorptive mechanism differs from that of phosphate in that Tm_{SO_4} is depressed by the infusion of hypertonic sodium chloride. The depression is unrelated to the resulting osmotic diuresis and thus appears to be a specific effect of the sodium or chloride ion. Because sulfate Tm is depressed to an equal extent by the infusion of sodium thiocyanate and sodium nitrate,

Fig. 6–7. — Reabsorption and excretion of sulfate as functions of filtered load. (From Lotspeich, W. D.: Am. J. Physiol. 151:311, 1947.)

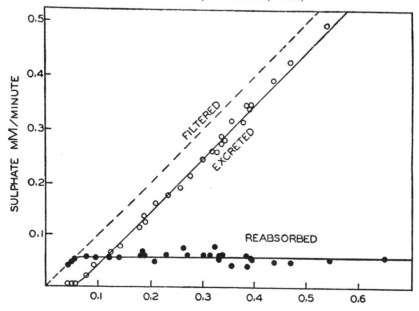

the presence of an excess of any readily transported anion in the tubular urine will probably depress the reabsorption of the less readily transported sulfate ion.

Thiosulfate is both reabsorbed and secreted by tubular cells. Secretion can be blocked with carinamide, a drug that has no effect on the reabsorption of either thiosulfate or sulfate. Under the influence of carinamide, sulfate and thiosulfate can be shown to compete for a single reabsorptive mechanism whose transport capacity for thiosulfate is about two thirds of that for sulfate. Strangely, sulfate depresses the secretion of thiosulfate, although it is not itself secreted (17).

AMINO ACIDS

The circulating amino acids of blood plasma are in dynamic equilibrium with intracellular amino acids, and these in turn are constantly interchanging with their counterparts in tissue proteins. Digestion of dietary protein and absorption of the fragments add to the amino acid pool of the body; deamination and formation of urea and ammonia subtract from the pool; and transamination converts one amino acid into another. These processes are so balanced as to maintain the plasma concentration of amino acids within limits of 2.5 – 3.5 mM/L. A major role of the kidney is that of conservation of the amino acids that enter the tubules in the glomerular filtrate; negligible quantities are excreted. However, the kidney extracts amide and aminonitrogen from renal arterial blood to produce the ammonia that is excreted in the urine in association with anions of strong acids. Excretion of ammonia permits the conservation of so-called fixed cations — sodium, potassium, etc. — and plays a major role in balancing acid-base requirements (see Chapter 11). The kidney also participates actively in transamination reactions — extracting certain amino acids from arterial blood and adding others to renal venous blood, most notably alanine and serine.

CLEARANCE OF AMINONITROGEN. — The clearance of aminonitrogen is normally very low but increases when plasma concentration is elevated twofold or more by the infusion of amino acids. A protein meal causes only a moderate increase in the plasma level of amino acids and does not result in aminoaciduria. The kidneys do not primarily regulate the plasma concentrations of amino acids. Like the glucose threshold, the aminonitrogen threshold is set sufficiently high so that urinary excretion is negligible under normal circumstances.

Because the urinary concentration of aminonitrogen can be reduced essentially to zero, reabsorption must be active. Doty observed that tyrosine and histidine are almost completely reabsorbed, N-methyltyrosine is less well reabsorbed and N-acetyltyrosine is poorly reabsorbed when each is administered singly in comparable dosage. The intravenous infusion of racemic mixtures of amino acids results in greater urinary losses than the infusion of similar mixtures of the naturally occurring forms. The L-isomers of alanine, methionine and histidine are reabsorbed more effectively than the D-isomers at the same plasma concentrations. Accordingly, it may be concluded that both structural and stereoisometric configurations influence rate of transport.

NUMBERS OF TRANSPORT MECHANISMS. — There are probably no fewer than three, and possibly there are more, renal mechanisms for the reabsorption of amino acids. One mechanism reabsorbs lysine, arginine, ornithine, cystine and, possibly, histidine; a second reabsorbs glutamic and aspartic acids; and a third and perhaps others reabsorb the remainder. The infusion of a single amino acid depresses, to the greatest extent, reabsorption of other amino acids transported by the same mechanism. However, it may also depress to a lesser extent reabsorption of certain amino acids presumably transported by a different mechanism. The infusion of histidine depresses the reabsorption of certain neutral amino acids as well as those of the basic group. The infusion of certain neutral and basic amino acids depresses histidine reabsorption. Because of such interactions between amino acids of different classes, the specificity of transport mechanisms and even the numbers of mechanisms are uncertain (17–21).

TITRATION CHARACTERISTICS. — Figures 6–8 and 6–9 illustrate the very dissimilar properties of the reabsorptive mechanisms for lysine (22) and for glycine (23) in the dog. The reabsorptive mechanisms for both amino acids exhibit Tm limitations of transport capacity. The threshold for lysine is relatively sharp; the titration curve exhibits little splay. The threshold for glycine is indefinite; the titration curve exhibits marked splay. The Tm for glycine is approximately 15 times that for lysine.

The titration curve for arginine is much like that for lysine, and the Tm value is roughly the same. The administration of large amounts of lysine blocks the reabsorption of arginine, and the administration of arginine blocks the reabsorption of lysine. A similar competitive interaction is observed among ornithine, cystine, histidine, lysine and arginine (19–21). It appears that all are reabsorbed by a single mechanism. The Tm value for histidine, if one exists, must be more than 10 times that for lysine; because of its toxicity, it has been impossible to infuse enough histidine to saturate the mechanism.

Glutamic acid also has a reasonably sharp

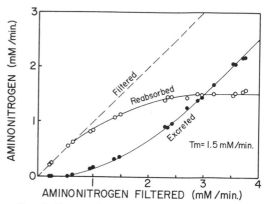

Fig. 6–9. — Reabsorption and excretion of aminonitrogen as functions of filtered load in experiments in which glycine was infused to increase plasma aminonitrogen concentration. (Adapted from Pitts, R. F.: Am. J. Physiol. 140:156, 1943.)

threshold and a relatively low Tm (24). Because Tm for D,L-alanine is only slightly less than that for glycine, it is probable that the value for L-alanine is much higher, because the D-isomer is relatively poorly reabsorbed. The characteristics of leucine reabsorption are somewhat similar to those of glycine and D,L-alanine. Other amino acids have not been studied at sufficiently high plasma levels to delineate their reabsorptive mechanisms adequately.

SPLAY. — The marked splay in the titration curve of glycine has been explained in terms of the kinetics of the combination of the amino acid with the membrane carrier (23), much as the minor splay of the glucose titration curve has been explained. If the dissociation constant of the carrier-glycine complex is relatively large, then a high concentration of glycine in the tubular urine will be required to saturate the transport mechanism, and excretion will begin long before Tm is achieved.

CREATINE. — Creatine, at normal plasma concentrations of 0.5–1.0 mg/100 ml, is reabsorbed completely from the glomerular filtrate. When creatine is infused, its clearance rises sharply with increasing plasma concentration (25). Reabsorption also increases; no Tm has been demonstrated. Reabsorption of creatine is completely blocked

Fig. 6–8. — Reabsorption and excretion of lysine as functions of filtered load. (Adapted from Wright, H. R., Russo, H. F., Skeggs, H. R., Patch, E. A., and Beyer, K. H.: Am. J. Physiol. 149:130, 1947.)

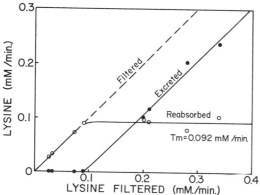

by saturation of the reabsorptive mechanism with glycine and with alanine. It is possible, therefore, that glycine, alanine and creatine are reabsorbed by a single mechanism.

SPECIFICITY OF AMINO ACID REABSORPTIVE MECHANISMS. — Amino acid reabsorption is unchanged by saturation of the glucose reabsorptive mechanism. It is also unaffected by the administration of phlorhizin in amounts that completely inhibit glucose reabsorption or by the administration of dinitrophenol in amounts that depress secretion of p-aminohippurate. However, as pointed out earlier in this section, reabsorption of phosphate and sulfate are moderately depressed by the infusion of large amounts of amino acids, perhaps as a result of competition for a limited supply of energy.

NATURE OF TRANSPORT MECHANISMS. — The nature of the transport mechanisms for amino acids has only partially been defined. Lotspeich (26) suggested, on the basis of Christiansen's work, that one step in transport may involve the formation of a stabilized

cells in considerable concentrations, for the mechanism is assumed to be responsible not only for the transport of amino acids across epithelial membranes but also for the entry of nutrient amino acids into cells of all tissues and organs. The system of enzymes, peptides and amino acid products is called the γ-glutamyl cycle.

An insoluble glycoprotein enzyme, bound to the cell membranes of the microvilli of proximal tubular cells, catalyzes the exchange of an amino acid within the tubular lumen for the cysteinyl-glycine of glutathione. Both the γ-glutamyl-amino acid and the cysteinyl-glycine are translocated to the interior of the cell, perhaps by a conformational change in the enzyme. This enzyme is γ-glutamyl-transpeptidase (γ-GTP); and its product, γ-glutamyl-amino acid, can be considered the carrier.

$$\gamma\text{-Glutamyl-cysteinyl-glycine} + \text{Amino acid} \xrightarrow{\gamma\text{-GTP}} \gamma\text{-Glutamyl-amino acid} + \text{Cysteinyl-glycine}$$

Within the cell a second soluble enzyme, γ-glutamyl-cyclotransferase (γ-GCT), catalyzes the conversion of γ-glutamyl-amino acid to free amino acid and 5-oxyproline:

$$\gamma\text{-Glutamyl-amino acid} \xrightarrow{\gamma\text{-GCT}} \text{Amino acid} + \text{5-Oxyproline}$$

Shiff's base between a metal chelate of an amino acid and pyridoxal. Such a reaction has been postulated to account for the uptake of amino acids by mouse ascites tumor cells against a concentration gradient. Ease of formation and stability of such a complex might account for differences in transport characteristics of different amino acids. Just how it could account for differences in group characteristics of basic, acidic and neutral amino acids is uncertain.

Recently a new thesis has been developed by Meister and his colleagues (personal communication), based on their observations of enzymes and reactions occurring within renal tubular cells. Incidentally, it accounts for the ubiquitous presence of glutathione in all

The final degradative step of the amino acid transport system is the splitting of cysteinyl-glycine to cysteine and glycine by cellular peptidases.

The restorative aspects of the cycle consist in the conversion of 5-oxyproline to glutamic acid by an ATP-powered catalysis dependent on 5-oxyprolinase. A second step involves the formation of γ-glutamyl-cysteine by its synthetase — also an ATP-powered catalysis. The final restorative step is the addition of glycine to γ-glutamyl-cysteine to reform glutathione. This reaction likewise involves ATP. Thus the reabsorption of 1 mol of amino acid involves the expenditure of 3 mol of ATP — a moderately expensive procedure, in view of the fact that, in man, about 0.5 mol of amino acid is reabsorbed per day. All of these enzymes are present in kidney in high concentration.

Whether this is the only mechanism of reabsorption of amino acid is unknown. Apparently proline is dependent on another mechanism, for it does not enter into the initial transpeptidase reaction. However, the mechanism can explain at least two of the characteristics of amino acid reabsorption: competition, and the affinity of the carrier for amino acids. If isozymes are present, it could explain group specificity. The mechanism also provides a major role for glutathione and explains its high cellular concentration in the kidney (4–5 mM), its low plasma concentration, the fact that it is largely synthesized within tissues including kidney, and its fairly rapid turnover.

ORGANIC ANIONS

A number of organic anions are normally excreted in the urine in small amounts. In general, rates of excretion are increased in alkalosis and reduced in acidosis. Cooke *et al.* (27) asserted that organic aciduria represents a mechanism for the conservation of chloride in alkalosis; i.e., chloride is reabsorbed and sodium is excreted in combination with organic anions. In acidosis, chloride ions, rather than organic anions, are excreted with sodium.

CITRATE. – Citrate is a normal constituent of human urine. It plays a specific role in solubilizing calcium by forming an undissociated complex, thereby lessening the possibility of precipitation of calcium phosphate stones in the urinary tract. Rate of excretion is greatly increased in metabolic alkalosis and is reduced in acidosis. The infusion of sodium citrate results in increases in both the rate of excretion and the rate of reabsorption of citrate; no Tm is demonstrable at plasma concentrations that can be tolerated by the intact animal. However, the titration curve exhibits marked splay, and its shape suggests the possibility that a Tm value might be attained if cardiac toxicity were not a factor

limiting the rate of administration of citrate (21).

It has long been known that citrate excretion is increased by the infusion of certain members of the tricarboxylic acid cycle, such as oxaloacetate, succinate, fumarate and malate. It is also increased by blocking the conversion of succinate to fumarate with malonate, presumably damming back all components of the cycle and leading to the accumulation of citrate in cells. These observations suggested to Lotspeich that citrate may not only be reabsorbed but also secreted by tubular cells. A critical study by Grollman *et al.* (28) showed that the infusion of the organic anions referred to above merely blocks reabsorption of citrate, the citrate clearance becoming equal to the rate of glomerular filtration but never exceeding it. They maintain that these components of the Krebs cycle compete with citric acid for a single reabsorptive mechanism. Another possibility is that citric acid synthesis is increased in tubular cells and that high intracellular citrate levels inhibit reabsorption. Citrate excretion is increased by estradiol and by the administration of calcium salts, presumably by reducing reabsorption.

MALATE. – Malate is reabsorbed by a Tm-limited system, which in the dog transports a maximum of 4–6 mg/min. The reabsorptive mechanism exhibits relatively little splay when the tubules are titrated by the infusion of sodium L-malate. Tm is increased by the administration of catalytic amounts of fumarate. Malate is synthesized within tubular cells from certain precursors of the Krebs cycle and secreted into the tubular urine. The infusion of citrate, α-ketoglutarate and succinate, all of which increase tubular synthesis of malate, stimulates its secretion. Under these circumstances, the malate clearance exceeds the rate of glomerular filtration. By reducing tubular synthesis, malonate blocks the secretion of malate that was induced by the infusion of these three precursors. Although good evidence exists for the bidirectional transport of malate – whether it represents the activities of a single mechanism, whose directional orientation is governed by relative concentrations of the anion in tubular urine and tubular cells, or the activities of separate reabsorptive and secretory mechanisms — the nature of the transport is uncertain (29).

α-KETOGLUTARATE. — In studies on the dog, Cohen (30, 31), Balagura (32, 33) and their associates have described the major characteristics of tubular transport of α-ketoglutarate, a substance that circulates in low concentration in plasma, yet is a highly important constituent of the metabolic cycle of all cells, including those that make up the renal tubules. Plasma concentration of α-ketoglutarate is normally quite low: less than 0.1 μmol/ml. Essentially all that enters the tubules in the glomerular filtrate is reabsorbed. Reabsorption is active, for transport across the luminal membranes from tubular fluid to the interior of tubular cells occurs against an electrochemical gradient. Furthermore, reabsorptive transport is Tm-limited, and saturation of the transport mechanism occurs at plasma concentrations more than 20 times normal. The reabsorptive mechanism exhibits relatively little splay. Accordingly, the kidneys do not regulate the plasma concentration of α-ketoglutarate: the renal plasma threshold is far higher than the plasma concentration, and reabsorptive transport serves mainly to prevent loss of the α-ketoglutarate that enters the renal tubules in the filtrate.

The tubules by no means transport α-ketoglutarate from filtrate to blood as an inert substance. When plasma concentration is increased and the amount reabsorbed is correspondingly raised, the kidneys use large amounts of α-ketoglutarate. Utilization includes metabolism via the Krebs cycle to CO_2 and water and conversion to glutamate, aspartate, glucose and possibly to other compounds as well, which may be stored in the kidney or added to renal venous blood. Little α-ketoglutarate is stored as such. Most of the α-ketoglutarate administered intravenously to a dog is used by the kidneys and liver; relatively little is used by the rest of the

body. Thus the kidneys, which constitute less than 1% of body weight, may use more than 50% of an intravenously administered load of α-ketoglutarate.

When plasma concentration is increased by the infusion of α-ketoglutarate, more is extracted from blood flowing through the kidney than is contained in the glomerular filtrate. Accordingly, α-ketoglutarate must be transported into tubular cells across their peritubular membranes, as well as across their luminal membranes. Peritubular transport, like luminal transport, is active, in that it occurs against an electrochemical gradient. Peritubular transport may also be Tm-limited, although this possibility has not been established as fact.

Although large amounts of α-ketoglutarate are extracted from blood and used when the compound is administered intravenously, no significant net amount is extracted when plasma concentration is within the low range of normal. At these low concentrations, only a small amount of α-ketoglutarate is delivered to the kidneys in arterial blood. Essentially the same amount leaves the kidneys in venous blood. However, the moiety that leaves the kidneys is not the same one that entered the kidneys. The Krebs cycle of tubular cells turns rapidly, producing α-ketoglutarate from precursors and using it with equal rapidity. The small amounts that are normally filtered, reabsorbed and enter cells across peritubular membranes are, at least in part, incorporated into this metabolic pool. From this pool, α-ketoglutarate re-enters renal venous blood in essentially equivalent amounts.

The capacity of the renal tubules of the dog to reabsorb α-ketoglutarate is markedly influenced by the acid-base state of the animal. Maximal reabsorptive capacity (Tm-α-ketoglutarate) of the normal dog (20 kg) averages 48 μmol/min. In acute respiratory acidosis, Tm is increased to 77 μmol/min and in chronic metabolic acidosis to 110 μmol/min. In acute metabolic alkalosis induced by the infusion of THAM (tris[hydroxymethyl]aminomethane) and in acute respiratory alkalosis. Tm is reduced to an average of $5-10$ $\mu mol/min$. Because alkalosis induced by infusion of sodium bicarbonate is less effective in depressing Tm-α-ketoglutarate than is infusion of THAM and respiratory alkalosis, it is probable that these effects of hydrogen ion concentration are mediated through changes in intracellular rather than extracellular pH (32). In any event, depression of net reabsorptive transport and occasional stimulation of net secretion of α-ketoglutarate account, in part, for the well-documented increase in excretion of organic acids in alkalosis.

Renal transport, extraction and use of α-ketoglutarate are further complicated by the fact that flux across both luminal and peritubular membranes of tubular cells is bidirectional. When Krebs cycle precursors of α-ketoglutarate, such as citrate, pyruvate and acetate, are infused intravenously in a normal dog, essentially complete reabsorption of filtered α-ketoglutarate is replaced by net secretion; i.e., rate of urinary excretion exceeds rate of filtration. Respiratory alkalosis routinely depresses reabsorption of α-ketoglutarate and occasionally induces net secretion, as noted above. Furthermore, alkalosis potentiates the net secretion induced by infusion of precursors. Secretion of α-ketoglutarate is passive, in the sense that transport occurs down an electrochemical gradient. Under those conditions, outlined above, that induce net secretion, α-ketoglutarate is also added to renal venous blood in net amounts.

Renal tubular cells are most simply described as dual-pump, dual-leak systems with respect to α-ketoglutarate. Pumps in both luminal and peritubular membranes actively transport α-ketoglutarate into tubular cells, from which it passively leaks back into peritubular blood and tubular urine. α-Ketoglutarate is both produced and used within tubular cells via the Krebs cycle and its several offshoots into pathways of carbohydrate, amino acid and fatty acid metabolism. An increase in cellular production of α-ketoglutarate or a reduction in its oxidation or use by other pathways favors its passive-leak discharge into urine and blood. Conversely, a decrease in production or an increase in use favors active uptake over passive back leak. Furthermore, as clearly indicated by the work of Balagura and Stone (33), an increase in plasma concentration of α-ketoglutarate accentuates cell uptake and use and converts net secretion, induced by citrate, to net reabsorption. The complexity of the renal handling of α-ketoglutarate, in comparison with substances such as glucose, no doubt derives from the following facts: (1) α-ketoglutarate is an important intermediate in the energy generating system of renal tubules; (2) the small quantities of α-ketoglutarate that are normally filtered and reabsorbed are, at least in part, incorporated into the energy and metabolic cycles of tubular cells; and (3) back diffusion of α-ketoglutarate, in a direction opposite to that of active pumping, occurs to an appreciable extent.

ACETOACETATE. — Acetoacetate is completely reabsorbed from the tubular urine under normal conditions. In starvation and in uncontrolled diabetes mellitus, plasma acetoacetate rises and excretion increases in proportion to plasma level. From experiments on dogs, it is evident that the reabsorption of acetoacetate is active and that the mechanism is Tm-limited. However, Tm is not stable; for, as plasma concentration is progressively increased, rate of reabsorption decreases moderately. This self-depression of reabsorption has been explained in terms of autoinhibition of some enzyme system involved in transport by excessive concentration of substrate (34). As pointed out earlier, some step in reabsorption is common to acetoacetate, phosphate, sulfate and glucose, for they all interact.

β-HYDROXYBUTYRATE. — β-hydroxybutyrate is also reabsorbed by an active mechanism of limited transport capacity. Tm in the dog averages $2-3$ mg/kg per minute. The titration curve exhibits marked splay: excretion is significant at a plasma concentration only slightly above normal, and saturation of the mechanism is attained only at relatively high plasma levels (35).

In man, the renal threshold is about 20 mg/ 100 ml.

LACTATE. – Lactate is reabsorbed more or less completely from the tubular urine, under normal conditions. The renal threshold in man is 60 mg/100 ml; above the threshold, lactate excretion varies in proportion to blood level. Whether or not a true Tm exists has not been determined. In the dog, the threshold is 100 mg/100 ml, and reabsorption is Tm-limited. Tm is the same for both D and L-isomers, although the plasma concentration required to saturate the mechanism is somewhat higher for the D- than for the L-form (36).

VITAMIN C

The mechanism of reabsorption of vitamin C in man and dog exhibits limited transport capacity. In man, Tm is 1.77 mg/min, and in the dog, 0.52 mg/min, both per 100 ml of glomerular filtrate. In both man and dog, the titration curves exhibit marked splay (37, 38).

In the dog, the administration of estradiol, the infusion of sodium chloride, saturation of the tubular secretory mechanism for p-aminohippurate and saturation of the tubular reabsorptive mechanism for glucose all depress Tm for vitamin C. The nature of these interactions is uncertain.

URIC ACID

The normal adult excretes each day 0.5 – 0.8 Gm of uric acid, which is derived from the metabolism of purine bases liberated in the degradation of ingested and endogenous nucleoproteins. Uric acid represents only 5% or so of the total urinary nitrogen; the bulk of the nitrogen is excreted as urea. Interest in uric acid in man stems largely from abnormalities in metabolism and excretion, which result in the formation of urate calculi in the urinary tract, renal damage from the deposition of urate crystals in the renal parenchyma, acute paroxysmal or chronic arthritis and the deposition of urate tophi in articular, periarticular and subcutaneous tissues.

The normal plasma concentration of urate is 4 – 6 mg/100 ml, and the uric acid clearance is 6 – 12 ml/min. Because urate is freely filterable from plasma, it may be concluded that the filtered load is 10 – 15 times the rate of excretion; hence, more than 90% of the filtered urate is reabsorbed.

Berliner et al. (39) observed that, when lithium urate is infused intravenously into normal man, both excretion and reabsorption increase with increasing plasma level. At plasma concentrations of 15 – 20 mg/100 ml, the reabsorptive mechanism saturates; the maximum rate of transport. Tm urate, averages 15 mg/min per 1.73 m² of surface area. The titration curve exhibits marked splay, and the extent of the splay, rather than the Tm, governs the excretion of urate.

The basic abnormality in gout is undefined. Some patients produce and excrete abnormally large amounts of urate; many do not. However, an elevated plasma concentration of urate is a characteristic finding in the disease. If the $U \cdot V$ urate is normal and the P urate is elevated, it is obvious that the clearance of urate must be less than normal. The reason for the reduced clearance is not entirely clear, and no doubt it is not the same in all patients. In many patients, the rate of glomerular filtration is moderately to markedly reduced; in some, the reduction is a manifestation of renal damage from urate deposits in the kidneys, and in others it is the result of advancing age or antecedent renal disease. However, the filtered load is frequently greater than normal, as a consequence of an increase in plasma urate level disproportionately large in comparison with the reduction in filtration rate. In these patients, tubular reabsorption must be increased. In a minority of instances, increased production of urate may be the major cause of increased plasma concentration. Thus, three factors may play a role in the production of the hyperuricemia of gout: (1) a reduction in filtration rate with maintained tubular reabsorption of urate, (2) increased reabsorption of urate and (3) increased production of urate (40).

Gutman maintained that uric acid is more or less completely reabsorbed by the renal tubules of both normal and gouty persons and that the uric acid that is excreted is added to the tubular urine by a secretory mechanism located more distally in the nephron than the reabsorptive mechanism. Evidence for complete reabsorption is by no means conclusive; that for secretion of urate is the following: G-28315 is a uricosuric agent that presumably depresses reabsorption of urate. In a selected group of patients who had low filtration rates, were undergoing mannitol diuresis and were being treated with G-28315, the urate clearance exceeded the inulin clearance by 4–20%. The conclusion was drawn that a partial blockade of the reabsorption of urate by the drug unmasked the secretion. Salicylate and certain other uricosuric drugs in small doses reduce, but in high doses increase, the excretion of urate. Yü and Gutman (41) interpreted this action as indicating (1) suppression of secretion by small doses, resulting in decreased excretion, and (2) suppression of both secretion and reabsorption by large doses, resulting in increased excretion.

Most mammals other than man, the apes, the New World monkeys and the Dalmatian dog rapidly oxidize urate to allantoin, excreting the major part of their purine nitrogen in this form. The plasma concentration of urate in mongrel dogs is low because of rapid conversion to allantoin; urinary excretion of urate is low because of nearly complete reabsorption from the tubular urine. When plasma urate is elevated by the infusion of lithium urate, both reabsorption and excretion increase; no Tm can be demonstrated.* Stop-flow experiments have shown that urate is reabsorbed in the proximal tubule and that probenecid, a moderately effective uricosuric agent, depresses reabsorption (42).

---

*Tm in the dog, if one exists, is much greater than in man. The relative insolubility of urate salts makes it impossible to elevate the plasma concentration sufficiently to saturate the reabsorptive mechanism.

The clearance of urate in the Dalmatian dog is high. Most of the purine nitrogen of this breed is eliminated as urate, not so much because of failure of oxidative enzymes to convert it to allantoin but because of failure of tubular reabsorption. Stop-flow experiments have demonstrated that urate is secreted in small amounts by the same segment of the nephron of the Dalmatian dog as that which reabsorbs urate in the mongrel dog (42). Furthermore, probenecid blocks the secretion of urate in the Dalmatian dog. However, conventional clearance experiments on Dalmatian dogs demonstrate no net secretory transport: the urate clearance is approximately equal to the filtration rate. It is possible that, in the Dalmatian dog, urate is transported in both directions in essentially equal amounts. Secretory transport may be absent or insignificant in the mongrel dog. Such observations at least suggest the possibility that bidirectional transport may occur in the renal tubules of man, although the matter is by no means definitely settled.

Although uric acid accounts for a minor fraction of the total nitrogen excretion in mammals, it is the major nitrogenous end product in birds and arid-living reptiles. In these forms, uric acid is secreted into the tubular urine in high concentration, forming a milky supersaturated solution. The urine refluxes from the cloaca into the lower bowel, where water is reabsorbed, leaving a paste of solid uric acid to be evacuated with the feces. Because of low solubility, the excretion of uric acid requires the elimination of only 10 ml of water per gram of nitrogen. In comparison, the excretion of urea by man requires the elimination of at least 40–60 ml of water per gram of nitrogen. Accordingly, the kidneys of birds and arid-living reptiles, neither of which can form urine significantly hypertonic to plasma, accomplish a far greater conservation of water per gram of nitrogen excreted than do the kidneys of man, which are capable of elaborating urine having an osmotic pressure 4 times that of plasma. The advantage of uricotelic metabolism to an organism with limited access to water is obvious. This biochemical adaptation has apparently evolved more than once, for insects also excrete most of their nitrogen as uric acid.

PROTEIN

In Chapter 4, it was pointed out that the glomerular capillaries behave as though they are perforated by pores 75–100 Å in diameter; i.e., of a size just adequate to permit the passage of plasma albumin. However, rate of filtration of protein is normally restricted to a minute fraction of rate of filtration of water

purified hemoglobin is infused slowly, none of the hemoglobin is excreted in the urine until the plasma concentration exceeds 150 mg/100 ml. Above this threshold concentration, excretion becomes a linear function of plasma concentration. The slope of the line relating the rate of excretion to plasma concentration is an expression of glomerular clearance of hemoglobin. On average, hemoglobin is filtered at a rate only 5% that of water: 95% of the hemoglobin molecules are sieved, and 5% enter the glomerular filtrate. Accordingly, when plasma concentration just equals the threshold value of 1.5 mg/ml, 9.38 mg of hemoglobin is filtered per minute:

$$\text{Quantity of Hb filtered} = C_{in} \cdot P_{Hb} \cdot 0.05 = 125 \cdot 0.05 = 9.38 \text{ mg/min}$$

by the combined factors of steric hindrance, viscous drag and electrical hindrance. The concentration of albumin in the filtrate is probably less than 30 mg/100 ml; thus, in comparison with plasma, in which the concentration is 4 Gm/100 ml, the filtrate can be considered essentially albumin-free. However, if 160 L of plasma water were filtered each day and if each liter of filtrate contained only 200 mg of albumin (20 mg/100 ml), 32 Gm would enter the tubules in 24 hours. But no more than 100 mg is normally excreted each day; therefore albumin must be reabsorbed. When the plasma albumin of normal dogs is elevated to 6–7 Gm/100 ml by daily infusions of plasma, albuminuria results, and the rate of excretion increases linearly with increasing plasma level (43). Such results have been interpreted to indicate that a minute fraction of the plasma albumin is filtered, that tubular reabsorptive capacity is limited and that the delivery of excess albumin into the tubules results in albuminuria. One may estimate that, in man, about 0.5–0.6% of the albumin of plasma is filtered, Tm albumin is about 30 mg/min, and the renal plasma threshold for albumin is 6–7 Gm/100 ml (44, 45).

When hemoglobin is liberated from red cells by intravascular hemolysis or when

Because no hemoglobin is excreted at the renal threshold, it has been assumed that reabsorptive capacity is 9.38 mg/min.

This argument has been shown by Lathem (46) to be incorrect, for the following reasons: Hemoglobin is tightly bound to an α_2-globulin to form a nonfilterable complex having a high molecular weight. On average, the hemoglobin-combining capacity of plasma is 128 mg/100 ml. Only when the plasma concentration of hemoglobin exceeds this value is there any filterable hemoglobin present in plasma. The Tm for hemoglobin is about 1 mg/min, rather than 9 mg/min; and, because of its very low value, it cannot be measured at all accurately. However, stopflow studies (47) have recently confirmed the long-held view that albumin, hemoglobin and proteins of smaller molecular dimensions are filtered and reabsorbed in the proximal segment of the nephron.

SITE OF REABSORPTION

The several reabsorptive mechanisms described in the preceding sections of this chapter are now known to reside in cells making up the proximal segments of the renal tubules. Evidence as to site of reabsorption of glucose and phosphate was first derived from micropuncture studies on nephrons of *Necturus* and the rat. More recently, proximal reabsorption of glucose (48), phosphate (49), sulfate (50), urate (42), amino acids (51) and hemoglobin (47) has been demonstrated by the stop-flow technic devised by Malvin, Sullivan and Wilde. This technic has also provided information as to the loci of certain secretory processes. Although localization by this method is at best gross, it has the virtue of being applicable in the dog, the species in which renal mechanisms of reabsorption and secretion have been most precisely defined.

The method, in brief, is the following: One ureter of an anesthetized dog is catheterized through a flank incision. Creatinine and *p*-aminohippurate are infused intravenously at rates sufficient to maintain plasma concentrations adequate for accurate measurement of clearances. The substance whose reabsorption or secretion is to be studied is also incorporated in this infusion. A second infusion, of hypertonic mannitol, is administered intravenously at a rate that causes the urine flow of the one kidney under study to increase to about 10 ml/min. When the urine flow stabilizes at such a value, the ureter is clamped. After 3–8 minutes, the clamp is released, and the urine, which gushes out under high pressure, is collected in a series of 30 or more samples of about 1 ml each. Some 15–30 seconds prior to release of the clamp, 1 Gm of sodium ferrocyanide or inulin is rapidly injected into a peripheral vein.

The rationale of this procedure is as follows: When the ureter is clamped, pressure within the system of ureter, pelvis, tubule and glomerular capsule rises rapidly, to approximately 90 mm Hg. Although filtration does not cease entirely, it is markedly reduced. An essentially stationary column of fluid is held in contact with the tubular epithelium for the period of clamping. As a result of prolonged contact, the tubular epithelium performs, in an exaggerated manner, those operations on the static column of fluid that it normally performs in lesser degree on

the moving column. When the clamp is released, urine spurts out under pressure, the first samples coming from pelvis and distal parts of the nephron and the later samples from more proximal parts. The final samples, which contain increasing amounts of ferrocyanide or inulin, are obviously derived from fluid filtered after release of the clamp.

The results of an experiment in which the site of reabsorption of glycine was studied are summarized in Figure 6–10. Creatinine, *p*-aminohippurate and glycine were administered in one infusion. Hypertonic mannitol was administerd in a second infusion. When urine flow reached 10 ml/min, three 3-minute control specimens were collected and the ureteral catheter was clamped. After 3.5 minutes, 1 Gm of inulin was injected intravenously; at the end of 4 minutes, the clamp was released; and over the succeeding 3 minutes a series of specimens of about 1 ml each was collected. Three additional 3-minute control urine specimens completed the experiment. Blood samples were drawn at the midpoints of the control specimens of urine, U 1–3 and U 4–6, and other necessary values were interpolated.

The ratios of urinary and plasma concentrations of creatinine (U/P ratios) are plotted at the bottom of the figure, with the first three control values to the right, the last three control values to the left and the values of the intervening fractional samples in between. The volumes of all fractional samples collected after release of the clamp, including the one containing the half-maximal concentration of inulin, were summed and arbitrarily assigned the value of 100%.

This volume is considered to represent that within the tubules at the moment of release of the clamp. The U/P ratio of creatinine for each fractional specimen is plotted at its proper position along the abscissa; specimens from more distal parts of the nephron are plotted to the right, and those from more proximal parts are plotted to the left. The U/P ratios of *p*-aminohippurate and those of α-aminonitrogen, each factored

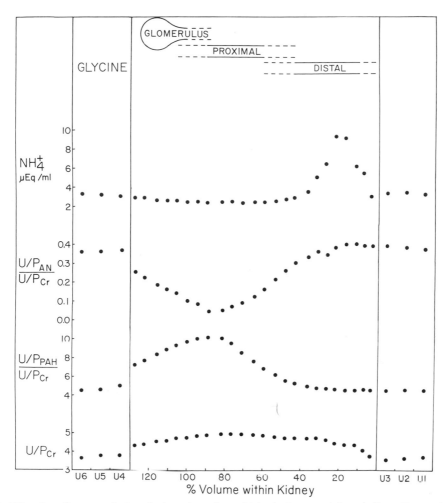

Fig. 6–10. — Stop-flow analysis of the site of aminonitrogen reabsorption in an experiment in which glycine was infused. (From Brown, J. L., Samiy, A. H., and Pitts, R. F.: Am. J. Physiol. 200:370, 1961.)

by the corresponding U/P ratio of creatinine, are plotted just above. This arithmetic device corrects for the reabsorption of water, which occurs at a variable rate along the nephron during the stoppage of flow. Such U/P ratios are equivalent to clearances of the substance in question divided by filtration rate. If the value exceeds 1, the substance is secreted; if the value is less than 1, it is reabsorbed. The ammonium ion concentrations of the control and fractional specimens are plotted as the first line of data. The schematic nephron is placed at the top of the figure to illustrate the sites at which the sev-

eral secretory and reabsorptive processes are presumed to occur.

Ammonia secretion* is most evident in the distal nephron — probably in the collecting ducts. Secretion of p-aminohippurate occurs in the proximal nephron. Aminonitrogen is reabsorbed almost completely from the proximal tubule at the site where p-aminohippurate secretion is most evident. Not only is the

———
*Plasma ammonia analyses were not performed; but, because plasma concentration is known to be vanishingly low, the U/P ratios must be extremely high. In this instance, urinary concentration alone is adequate to indicate the site of secretion.

$\dfrac{U/P_{AN}}{U/P_{Cr}}$ ratio very low in this portion of the nephron, but the U/P_{AN} ratio itself approaches zero, indicating active tubular reabsorption against a concentration gradient. Similar experiments have shown that alanine, glutamic acid, arginine, lysine and ornithine are all reabsorbed within the same portion of the proximal tubule.

For several reasons, the stop-flow technic is capable of defining only grossly the site of reabsorption or secretion. The several nephrons vary significantly in length. Therefore, any given sample of urine is not derived from exactly the same segment of all nephrons. Filtration does not cease when the ureter is clamped; fluid continues to shift along the tubule. Therefore, a given sample of urine has not remained in contact with a specific portion of the tubule for the entire period of clamping. Finally, any so-called proximal sample of fluid must pass through the distal nephron when the clamp is released. Its composition, therefore, will be modified in the process of collection. Despite the limitations of the method, it has provided qualitative information of considerable value.

Characteristics of Passive Reabsorptive Mechanisms

No less than three components of the glomerular filtrate are reabsorbed passively by diffusion: water, urea and chloride. The reabsorption of water and urea is passive throughout the length of the nephron. The reabsorption of chloride is passive in the proximal tubule and, probably, active in the distal nephron. These components diffuse from lumen to peritubular fluid down osmotic, concentration and electrical gradients, respectively. In each instance, no work is performed directly on the substance in question to move it from lumen to peritubular fluid. Rather, energy is expended in reabsorbing sodium, the transport of which develops the three gradients down which passive diffusion occurs. The passive re-

absorption of chloride and water will be considered in Chapter 7; that of urea will be considered below.

UREA

UREA CLEARANCE. — The clearance of urea averages 75 ml/min in normal man at urine flows in excess of 2 ml/min (see Chapter 5). Inasmuch as glomerular filtration rate averages 125 ml/min, it is evident that the urea contained in 50 ml of glomerular filtrate must be reabsorbed each minute. The expression $1 - C_u/C_{in}$ permits calculation of the fraction of the filtered urea that is reabsorbed. Substituting average values, $1 - 75$ ml/min $\div 125$ ml/min $= 1 - 0.6 = 0.4$. Four 10ths, or 40%, of the filtered urea is normally reabsorbed by the tubules of man under conditions of polyuria.

Figure 6–11 illustrates the relationship in man between the urea/inulin clearance ratio and urine flow over a range of flows extending from moderate oliguria to marked polyuria (52). Below 2 ml/min, the urea clearance falls off sharply with decreasing urine flow; above 2 ml/min, the urea clearance increases only moderately with increasing urine flow. For this reason, Austin, Stillman and Van Slyke (53) designated a flow of 2 ml/min as the urea augmentation limit. Below this value, the urea clearance augments profoundly

Fig. 6–11. — Variation of urea/inulin clearance ratio with urine flow in man. (Adapted from Chasis, H., and Smith, H. W.: J. Clin. Invest. 17:347, 1938.)

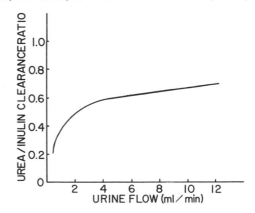

with increasing flow; above this value, the urea clearance augments but little with increasing flow.

MAXIMUM AND STANDARD UREA CLEARANCES. — Because the urea clearance varies so markedly with urine flow at flows below 2 ml/min, Van Slyke and his colleagues suggested that the urea clearance should be calculated in two ways: (1) by the usual, or "maximum clearance," formula, $U \cdot V/P$, if the flow is above 2 ml/min; and (2) by the "standard clearance" formula, $U \cdot \sqrt{V}/P$, if the flow is below 2 ml/min. The average normal value of the standard urea clearance is 57 ml/min, rather than the 75 ml/min referred to in all previous discussions. The student should understand that the standard clearance formula uses a mathematical trick to secure an empiric constant from data that are inherently variable. Because the true or maximum urea clearance varies so markedly with urine flow over a range of $0.10-2.0$ ml/min, it is obvious that no true constant value of clearance exists. Indeed, the term "standard clearance" is a misnomer—it is not a clearance at all. However, if one multiplies the square root of a volume between 1 and 2 ml/min by the U/P ratio for urea, the standard clearance value obtained (57 ml/min) is less than the observed true clearance of urea. On the other hand, if one multiplies the square root of a volume between 0.1 and 1.0 by the U/P ratio for urea, the standard clearance value obtained (57 ml/min) is greater than the observed true clearance of urea. The standard and maximum urea clearances are equal at a urine flow of 1.0 ml/min for $\sqrt{1} = 1$. The urea clearance calculated by the classic or maximum clearance formula, therefore, averages 57 ml/min at a urine flow of 1.0 ml/min and 75 ml/min at a urine flow of 2.0 ml/min.

Ideally, one should measure the urea clearance at urine flows above 2 ml/min and calculate a true (maximum) value. Practically, one cannot always attain this ideal. Frequently, polyuria cannot be induced in those patients in whom one most wishes to assess renal function. The standard clearance formula enables the clinical investigator to assess the extent of renal dysfunction even in oliguria. However, standard clearances have no physiologic significance; the kidney takes no square roots. The square root formula partially corrects, in an empiric manner, for back diffusion of urea. It should be applied only in the calculation of urea clearances, only in the clinical assessment of renal function and only if it is impossible to induce diuresis.

EVIDENCE FOR PASSIVE REABSORPTION OF UREA. — The evidence for passive reabsorption of urea is derived from two types of observations: (1) that the urea clearance is independent of plasma urea over a wide range of concentration; and (2) that the urea clearance varies with urine flow, especially at flows less than 2 ml/min.

Independence of plasma urea concentration and urea clearance suggests, although it does not prove, that the reabsorption of urea is passive. The plasma concentration of urea can be reduced to a few milligrams per 100 ml by maintenance on a low-protein diet and by forced water diuresis. It can be increased acutely to several hundred milligrams per 100 ml by the ingestion or infusion of large amounts of urea. The rate of excretion of urea varies in direct proportion to plasma concentration; clearance remains unchanged. The fraction of the filtered urea reabsorbed, $1 - C_u/C_{in}$, is likewise unchanged. Therefore, the absolute amount of urea reabsorbed, in milligrams per minute, varies in direct proportion to plasma concentration. One hundred times more urea may be reabsorbed at high plasma levels than at low plasma levels. This suggests that no limit to reabsorption exists and, therefore, that reabsorption depends on passive diffusion, not on an active energy requiring transport mechanism.

Variation of urea clearance with urine flow also suggests that passive diffusion determines reabsorption. Hypothetical data to illustrate this concept are presented in Table 6–1. If it were possible to induce such a massive diuresis that urine flow would increase

TABLE 6–1.—HYPOTHETICAL DIFFUSION
GRADIENTS FOR UREA IF GFR EQUALS 100 ML/
MIN. AND IF URINE FLOW VARIES FROM 100 TO 0.1
ML/MIN.

URINE FLOW	U/P UREA
100	1
50	2
10	10
5	20
2	50
1	100
0.5	200
0.2	500
0.1	1,000

to 100 ml/min and become equal to glomerular filtration rate, no difference in concentration of urea would exist across any portion of the renal tubule. The urea U/P ratio would be 1.0. In the absence of a diffusion gradient, no reabsorption of urea should occur. At a urine flow of 50 ml/min, the urea U/P ratio would be 2.0; at a flow of 10 ml/min, the urea U/P ratio would be 10. The lower the urine flow and the higher the U/P ratio, the greater would be the tendency for urea to diffuse from lumen to peritubular fluid. It is evident that, for any given absolute change in urine flow, the urea U/P ratio changes much more markedly when flow is less than 2 ml/min than when it is greater than 2 ml/min. The existence of an augmentation limit for urea is no doubt related to this fact.

Figure 6–12 describes the relationship between C_u/C_{Cr} and the creatinine U/P ratio in the dog. The creatinine U/P ratio varies inversely with urine flow; values of 400–600 are observed in oliguric animals deprived of water. With water loading and increasing urine flow, U/P ratios for creatinine decline to 8–10 in maximum water diuresis. If osmotic diuretics such as hypertonic mannitol, sodium sulfate or glucose are now infused intravenously at high rates, urine flow can be further increased to values roughly half that of the rate of glomerular filtration. It is evident that extrapolation to a creatinine U/P ratio of 1.0 yields a urea/creatinine clearance ratio of 1.0. In other

words, if the diffusion gradient for urea is abolished by abolishing water reabsorption, the reabsorption of urea ceases.

The rather marked difference in slopes of the two lines of Figure 6–12 has been explained by Shannon (54) as indicating greater permeability of the proximal tubule than of the distal nephron to urea. This follows from the accepted fact that variations in creatinine U/P ratio from 10 to 600 or so are related to variable reabsorption of water in the distal tubules and collecting ducts. Because the slope of the line relating C_u/C_{Cr} to creatinine U/P over this range is rather flat, the distal nephron must be relatively impermeable to urea. On the other hand, variations in creatinine U/P ratio over the range of 2–10 are related to variable reabsorption of water in the proximal tubules (see Chapter 7). In profound osmotic diuresis, the contribution of the distal tubules and collecting ducts to water reabsorption is quantitatively insignificant. Because the slope of the line relating C_u/C_{Cr} to creatinine U/P over this range is steep, the proximal nephron must be more permeable to urea than the distal nephron.

The above description of the tubular handling of urea in dog and man may be somewhat oversimplified. In ruminants, the urea clearance, relative to filtration rate at any given urine flow, is less in animals maintained on a low-protein diet than in those maintained on a high-protein diet (55). Thus, urea is conserved when protein intake is reduced. Because the urea U/P ratio is always greater than 1.0, no evidence for active reabsorption against a concentration gradient exists; reduced clearance may only be a consequence of increased tubular permeability to, and increased back diffusion of, urea. The biologic import of urea conservation by the ruminant is evident from the following considerations: Urea nitrogen, entering the rumen in the ingesta or through the mucosa from the blood, is incorporated into bacterial protein and subsequently absorbed as amino nitrogen in the lower digestive tract. Thus, in protein deficient ruminants, the urea nitrogen that is not excreted is po-

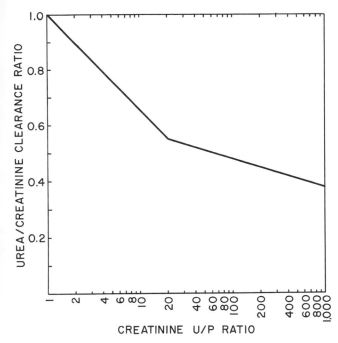

Fig. 6—12. — Variation of urea/ creatinine clearance ratio with degree of urinary concentration in the dog. (Adapted from Shannon, J. A.: Am. J. Physiol. 123:182, 1938.)

tentially available as a source of protein nitrogen. Renal conservation of urea is most evident in pregnant camels maintained on a low-protein diet. If a similar conservation of urea exists in other mammals, it is much less apparent than in ruminants.

In sharks and rays, urea is actively reabsorbed from the glomerular filtrate; i.e., the urea U/P ratio is well below 1 (range, 0.1 – 0.4). As a consequence of active conservation, the concentration of urea in the body fluids is maintained at phenomenally high levels: 200 – 300 mM/L. Because cells of elasmobranchs are as permeable to urea as are those of other animals, the substance exerts no osmotic force to condition the distribution of water within the body. However, because the gills, mucosa and integument are impermeable to urea, its full osmotic force is exerted to attract water into the body from the saline environment (56). In sharp contrast, frogs actively secrete urea into the tubular urine; the urea clearance is normally some 5 – 10 times the filtration rate (57). Although there is no evidence for active reabsorptive or secretory transport of urea in the mammalian kidney, the possibility exists that

either or both may occur. However, if they occur at all, it is certain that their contributions to the renal disposition of urea in man and dog are of minor significance.

Summary

The many valuable constituents of the glomerular filtrate are reabsorbed by a variety of independent or semi-independent transport mechanisms. They may be grossly categorized as active mechanisms that exhibit absolute limitation of transport capacity, active mechanisms that exhibit gradient-time limitation of transport capacity and passive mechanisms that depend on diffusion down osmotic or electrochemical gradients.

Mechanisms that are Tm-limited include those concerned with the reabsorption of glucose, phosphate, sulfate, amino acids, certain organic acids of the Krebs cycle, uric acid and proteins. If a given mechanism transports more than one substance, competition for the carrier occurs. The substance having the greatest affinity for the carrier, especially if it is present in high concentration in the tubular urine, is reabsorbed to the exclusion of others. Glucose, xylose, fructose and galactose are all reabsorbed by a single mechanism; glucose has the highest affinity for the carrier. Phlorhizin blocks the reabsorption of all, possibly by combining with the common carrier to form a relatively stable and slowly dissociating complex. Less striking competition in transport occurs among substances reabsorbed by basically different mechanisms that have some step in common. Glucose and phosphate, glucose and sulfate, etc., compete in this manner, perhaps for a limited supply of cellular energy.

Gradient-time limitation of transport capacity is exhibited by mechanisms that reabsorb the major ions of extracellular fluid, namely, sodium, chloride and bicarbonate. The rates of reabsorption of these ions are determined by the gradients that can be established between tubular urine and blood and by the time of contact of urine with tubular epithelium. Chapters 7 and 11 will be devoted to a discussion of such mechanisms.

Water, chloride and urea are reabsorbed passively along gradients of osmotic activity, electrical potential and concentration, respectively. No energy is expended directly in effecting transport of the substance in question. However, energy is expended in establishing the gradient along which diffusion occurs. Fundamentally, the passive reabsorption of water, chloride and urea is dependent on, and determined by, the active transport of sodium.

REFERENCES

1. Shannon, J. A., and Fisher, S.: The renal tubular reabsorption of glucose in the normal dog, Am. J. Physiol. 122:765, 1938.
2. Shannon, J. A., Farber, S., and Troast, L.: The measurement of glucose Tm in the normal dog, Am. J. Physiol. 133:752, 1941.
3. Shannon, J. A.: Renal tubular excretion, Physiol. Rev. 19:63, 1939.
4. Smith, H. W.: *Lectures on the Kidney* (Lawrence: University of Kansas Press, 1943).
5. Steinitz, K.: Studies on the conditions of glucose excretion in man, J. Clin. Invest. 19: 299, 1940.
6. McCance, R. A., and Widdowson, E. M.: Functional disorganization of the kidney in disease, J. Physiol. 95:36, 1939.
7. Reubi, F. C.: Glucose Titration in Renal Glycosuria, in *Ciba Foundation Symposium on the Kidney* (Boston: Little, Brown & Company, 1954).
8. Mudge, G. H.: Clinical patterns of tubular dysfunctions, Am. J. Med. 24:785, 1958.
9. Mudge, G. H., and Taggart, J. V.: Effect of 2,4-dinitrophenol on renal transport mechanisms in the dog, Am. J. Physiol. 161:173, 1950.
9a. Chinard, F. P., Taylor, W. R., Nolan, M., and Ennis, T.: Renal handling of glucose in the dog, Am. J. Physiol. 196:535, 1959.
10. Shannon, J. A.: The tubular reabsorption of xylose in the normal dog, Am. J. Physiol. 122:775, 1938.
11. Pitts, R. F., and Alexander, R. S.: The renal absorptive mechanism for inorganic phosphate in normal and acidotic dogs, Am. J. Physiol. 142:648, 1944.
12. Albright, F.: The parathyroids — physiology and therapeutics, J.A.M.A. 117:527, 1941.
13. Hiatt, H. H., and Thompson, D. D.: The effects of parathyroid extract on renal function in man, J. Clin. Invest. 36:557, 1957.
14. Thompson, D. D., and Hiatt, H. H.: Renal reabsorption of phosphate in normal human subjects and in patients with parathyroid disease, J. Clin. Invest. 36:550, 1957.
15. Thompson, D. D., and Hiatt, H. H.: Effects of phosphate loading and depletion on the renal excretion and reabsorption of inorganic phosphate, J. Clin. Invest. 36:566, 1957.
16. Lotspeich, W. D.: Renal tubular reabsorption of inorganic sulfate in the normal dog, Am. J. Physiol. 151:311, 1947.
17. Beyer, K. H., Wright, L. D., Skeggs, H. R., Russo, H. F., and Shaner, G. A.: Renal clearance of essential amino acids: Their competition for reabsorption by the renal tubules, Am. J. Physiol. 151:202, 1947.
18. Kamin, H., and Handler, P.: Effect of infusion of single amino acids upon excretion of other amino acids, Am. J. Physiol. 164:654, 1951.
19. Webber, W. A., Brown, J. L., and Pitts, R. F.: Interactions of amino acids in renal tubular transport, Am. J. Physiol. 200:380, 1961.
20. Dent, C. E., and Rose, G. A.: Amino acid metabolism in cystinuria, Quart. J. Med. 20: 205, 1951.
21. Robson, E. B., and Rose, G. A.: The effect of intravenous lysine on the renal clearances of cystine, arginine, and ornithine in normal subjects, in patients with cystinuria and Fanconi's syndrome and their relatives, Clin. Sc. 16:75, 1957.
22. Wright, H. R., Russo, H. F., Skeggs, H. R.,

Patch, E. A., and Beyer, K. H.: The renal clearance of essential acids: Arginine, histidine, lysine, and methionine, Am. J. Physiol. 149:130, 1947.

23. Pitts, R. F.: A renal reabsorptive mechanism in the dog common to glycin and creatinine, Am. J. Physiol. 140:156, 1943.

24. Pitts, R. F.: A comparison of the renal reabsorptive processes for several amino acids, Am. J. Physiol. 140:535, 1944.

25. Pitts, R. F.: The clearance of creatinine in dog and man, Am. J. Physiol. 109:532, 1934.

26. Lotspeich, W. D.: *Metabolic Aspects of Renal Function* (Springfield, Ill.: Charles C Thomas, Publisher, 1959).

27. Cooke, R. E., Segar, W. E., Reed, C., Etzweiler, D. D., Vita, M., Brusilow, S., and Darrow, D. C.: The role of potassium in the prevention of alkalosis, Am. J. Med. 17:180, 1954.

28. Grollman, A., Harrison, H. C., and Harrison, H. E.: The renal excretion of citrate, J. Clin. Invest. 40:1290, 1961.

29. Vishwarkarma, P., and Lotspeich, W. D.: The excretion of L-malic acid in relation to the tricarboxylic acid cycle in the kidney, J. Clin. Invest. 38:414, 1959.

30. Cohen, J. J., and Wittman, E.: Renal utilization and excretion of α-ketoglutarate in dog: Effect of alkalosis, Am. J. Physiol. 204:795, 1963.

31. Selleck, B. H., and Cohen, J. J.: Specific localization of α-ketoglutarate uptake to dog kidney and liver in vivo, Am. J. Physiol. 208:24, 1965.

32. Balagura, S., and Pitts, R. F.: Renal handling of α-ketoglutarate by the dog, Am. J. Physiol. 207:483, 1964.

33. Balagura, S., and Stone, W. J.: Renal tubular secretion of α-ketoglutarate in the dog, Am. J. Physiol. 219:1319, 1967.

34. Schwab, L., and Lotspeich, W. D.: Renal tubular reabsorption of acetoacetate in the dog, Am. J. Physiol. 176:195, 1954.

35. Visscher, F. F.: Renal clearance of β-hydroxybutyric acid in the dog, Proc. Soc. Exper. Biol. & Med. 60:296, 1945.

36. Craig, F. N.: Renal tubular reabsorption, metabolic utilization and isomeric fractionation of lactic acid in the dog, Am. J. Physiol. 146:146, 1946.

37. Ralli, E. P., Friedman, G. J., and Rubin, S. H.: The mechanism of excretion of vitamin C by the human kidney, J. Clin. Invest. 17:765, 1938.

38. Sherry, S. G., Friedman, J., Paley, K., Berkman, J., and Ralli, E.: The mechanism of excretion of vitamin C by the dog kidney, Am. J. Physiol. 130:276, 1940.

39. Berliner, R. W., Hilton, J. G., Jr., Yü, T. F., and Kennedy, T. J., Jr.: The renal mechanism for urate excretion in man, J. Clin. Invest. 29:396, 1950.

40. Gutman, A. B., and Yü, T. F.: Renal function in gout, Am. J. Med. 23:600, 1957.

41. Yü, T. F., and Gutman, A. B.: Paradoxical retention of uric acid by uricosuric drugs in low dosage, Proc. Soc. Exper. Biol. & Med. 96:264, 1957.

42. Kessler, R. H., Hierholzer, K., and Gurd, R. S.: Localization of urate transport in the nephron of mongrel and Dalmatian dog kidney, Am. J. Physiol. 197:601, 1959.

43. Terry, R., Hawkins, D. R., Church, E. H., and Whipple, G. H.: Proteinuria related to hyperproteinemia in dogs following plasma given parenterally, J. Exper. Med. 87:561, 1948.

44. Malmendier, C., and Lambert, P. P.: Étude sur la concentration en sérum albumine du filtrat glomérulaire, J. urol., Paris 61:327, 1955.

45. Lambert, P. P., Gregoire, F., and Malmendier, C.: La permeabilité glomérulaire aux substances protidiques, Rev. franç. clin. et biol. 2:15, 1957.

46. Lathem, W.: The renal excretion of hemoglobin: Regulatory mechanisms and the differential excretion of free and protein bound hemoglobin, J. Clin. Invest. 38:652, 1959.

47. Lathem, W., Davis, B. B., Zweig, P. H., and Dew, R.: The demonstration and localization of renal tubular reabsorption of hemoglobin by stop flow analysis, J. Clin. Invest. 39:840, 1960.

48. Malvin, R. L., Wilde, W. S., and Sullivan, L. P.: Localization of nephron transport by stop flow analysis, Am. J. Physiol. 194:135, 1958.

49. Pitts, R. F., Gurd, R. S., Kessler, R. H., and Hierholzer, K.: Localization of acidification of urine, potassium and ammonia secretion and phosphate reabsorption in the nephron of the dog, Am. J. Physiol. 194:125, 1958.

50. Hierholzer, K., Cade, R., Gurd, R., Kessler, R., and Pitts, R.: Stop-flow analysis of renal reabsorption and excretion of sulfate in the dog, Am. J. Physiol. 198:833, 1960.

51. Brown, J. L., Samiy, A. H., and Pitts, R. F.: Localization of aminonitrogen reabsorption in the nephron of the dog, Am. J. Physiol. 200:370, 1961.

52. Chasis, H., and Smith, H. W.: The excretion of urea in man and in subjects with glomerulonephritis, J. Clin. Invest. 17:347, 1938.

53. Austin, J. H., Stillman, E., and Van Slyke, D. D.: Factors governing the excretion of urea, J. Biol. Chem. 46:91, 1921.

54. Shannon, J. A.: The renal reabsorption and excretion of urea under conditions of extreme diuresis, Am. J. Physiol. 123:182, 1938.

55. Schmidt-Nielsen, B.: Urea excretion in mammals, Physiol. Rev. 38:139, 1958.
56. Kempton, R. T.: Studies on the elasmobranch kidney. II. Reabsorption of urea by the smooth dogfish, *Mustelis canis*, Biol. Bull. 104:45, 1953.
57. Forster, R. P.: Active cellular transport of urea by frog renal tubules, Am. J. Physiol. 179:372, 1954.

7

Mechanisms of Reabsorption and Excretion of Ions and Water

Revised by Erich E. Windhager, M.D.

THE KIDNEY is a mysterious organ, not only with respect to what it does and how it does it, but also with respect to why it does it that way. A biologic engineer, assigned the task of designing an excretory organ, would certainly not follow the pattern laid down in the kidney of man. Why in excreting a liter or so of urine containing 10–15 Gm of urea nitrogen, a few grams of sodium chloride and other assorted excretory products, is it necessary to filter 180 L of plasma, containing more than 1 kg of sodium chloride and large quantities of many other valuable constituents, and then face the problem of having to salvage them all? The kidney that an engineer would design would be a simple secretory gland; it certainly would not involve such wasteful processes as filtration and reabsorption. It would be an excretory, rather than a regulatory, organ, and for that reason it might not work very well. However, it would be a lot easier for the student of renal physiology to understand.

Evolution of Renal Functions

Some appreciation of the apparent foibles and inconsistencies of the kidney of man may be obtained from a review of its evolutionary development, a subject most engagingly treated by H. W. Smith in his Porter

Lectures (1) and in his book *From Fish to Philosopher* (2). A much abridged schema of evolution is illustrated in Figure 7–1.

Our protovertebrate ancestors evolved in a sea of moderate salinity, which had a composition somewhat akin to that of our own extracellular fluid. Excretion of wastes was a simple matter. These animals could drink freely of the fluid surrounding them, pump it through their vascular systems, allow it to permeate their tissues, secrete it into their body cavities and then propel it and its dissolved wastes to the outside through simple ciliated conduits.

But, driven by some wanderlust and perhaps to escape their enemies, these early ancestors migrated into freshwater streams. Their osmotic superiority to their environment created a major problem, for they tended to soak up large quantities of water. To avoid fatal dilution, they developed a relatively impermeable integument and invented, in association with their simple excretory conduits, a vascular tuft that enabled them to filter off the excess fluid from their blood stream. However, filtration created the problem of conservation of valuable solutes present in the filtrate. Salt loss was an especially critical factor in a freshwater environment. The development of a proximal convoluted tubule having the capacity to reabsorb salt,

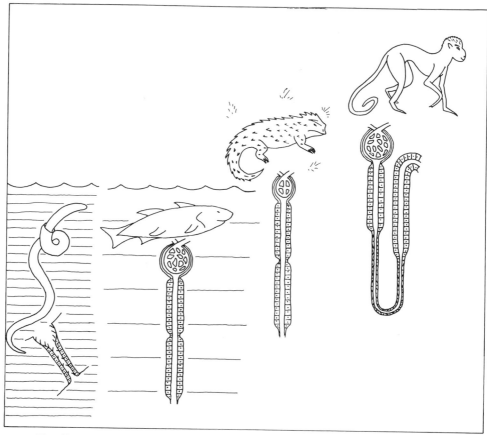

Fig. 7–1. —The development of the nephron in relation to habitat. (Modified from Smith, H. W.: *Lectures on the Kidney* [Lawrence: University of Kansas Press, 1943].)

glucose and amino acids and of a distal convoluted tubule capable of diluting the urine — i.e., reabsorbing salt while rejecting water — were answers to these self-created problems.

Crawling out on dry land some millions of years later, terrestrial forms were faced with the opposite problem, at least with respect to water. Fluid conservation, rather than fluid elimination, was the major concern. Instead of discarding their now unnecessary pressure filters and redesigning their kidneys as efficient secretory organs,* the terrestrial vertebrates modified and amplified their existing systems to salvage the precious water of the

*This course has been followed by certain marine fish, which have developed aglomerular kidneys: the pipefish, sea horse, goosefish, toadfish, etc. These forms were the first to return to the sea and have resided in a medium of increasing salinity for the longest period of time.

filtrate. Salt was also at a premium; hence, the salt-conserving mechanisms of the kidneys of fresh-water forms had to be retained and developed even further.

Reptiles, birds, and mammals, including man, are essentially arid-living forms. The birds and reptiles have de-emphasized pressure filtration by reducing the number of capillary loops in glomerular tufts, by developing tubular secretory systems to eliminate nitrogenous wastes efficiently, thereby avoiding the necessity for high rates of filtration, and by changing over their nitrogen metabolism to end up with a relatively insoluble end product, uric acid, which can be excreted in supersaturated solution with minimal water loss.

The mammals have kept their high-pressure filters operating full blast and have de-

TABLE 7−1.—FILTRATION, REABSORPTION AND EXCRETION OF IONS AND WATER BY MAN

	PLASMA CONCENTRATION (mEq/L)	RATE OF GLOMERULAR FILTRATION (L/24 hr)	GIBBS-DONNAN FACTOR	QUANTITY FILTERED (mEq/24 hr)	QUANTITY EXCRETED (mEq/24 hr)	QUANTITY REABSORBED (mEq/24 hr)	PER CENT REABSORBED
Sodium	140	180	0.95	23,940	103	23,837	99.6
Chloride	105	180	1.05	19,845	103	19,742	99.5
Bicarbonate	27	180	1.05	5,103	2	5,101	99.9+
Potassium	4	180	0.95	684	51	633	92.6
	(L/L)			(L/24 hr)	(L/24 hr)	(L/24 hr)	
Water	0.94	180	...	169.2	1.5	167.7	99.1

veloped an entirely new system, a countercurrent multiplier system, to salvage water by concentrating the urine highly. They likewise have developed, to a fine point, an osmoregulatory mechanism of control of water reabsorption, operating through the hypothalamus and the posterior lobe of the pituitary gland, and a volume-regulating mechanism based on control of salt reabsorption by the adrenal cortex. The mechanisms of salt and water reabsorption will be considered in this chapter; the operation of regulatory mechanisms will be described in Chapter 12.

Magnitude of the Problem of Salt and Water Reabsorption

In a quantitative sense (i.e., in terms of moles per day), the filtration and reabsorption of ions and water are by far the most significant operations of the mammalian kidney. Excretion of only minute fractions of the filtered quantities is sufficient to balance daily intake. The quantitative aspects of filtration, reabsorption and excretion of ions and water by the kidney of man are illustrated in Table 7 − 1. If the rate of glomerular filtration is 125 ml/min, 180 L of plasma are filtered each day. The product of the rate of glomerular filtration (in liters per day), the plasma concentration of a given ion (in milliequivalents per liter) and the appropriate Donnan factor* yields the quantity of that

*The Donnan factor for univalent cations is approximately 0.95; for univalent anions, 1.05.

ion filtered each day. If the daily diet contains 6 Gm of sodium chloride and 2 Gm of potassium, then a person need excrete only these amounts in order to maintain balance, namely, 103 mEq each of sodium and chloride ions and 51 mEq of potassium ions, per day. Normally, only 1 − 2 mEq of bicarbonate ions are excreted each day. Accordingly, reabsorption of the major ions of the extracellular fluid, with the exception of potassium, is more than 99% complete. If 1.5 L of urine is excreted each day, over 99% of the filtered water† is also reabsorbed. Much of the energy turnover of the kidney is concerned with these reabsorptive activities.

The tubular reabsorption of sodium, potassium and chloride ions and of water will be considered together in this chapter, because their mechanisms are inseparably linked. The reabsorption of bicarbonate ions and the effect of potassium on bicarbonate reabsorption will be dealt with in Chapter 11.

Reabsorption of Ions and Water in the Proximal Tubule

Reabsorption of ions and water in the proximal segment of the renal tubule may be characterized as follows:

1. *Reabsorption is isosmotic*: both the fluid reabsorbed and that remaining in the tubular lumen have the same osmotic pres-

†The rate of glomerular filtration is expressed as milliliters per minute or liters per day of plasma. Because plasma is roughly 94% water (6% protein), the rate of glomerular filtration of water is calculated as GFR · (100 − % protein in plasma)/100.

sure as the plasma. Because the major ions — sodium, chloride and bicarbonate — account for 90–95% of the osmotic activity of the plasma and glomerular filtrate, it is evident that ions and water must be reabsorbed at osmotically equivalent rates. The proximal tubule performs no osmotic work; it neither dilutes nor concentrates the tubular urine.

2. *Reabsorption of sodium is active.* By active reabsorption is meant reabsorption that cannot be accounted for by an electrochemical potential gradient but which requires energy derived from metabolic processes within the cell.

3. *Reabsorption of potassium is active.* Essentially all the filtered potassium is actively reabsorbed in the proximal tubule.

4. *Reabsorption of chloride is passive*, for transport takes place down an electrochemical gradient. Accordingly, no energy need be expended directly in salvaging this ion.

5. *Water is reabsorbed passively* as the result of the osmotic force created by the active reabsorption of sodium ions and the passive diffusion of chloride ions. Because under all conditions, water diffuses readily in both directions across the proximal tubular epithelium, the osmotic pressure of the tubular contents remains equal to that of the blood plasma.

6. *From two thirds to seven eighths of the glomerular filtrate is normally reabsorbed in the proximal tubule.* Only one third to one eighth passes on to, and is processed in, the remainder of the tubule.

Isosmotic Reabsorption of Proximal Tubular Fluid

Isosmotic reabsorption of proximal tubular fluid was first demonstrated in the nephron of the frog and *Necturus* by Walker, Hudson, Findley and Richards (3), in that of the rat by Walker, Bott, Oliver and MacDowell (4) and in the dog kidney by Clapp, Watson and Berliner (5). The experiments illustrated in Figure 7–2 are those of Gottschalk and Mylle (6, 7) on the rat. Fluid was

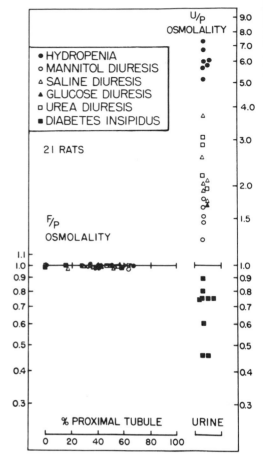

Fig. 7–2. — Isosmotic nature of proximal urine of the rat under a variety of conditions in which the final ureteral urine is either hypertonic or hypotonic. (From Gottschalk, C. W.: Physiologist 4:35, 1961.)

collected by puncturing surface convolutions of proximal tubules and withdrawing minute samples of fluid (0.001 – 0.1 μl) into a micropipet. From freezing-point depressions of tubular fluid and blood plasma, determined by a microcryoscopic technic, total osmolar concentrations were calculated. Dye was injected at the site of puncture, the kidney was macerated and the entire tubule was dissected free. Only the first 60% of the proximal tubule coils near the surface and can be punctured; the other 40% plunges deep through the cortex as the pars recta or descending thick limb of Henle's loop and is inaccessible. It is apparent from Figure 7–2 that the proximal fluid is isosmotic with plasma (F/P osmolal ratio = 1.0) under a variety of conditions in which the final urine collected from the ureter is hypotonic (U/P osmolal ratio = 0.45) or variably hypertonic (U/P osmolal ratio as high as 7.0). The proximal tubule, therefore, reabsorbs ions and water in osmotically equivalent proportions; it neither concentrates nor dilutes the urine with respect to the plasma in the process.

ACTIVE TRANSPORT OF SODIUM IN THE PROXIMAL TUBULE

The active transport of sodium in the proximal tubule was first strongly suggested by experiments of Wesson and Anslow (8). Dogs were infused with hypertonic mannitol to establish a profound osmotic diuresis. When 60% of the filtered water was excreted, only 33% of the filtered chloride, 28% of the filtered sodium and 10% of the filtered bicarbonate were excreted. The urine was isosmotic* with plasma and probably represented proximal tubular fluid relatively unmodified during its rapid transit through the more distal parts of the nephron. Because a

---

*The deficit of concentration of ions in the urine with respect to the plasma was exactly balanced by an increase in the concentration of mannitol.

much greater proportion of the filtered water than of the filtered ions was excreted, ions must have been reabsorbed against concentration gradients. This strongly suggests that one or more of these ions is reabsorbed actively.

Solomon and his associates (9, 10) have provided additional evidence of active transport of sodium chloride by the method of stop-flow perfusion of the *Necturus* tubule. As shown in Figure 7–3, a glomerulus is punctured and the tubule is partly filled with stained oil. The tubule is then punctured and a solution of known composition is introduced, splitting the oil drop. After 20 minutes, the tubule is punctured distally and the fluid is collected into a micropipet. If a small amount of radioactive (${}^{14}C$-labeled) inulin is added to the perfusate, one can calculate the percentage of the water reabsorbed by the degree of radioinulin concentration.

The results of an experiment in which four different perfusion fluids were introduced into the tubule are shown in Figure 7–4. Although the fluids contained differing amounts of sodium chloride, all were made isosmotic to *Necturus* plasma by the addition of appropriate amounts of mannitol. Accordingly, any movement of water observed during the experiment could not be ascribed to a pre-

Fig. 7–3. — Technic of stop-flow perfusion of the proximal tubule of *Necturus*. (From Shipp, J. C., Hanenson, I. B., Windhager, E. E., Schatzmann, H. J., Whittembury, G., Yoshimura, H., and Solomon, A. K.: Am. J. Physiol. 195:563, 1958.)

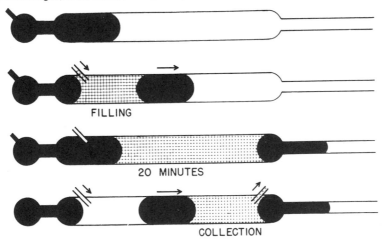

FILLING

20 MINUTES

COLLECTION

CORRECTED WATER MOVEMENT

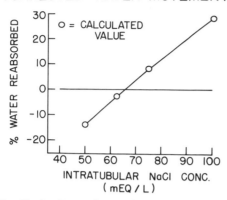

Fig. 7—4.—Dependence of water reabsorption on sodium chloride reabsorption in the nephron of *Necturus*. The limiting gradient against which salt can be reabsorbed in 66—100 mEq/L. (Modified from Windhager, E. E., Whittembury, G., Oken, D. E., Schatzmann, H. J., and Solomon, A. K.: Am. J. Physiol. 197:313, 1959.)

existing osmotic force acting across the renal tubule. Because the sodium concentration of *Necturus* plasma is 100 mEq/L, no mannitol was added to the solution of highest sodium chloride concentration. It is evident that water was reabsorbed from the two solutions of higher sodium chloride content but that water moved into the tubule and volume increased when the two solutions of lower sodium chloride content were perfused. This experiment tells us that sodium chloride can be reabsorbed from a solution containing more than 66 mEq/L into plasma containing 100 mEq/L. Water follows in proportion to the salt reabsorbed. However, if the gradient is greater than 34 mEq/L, sodium chloride diffuses into the tubule, along with sufficient water to re-establish this limiting gradient. If water were actively transported, there is no reason why it should not be reabsorbed from the solution of low, as well as from that of high, sodium chloride concentration, for the osmotic pressures of the two solutions were the same. This experiment also emphasizes the fact that the tubule is significantly permeable to sodium and chloride ions in both directions and that reabsorption is merely the result of greater outflux than of influx of these ions. Similar perfusion experiments

have been performed on the rat proximal tubule (11, 12), which, within a few seconds, can establish a limiting gradient of 30–50 mEq/L between the tubular contents and blood plasma. Net sodium reabsorption in proximal tubules of rats amounts to some $70–90 \cdot 10^{-12}$ Eq/cm² sec. (11). Several investigators (13, 14), using conventional micropuncture technics, have also shown that the intact kidney of the rat can reabsorb sodium chloride against a concentration gradient under conditions of osmotic diuresis induced by the infusion of mannitol. However, such experiments indicate only that either sodium or chloride ions, or perhaps both, are reabsorbed actively; they do not indicate which ion is actively reabsorbed.

ELECTRICAL POTENTIALS

A knowledge of the electrical potentials across the tubular membrane is necessary in order to decide which ion is actively transported. Giebisch (15, 16), with his work on *Necturus*, has contributed most to the knowledge along these lines. Minute capillary electrodes with a tip diameter of 1 μ or less can be inserted into single proximal tubular cells without evident impairment of their function. On average, the *membrane potential* so recorded in *Necturus* is 72 mV; the interior of the cell is negative to the surrounding peritubular fluid. If the electrode is pushed on through the tubular cell and into the tubular lumen, a *transtubular potential* is recorded. The tubular lumen is, on average, 20 mV negative to the peritubular fluid. This latter observation clinches the argument that the reabsorption of sodium is active, for this ion is transported not only against a concentration gradient but also against a potential gradient (negative lumen to positive peritubular fluid). Quantitative agreement has been observed by Spring and Paganelli (17) between net sodium reabsorption and the transepithelial electrical current flowing from tubular lumen to peritubular fluid under experimental conditions when all passive driving forces for ion movement had been eliminated. This proves that all net reabsorption of sodium by *Necturus* proximal tubule is active in nature.

Recent studies by Boulpaep and Seely (18) and by Burg and Orloff (19) have demonstrated that the electrical potential difference across the proximal tubular wall of mammalian kidneys is only 3 – 4 mV (lumen negative). This does not mean that mammalian proximal tubular salt transport operates on a principle different from that in the amphibian. Intercellular ion-shunting is possibly responsible for the lower potential difference found in rats and rabbits. The work of Lutz *et al.* (20) on isolated perfused proximal tubules of rabbits proves that sodium transport is active. By using fluids of identical ionic composition inside and outside the tubule, all chemical potential gradients were eliminated, in these experiments. Simultaneously, any pre-existing transepithelial electrical potential difference was abolished by supplying the appropriate counter-electromotive force via an external voltage source. The transepithelial electrical current measured under these circumstances was nearly equal to the average absorptive net flux of sodium. Thus, sodium transport is an energy-requiring process, and active transport of other ions, such as potassium, constitutes only a small fraction of the total ionic net flux across the proximal tubular wall.

Bloomer *et al.* (21) observed extensive reabsorption of potassium in proximal tubules of rats. The intratubular concentration of potassium is less than in plasma, but this part of the nephron cannot maintain concentration ratios lower than 0.7. Malnic *et al.* (22) found the limiting potassium concentration gradient during stop-flow microperfusion to be similar to that under free-flow conditions. Potassium, therefore, is actively reabsorbed by mammalian proximal tubules, and solvent drag does not constitute a significant driving force for proximal tubular potassium transfer.

Giebisch and Windhager (23) measured the bidirectional fluxes of chloride across the proximal tubule of *Necturus*. Both outflux and influx are relatively high. The excess of outflux over influx (i.e., the flux asymmetry or net reabsorption) can be adequately accounted for on the basis of the transtubular potential of 20 mV. Chloride, therefore, diffuses passively from negative lumen to positive peritubular fluid down a potential gradient. Furthermore, throughout most of the proximal tubule there is a slight concentration gradient, which also favors the outflux of chloride. Reabsorption is passive: no work need be performed on the chloride ion to move it from lumen to peritubular fluid.

ORIGIN OF TUBULAR POTENTIALS

In the past, both the transtubular potential and the cell membrane potential were thought to be basically potassium diffusion potentials, much like those of muscle and nerve. Boulpaep (24) has confirmed this view with respect to the peritubular cell membrane. His studies of the luminal cell membrane indicate, however, that the electrical gradient at this site is generated by a more complex mechanism than passive diffusion of potassium. Because the *Necturus* kidney can be doubly perfused, the composition of the fluid bathing the peritubular membrane and that of the fluid bathing the luminal membrane of tubular cells can be altered. It is for this reason that most of the available information on the origin of potentials pertains to amphibian kidneys.

If one perfuses the renal portal system and the aorta with solutions of increasing potassium concentration, the potential measured across the peritubular membrane decreases from its normal value of 72 mV to zero (Fig. 7 – 5). The slope of this function is −55mV per 10-fold change in concentration over its linear portion. If the peritubular membrane were perfectly potassium perm-selective,* the slope should be 58 mV at room temperature. These studies were performed at constant $(K) \cdot (Cl)$ product, in order to avoid

---

*The relationship between potential and potassium concentrations on the two sides of the membrane permeable only to potassium is given by the Nernst equation: where (K_i) and (K_o) represent, respectively, the concentrations of potassium on the two sides of the membrane.

$$E(mV) = -58 \log (K_i)/(K_o)$$

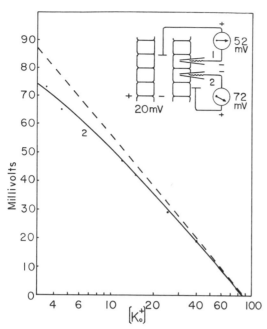

Fig. 7—5.—Variations in peritubular cell membrane potential with potassium concentration of the contraluminal bathing medium (K^+). The insert illustrates the potential differences found across luminal and peritubular cell membranes of *Necturus* kidney in vivo. The cell interior is -52 mV with respect to the tubule lumen (1) and -72 mV when referred to the peritubular fluid environment (15, 24).

volume changes or changes in intracellular concentration. Therefore, it was not possible to evaluate the relative contribution of K and Cl in generating the potential difference. Boulpaep measured the effect of sudden changes of concentration gradients of K and Cl alone. The kidney was flushed on its surface by means of double-barreled pipets, with each barrel connected to a syringe filled with a solution of different composition. The transient changes in potential were recorded and related to instantaneous K and Cl concentrations. A slope of 31.6 mV obtains for a sudden 10-fold change in $(K)_0$ and a slope of 11.6 mV for $(Cl)_0$. The peritubular membrane is permeable to potassium and chloride ions, and the membrane potential at this site of the cell can be explained largely on the basis of diffusion potentials of these ions.

If one perfuses single proximal tubules through a double-barreled pipet, allowing rapid changes in composition of intraluminal fluid while maintaining a normal ionic environment at the peritubular surface, information on the permeability characteristics of the luminal membrane can be obtained. In such experiments, a differential input between an intraluminal and an intracellular microelectrode provides a measure of the luminal potential difference. The intracellular electrode can be used simultaneously to record the peritubular potential with respect to an indifferent electrode in the extracellular fluid compartment. When transient changes in luminal potential produced by sudden alterations in intraluminal concentration of K or Cl were analyzed, a slope of only 10 mV per 10-fold change of KCl was found. This slope is much less than that at the peritubular membrane. Perfusion of the lumen with choline, in the absence of sodium, led to an increase in the luminal membrane potential from about -55 mV to -75 mV. This indicates a rather significant degree of sodium permeability of the luminal cell border. A high Na/K permeability ratio might be thought to be the explanation for the low slope value observed in potassium substitution experiments. Sodium diffusing into the cell could, in part, counteract the diffusion potential set up by potassium leaking from cell to lumen. However, a very high Na/K permeability ratio would lead to small luminal potential differences under normal circumstances when sodium is at a high concentration in tubular fluid. Therefore, the luminal potential step of some -55 mV cannot be explained as a diffusion potential of K or Cl. Boulpaep has also tested the role of other anions. No difference was observed in Ringer's solution buffered with bicarbonate or with phosphate.

Electrical shunting between lumen and peritubular fluid via intercellular routes offers an explanation for the magnitude of the luminal potential. Intercellular ion shunts were first proposed by Ussing and Windhager (25) in the studies on frog skin. It is well known that frog skin epithelium bathed in SO_4-Ringer can maintain potential differences as high as 140 mV. Half of this potential is due to a potassium diffusion potential across the inward-facing cell membrane, analogous to the peritubular potential of proximal tubules. The remaining 70 mV of the difference is caused by a sodium diffusion potential across the outer cell boundary (26). There is normally little ion movement through extracellular spaces of the epithelium. Frog skin, toad bladder and distal convoluted tubules are examples of epithelia with negligible ion permeability of the tight junctions. The situation changes, however, when the outside of frog skin is exposed to hyperosmotic solutions. Tight junctions become quite permeable to passive ion movement, shunting the transepithelial potential difference from 140 mV to values approaching zero. A microelectrode advancing from the outside through the frog skin epithelium encounters first a potential step of about 50 to 70 mV (cell negative to outside); one advancing from the inside encounters 70 mV (cell negative to inside bathing solution). This potential profile is nearly identical to that formed across proximal tubular epithelium.

Subsequently, Windhager *et al.* (27) demonstrated that, in *Necturus* proximal tubules, a major fraction of the total passive ion movement across proximal tubules occurs via extracellular shunts. This conclusion was reached because the electrical resistance between lumen and peritubular space is much less than the membrane resistance between cell interior and lumen or peritubular fluid. The junctional complex described by Farquhar and Palade (28), which connects neighboring cells at their luminal sides, does not act as a perfect seal. "Tight junctions" are known to be shorter in proximal tubular epithelium than in distal tubules, and proximal tubules are much more permeable to ions and to water than the distal tubular wall. Ionized lanthanum can be seen within "tight junction" in electron micrography of renal tubular epithelium (29).

Recent measurements of electrical resistances between neighboring proximal tubule cells in *Necturus* indicate that low-resistance pathways connect adjoining cells. The resistance found in renal epithelium was 16 ohm · cm² , which is of similar magnitude to the resistances between neighboring cells in syncytial cardiac muscle. Thus, ionic exchange between cells and possibly cross-information can occur in renal epithelial tissue.

SCHEMATIC REPRESENTATION OF THE PROXIMAL TUBULAR CELL

Figure 7–6 presents a model of a proximal tubular cell. The potassium content of the cell is high; the sodium and chloride content is low (30–40 mEq/L). The cell is electrically negative with respect to lumen and peritubular fluid. Sodium ions can diffuse along an electrochemical gradient from lumen to cell. To keep the sodium content of the cell low, the sodium that diffuses in from the lumen is pumped out into the intercellular spaces of the epithelium. Diffusion of potassium and chloride is the major determinant of the potential across the peritubular membrane. The potential across the luminal cell membrane is not a diffusion potential in the common sense of being determined by the ratio of transmembrane concentration gradients; it is produced by the current × resistance drop that occurs as current flows from lumen into the cell. The electromotive force in this circuit is the diffusion potential, and possibly the sodium pump in the peritubular membrane; the circuit is closed by the existence of intercellular channels in parallel with the cellular pathway.

Chloride ions are reabsorbed passively in proximal tubules, but the exact nature of chloride entry across the luminal cell border is, at present, only poorly understood. The chloride concentration gradient from lumen to cell favors passive entry but is too small to balance the opposing electrical potential gradient of 50–70 mV. Passive entry by ionic diffusion would, therefore, require that either a fraction of the intracellular chloride is bound or that the intracellular space is inhomogeneous with respect to chloride activ-

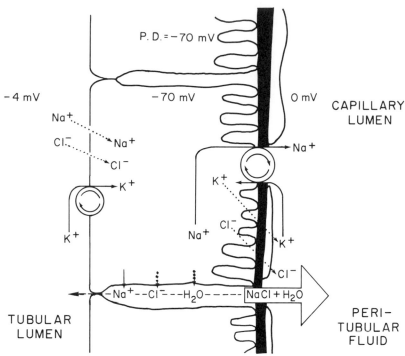

Fig. 7–6. — Schematic representation of ion transport in a proximal tubular cell. *Dashed lines*, passive diffusion down electrochemical gradients; *solid lines*, active transport; *open arrow*, filtration across epithelial basement lamina. Although indicated as passive in this diagram, the mechanism of chloride entry into the cell is presently not clearly defined. Active sodium transport occurs not only across the peritubular membrane but also across the cell membranes facing the lateral interspaces, with chloride and water following passively. The same mechanism of salt and water movement that is shown in one lateral interspace is thought to occur in all intercellular spaces, as well as in the spaces created by the basal infoldings. Back leakage of salt and water into the tubule lumen occurs across the "tight" junctions.

ity. As an alternative, chloride ions may traverse the luminal membrane in combined form; e.g., as neutral sodium chloride. Such a mechanism, in which transport of one sodium ion is directly coupled to the transport of one chloride ion by a single carrier, has been proposed as responsible for salt transport in the gallbladder (30). In proximal tubules, this type of transfer is hypothetical but is suggested by the diuretic effect of poorly permeating anions. Diuresis occurs without change in the electrical potential. A double carrier, crossing the membrane only when combined with Na and Cl, would not be expected to transport as rapidly if Cl were replaced by anions for which carrier affinity is low. In contrast to the luminal membrane, chloride reabsorption from cell to blood consists in ionic diffusion along the electrochemical potential gradient.

Net reabsorption of potassium occurs against an electrochemical potential difference across the luminal cell boundary; therefore, a potassium pump must be postulated to act at this site. At the peritubular membrane, potassium may also be pumped into the cell, partly in exchange for sodium (31). However, net movement across the peritubular cell border occurs by passive diffusion.

ENERGY SUPPLY OF ACTIVE TRANSPORT OF SODIUM

The extrusion of sodium from the cell against an electrochemical potential gradient requires the continuous expenditure of metabolic energy. Consonant with this view are the results of several investigators (32–34), who observed a linear relationship between the rate of oxygen consumption and that of tubular sodium reabsorption. About 20–30 sodium ions are reabsorbed per molecule of extra oxygen consumed (compare p. 147).

From Table 7–1 (p. 96), it is evident that nearly 1 mol of sodium is reabsorbed by the renal tubules per hour. Considering $\Delta Na/\Delta O_2$ to be 28, it follows that 1/28 mol, or 0.8 L, of oxygen per hour would be used in sodium transport. Assuming 4.83 Cal/L of oxygen, 3.86 Cal/hr, or approximately 6% of the resting metabolism of man, would be devoted to sodium, chloride and water reabsorption in the renal tubules. This might seem to be an inordinately high proportion of the resting energy metabolism. However, one must remember that the renal blood flow amounts to about one fourth of the resting cardiac output. Furthermore, the reabsorption of sodium, chloride and water is of major importance for the survival of the organism.

NATURE OF SODIUM PUMP

The nature of the sodium pump is poorly understood; at present, one can only speculate concerning its biochemical characteristics. Most investigators envision the pump as a carrier molecule that combines with a sodium ion at the cytoplasmic border of the peritubular membrane and releases it at the extracellular fluid border. The carrier molecule may rotate within the membrane, diffuse within the membrane or undergo elongation and contraction within the membrane. Conversely, the carrier molecule may remain fixed within the membrane and pass the sodium ion along a chain of carboxyl groups extending from cytoplasm to exterior. In any event, the transport distance is small: it does not exceed 50 Å, the thickness of the membrane. Energy is cycled into the system either to initiate combination of the carrier molecule with the sodium ion at the cytoplasmic border or to split the combination at the extracellular border.

A digitalis-sensitive, Na–K-activated ATPase, first detected by Skou (35), has been shown to be closely related to the active Na–K transport system in several tissues. High levels of activity of this enzyme have been found in renal tissue, and cardiac glycosides are known to inhibit renal tubular Na reabsorption. However, further studies are needed to elucidate the physiologic significance of Na–K-activated ATPase for transtubular net reabsorption of sodium in the kidney.

The student should not regard ATP as the sole energy source of sodium transport; in fact, there is evidence against this concept. Dinitrophenol (DNP) infused directly into one renal artery of a dog does not inhibit Na reabsorption. Because DNP is thought to uncouple oxydation and phosphorylation and to reduce the available supply of ATP, one might infer that Na transport is not obligatorily dependent on a continuous supply of high-energy phosphate bonds.

FLUID REABSORPTION IN THE PROXIMAL TUBULE

The volume of fluid reabsorbed in the proximal tubule is of the order of two thirds to seven eighths of that filtered through the glomerulus. Because, under all conditions, the proximal epithelium is highly permeable to water, the reabsorption of two thirds to seven eighths of the filtered ions creates an osmotic force, which accounts for the reabsorption of an equivalent fraction of the filtered water. Because reabsorption of water and ions occurs at an equal rate, proximal tubular fluid remains isosmotic with blood plasma. The figure "two thirds" was derived from micropuncture studies (36). Because only the first 60% of the tubule is accessible for micropuncture, the value for 100% of proximal tubule length must be estimated by extrapolation. The variability of data makes extrapolation uncertain, and the figure "two thirds" is only a gross approximation. Smith (37), derived the figure "seven eighths" from data on water diuresis in man. In maximum water diuresis, no more than one eighth of the filtered water is excreted in the urine; seven eighths is reabsorbed by an obligatory mechanism, presumably operating in the proximal tubule and dependent on the reabsorption of seven eighths of the filtered ions.

The reabsorption of fluid in proximal tubules varies directly with, and nearly in exact proportion to, the rate of glomerular filtration. The rate of glomerular filtration in man is reasonably stable; in the dog and the rat it is more variable. The fact that sodium reabsorption is not Tm-limited but adjusted to the glomerular load is, therefore, more clearly apparent in studies on dogs and rats than in those on man. Teleologically, adjustment of reabsorptive capacity of tubular epithelium fulfills the role of regulating the plasma concentration and the total body store of sodium far more than would a Tm-limited system.

The carnivorous animal in the wild makes infrequent kills and gorges on each kill. In the hours immediately following the ingestion of protein, urea formation increases markedly over its basal level. The rate of glomerular filtration increases concomitantly, and urea excretion is facilitated at the time of maximum production. In the interval between kills, when the load of excretory products is minimal, filtration rate declines. Man, long accustomed to more frequent meals and to a mixed diet, has largely lost this renal response to protein ingestion.

The glomerular filtration rate of a fasting dog may be 50 ml/min. Three hours after the ingestion of 2 lb. of lean beef, filtration rate may nearly double. While the dog fasts, the plasma sodium concentration is normal (145 mEq/L) and the rate of excretion of sodium is low (perhaps $2-10$ μEq/min). If the plasma sodium level were poised at the renal plasma threshold and if reabsorption were Tm-limited, doubling the filtration rate would deliver into the renal tubules twice the amount of sodium they could reabsorb.* Sodium loss would increase from 10 μEq/min to more than 7,000 μEq/min, a rate that would rapidly exhaust body stores. Instead, reabsorption of sodium increases

nearly in proportion to the increase in filtration of sodium; little loss ensues.

The increase in reabsorptive capacity largely resides in the proximal tubule. Some evidence suggests that the distal tubules and collecting ducts cannot fully reabsorb the increased load, despite some adaptive augmentation of transport. The small increase in sodium loss that occurs when glomerular filtration increases may be a consequence of the delivery into the distal tubules of quantities of sodium in excess of their reabsorptive rate.

When filtration rate is reduced to 50% of normal by a reduction of renal arterial pressure, sodium is completely reabsorbed from the urine. Under such conditions, perhaps more than the normal fraction of the filtered load is reabsorbed proximally. Less than saturation quantities are delivered into the distal nephron, and all is reabsorbed.

The nearly perfect proportionality between glomerular sodium load and proximal tubular reabsorption has been termed "glomerulotubular balance." It pertains not only to sodium but also to water reabsorption in proximal tubules. Its existence has been demonstrated in micropuncture studies on rats and dogs under conditions of marked variations in filtration rate. Only minor deviations from perfect balance have been observed during acute reductions or elevations of glomerular filtration rate. A high degree of proximal glomerulotubular balance has been found during acute reductions in GFR brought about by partial clamping of the renal vein (38), the renal artery (39, 40) or the ureter (41), as well as during spontaneous changes in glomerular filtration rate of laboratory animals (42).

A possible clue as to the underlying common factor relating proximal tubular reabsorption to changes in glomerular load of salt and water may be found in the effect of peritubular capillary absorption on epithelial transport processes. In micropuncture studies on rats, a direct relationship between filtration fraction (glomerular filtration rate/renal plasma flow) and the half-time of

---

*Good evidence exists that all nephrons are functional at all times and that twice the volume of filtrate is formed per glomerulus following a protein meal.

proximal tubular reabsorption was observed (38). Because the filtration fraction is a relative measure of the oncotic pressure of peritubular capillary blood, it appears likely that capillary absorption of tubular reabsorbate influences the rate of epithelial transport. An increase in filtration fraction would lead to an increase in peritubular oncotic pressure, which in turn enhances salt and water reabsorption by proximal tubules. A reduction in filtration fraction would lead to the opposite result.

Direct evidence for the view that an elevation of the oncotic pressure in postglomerular capillaries leads to augmentation of proximal reabsorption has been obtained in capillary perfusions (43–45). In the absence of colloids in the capillaries, reabsorption is about one half of normal; i.e., it is reduced from 3.78 nl/min per millimeter of tubule length to 1.86 nl/min per millimeter of tubule length. Between 0 and 90 mm Hg of oncotic pressure in capillary fluid reabsorption changes by 0.03 nl/min per millimeter length of tubule per 1 mm Hg of oncotic pressure.

Strong support for a regulatory function of postglomerular and hydrostatic pressure has come from the laboratories of R. W. Berliner and B. Brenner. Brenner et al. (46) demonstrated that reabsorption by proximal tubules varies directly with peritubular protein concentration when the latter is altered by bolus infusion of saline, iso-oncotic or hyperoncotic solutions. Falchuk et al. (47) studied glomerulotubular balance during partial occlusion of the renal vein, the renal artery, carotid artery occlusion with vagotomy, and the infusion of 6% of 15% albumin. In all these conditions, changes in colloid oncotic pressure and hydrostatic pressure were in a direction required by the hypothesis that capillary uptake regulates reabsorption of sodium and water by the proximal tubule.

The view that capillary fluid reabsorption may partly determine tubular salt and water transport does not mean that the force responsible for tubular reabsorption is the colloid osmotic pressure of peritubular blood.

Studies by Giebisch et al. (11) have shown that a reversal of the oncotic pressure gradient produced by intraluminal injection of protein solutions does not significantly affect tubular reabsorptive capacity. Furthermore, because of the low water permeability of the proximal tubular wall (45) the colloid osmotic pressure can, at best, account for reabsorption of about 1% of the filtrate. Hence, the driving force for reabsorption is active transport of sodium, with peritubular factors in part determining the rate of net reabsorption by the transporting epithelium.

Any attempt to explain and integrate peritubular factors in the general concept of tubular epithelial transport can, at present, be based only on speculation. Perhaps the sodium ions that have entered the cellular transport pool are actively transported into the basilar and lateral interspaces of the epithelium; i.e., into the basal labyrinth located between cell membranes proper and basement membrane. Water follows passively across the almost semipermeable cell membrane, thus elevating hydrostatic pressure in the basal labyrinth. A small hydrostatic pressure gradient leads to ultrafiltration across the tubular basement membrane. The reabsorbate is finally moved from the interstitium across the capillary wall by the force defined by the net balance of hydrostatic and oncotic pressure gradients across this barrier. Some back flux of solute and water might also occur, mostly through intercellular channels. The basal labyrinth thus might act as the middle compartment of the model proposed by Curran and MacIntosh (49), with the addition of some back leakage. Any reduction in capillary fluid reabsorption might then lead to volume expansion of the compartments interposed between transporting cell membranes and capillary endothelium. Volume expansion in the basal labyrinth may either widen intercellular channels or increase cell membrane permeability by stretching. If sodium pumping continues normally, one of several possible consequences may be envisioned. First, increased back flux of sodium and water may occur through widened intercellular channels, leading to decreased net flux. A second possibility is an increase in the membrane permeability to sodium, leading to augmented sodium back flux from basal labyrinth into the cell interior. Thus, the rate of net movement of sodium and water across the cell membrane proper would be diminished. Another possibility is that diffusion of sodium is importantly involved in the movement of this ion from transporting cell membranes to capillary walls. Volume expansion of this unstirred compartment must increase the length of the diffusional pathway. If the rate of diffusion is thus reduced, sustained active transport might lead to sodium concentrations higher than normal within the unmixed layer immediately adjacent to the transporting cell boundary. This, in turn, could lead to increased back leakage of sodium across the tight junction, thus reducing net reabsorption of salt and water.

Some of these views have received experimental verification. Boulpaep (50) found that intercellular electrical conductivity (lumen to blood) is markedly increased in *Necturus* undergoing saline loading, a condition in which peritubular oncotic pressure is reduced. Analysis of split-drop experiments in extracellular-volume-expanded *Necturus* has demonstrated that the passive permeability of proximal tubules is greatly enhanced, for nonelectrolytes as well as for NaCl. Active transport of sodium is not diminished. Hence, the reduction in proximal tubular salt reabsorption during saline loading is due to increased back flux of salt and water. Studies on mammalian proximal tubules under conditions of reduced peritubular oncotic pressure (51–54) are generally in support of this conclusion.

The effect of peritubular capillary absorption on epithelial transport may be relevant to the phenomenon of glomerulotubular balance, inasmuch as filtration load and peritubular oncotic pressure may be set at an equal rate by changes in the resistance of efferent arterioles. Thus, a relative increase in GFR will be paralleled by increased peritubular colloid osmotic pressure, decreased intersti-

tial volume, increased rate of tubular reabsorption and increased tubular volume. Relative reductions in GFR would result in the opposite effects. Glomerulotubular balance might thus be achieved by the simultaneous setting of load (GFR) and oncotic pressure (GFR/RPF), with concurrent changes in interstitial volume and epithelial transport.

ISOTONIC SALINE DIURESIS

De Wardener *et al.* (55) demonstrated that renal tubular sodium reabsorption is decreased in dogs infused with large amounts of saline solution. The effect of the solution was not curtailed by corticoids or vasopressin, and it occurred in the presence of reduced glomerular filtration rate. More recently, micropuncture studies have shown that the observed natriuresis in both rats (56, 57) and dogs (58) infused with isotonic saline solution is largely the result of a reduction in proximal tubular reabsorption. It was first suggested by De Wardener and his associates that an unknown humoral factor may be involved in the renal response to saline loading. This view has been strengthened considerably by the observation that cross-circulation of blood from a saline-loaded donor dog to a normal recipient dog produced a significant natriuresis in the recipient, even when the filtered sodium load was reduced by aortic constriction (59). It is presently unknown whether and to what extent a humoral factor may be involved in "glomerulotubular balance" for salt and water. Most proponents of the humoral hypothesis believe in the existence of a natriuretic hormone of unknown chemical composition. The strongest evidence for the existence of such a compound is the inhibitory effect of plasma from volume-expanded animals on sodium transport by the toad bladder (61).

PERMEABILITY OF RENAL TUBULES

In the past, renal physiologists have believed that the tubules were highly impermeable to all components of the glomerular filtrate other than water and urea. Sodium and chloride ions were considered to move in only one direction: from lumen to peritubular fluid. This view was first shaken by the observations of Hoshiko et al. (62), who demonstrated a significant influx of sodium, chloride and water from peritubular fluid to tubular lumen in frogs perfused through the renal portal system with radioisotopic ions and deuterium oxide. Subsequent observations have confirmed the view that mammalian renal tubules are also moderately "leaky" rather than "tight," as originally thought. Not only sodium, chloride and water but also sulfate, magnesium and calcium diffuse in both directions across the renal tubule. However, such movement from peritubular fluid to tubular lumen should not be misconstrued as tubular secretion. Instead, it represents influx down an electrochemical gradient and is passive in nature.* The term "secretion" should be reserved to describe net transport into the tubular lumen.

Ion and Water Reabsorption in Loop of Henle

Reabsorption of salt in excess of water by Henle's loop serves the dual purpose of conserving salt and providing the mechanism that is ultimately responsible for osmotic concentration or dilution of the urine. This aspect of loop function will be discussed subsequently. Henle's loop also participates in "glomerulotubular balance." Salt reabsorption by the loop varies in direct proportion to changes in the sodium load leaving

---

*If an isotopic ion, such as $^{35}SO_4$, and creatinine and inulin are injected instantaneously into one renal artery of a dog and if urine is collected in small samples from the ureter at frequent intervals, $^{35}SO_4$ appears in the urine before the creatinine and inulin appear. Because these latter substances do not penetrate the tubule in either direction and because they appear in the urine only in consequence of their filtration through glomeruli, precession of $^{35}SO_4$ must mean that this ion traverses the renal tubular epithelium downstream from the glomerulus; therefore, it is excreted earlier. This alone does not indicate that the ion is secreted. Because blood flows in vessels alongside the renal tubules more rapidly than filtrate flows in the lumen, a concentration gradient exists that favors diffusion of $^{35}SO_4$ from peritubular fluid to lumen. Diffusion alone can account for precession of chloride, sodium, magnesium, sulfate and calcium; secretion need not be invoked.

the end of the convoluted proximal tubule. In general, some 50% of the quantity of sodium entering the pars recta of the proximal tubule (i.e., the loop of Henle) is reabsorbed by the time the tubular fluid reaches the first surface convolution of the distal tubule (corresponding to 20% of the distal tubular length). During expansion of the extracellular fluid volume by saline loading, increased delivery of salt and water into the loop occurs, and the absolute quantities of salt and water reabsorbed increase (56, 57). On the other hand, when the delivery of salt and water to the loop is diminished during partial occlusion of the renal artery or the renal vein, a reduction in net reabsorption of salt and water along the loops of Henle is observed. Thus, in both the proximal tubules and the loops of Henle a direct proportionality exists between load delivered and amounts of salt reabsorbed. The factor of proportionality, however, is smaller with respect to water reabsorption. For example, when the absolute rate of net sodium reabsorption increases threefold in response to an increased load, the absolute rate of water reabsorption is only doubled.

Recently, it has been demonstrated that salt reabsorption by the ascending limb of Henle's loop is mainly due to active transport of chloride ions (64). Ascending limbs of the loop are located in the outer zone of the renal medulla and therefore are not accessible to renal micropuncture in vivo. Only the development and perfection of a technic for in vitro microperfusion of single, isolated tubules, by Burg (65), has made it possible to evaluate transport properties of these normally "hidden" nephron segments.

In contrast to previous speculations, Burg's direct observations and also those of Kokko (66) indicate that the tubular lumen of ascending limbs is electrically positive with respect to peritubular fluid by some 3–9 mV. This potential is eliminated by adding ouabain or by substitution of sulfate for chloride in the perfusion fluids. Furosemide, a potent diuretic, inhibits chloride transport in this nephron segment. Active chloride transport seems to provide the major driving force for sodium reabsorption in ascending limbs, although some additional component of active transport of sodium can presently not be excluded.

Ion and Water Reabsorption in the Distal Nephron

The proximal tubule reabsorbs the bulk of the valuable components of the glomerular filtrate in a somewhat stereotyped manner. In contrast, the distal nephron reabsorbs a small fraction of the filtrate—roughly one fifth to one eighth of the total—in a highly variable manner suited to the needs of the moment. By "distal nephron" is meant distal convoluted tubule and collecting duct.

The reabsorption of ions and water in the distal nephron is described as follows:

1. The epithelium of the distal nephron can establish relatively high ion concentration gradients between blood and urine. In salt deprivation, the urine may contain only a few milliequivalents of sodium ion per liter. When salt intake is high and water intake is low, urine sodium can be concentrated as much as twofold with respect to blood plasma.

2. The distal nephron can also establish relatively high osmolar concentration gradients between tubular urine and blood plasma. In water diuresis, the osmolality of the urine of man may be only one 10th or less that of blood plasma. In water deprivation, osmolality may exceed 1,200 mOsm/kg, a value 4 times that of blood plasma.*

3. The permeability of the distal nephron to water is variable and is controlled by the titer of circulating antidiuretic hormone (ADH). In water diuresis, a state of functional diabetes insipidus exists, in which the ADH titer approaches zero and tubular permeability to water is low. In hydropenia, the ADH titer is high, and the distal nephron becomes freely permeable to water. In addi-

tion, ADH may stimulate the pumping of sodium in the loops of Henle.

4. However, in both proximal and distal tubules, and in the loops of Henle and collecting ducts as well, reabsorption of water is passive and is determined by osmotic forces created by the reabsorption of ions.

FUNCTIONS OF DISTAL TUBULES AND COLLECTING DUCTS

In thirsting rats, in which the osmolar concentration of the final urine is 3–9 times that of blood plasma, the fluid entering the distal tubule is hypotonic. This fact, first observed by Walker *et al.* (4) in 1941, is illustrated by the data of Gottschalk and Mylle (6, 7) summarized in Figure 7–7. The urine rapidly becomes isotonic, its osmolar concentration equaling that of the plasma by the time it reaches the middle of the distal convolution. However, the tubular fluid never becomes hypertonic in the distal tubule. These observations tell us three things: (1) more salt than water must have been reabsorbed in the loop of Henle; (2) under conditions of hydropenia, water equilibrates rapidly across the distal tubule—i.e., the epithelium is permeable to water; and (3) the urine must be concentrated in the collecting ducts.

Wirz (67) was the first to demonstrate that, in water diuresis, the urine that leaves the loop of Henle is hypotonic and remains so as it flows along the distal tubule and collecting ducts. Figure 7–8 compares the changes in osmolality of distal tubular fluid in intact hydropenic rats and in rats with diabetes insipidus* exhibiting water diuresis. The water permeability of the distal tubules and collecting ducts of rats with diabetes insipidus is far less than that of intact hydropenic rats, for in the former the hypotonicity devel-

---

*The maximum osmolality of the urine of the dog is 5–6 times, of the rat 7–9 times, and of the desert rat 16–20 times, that of the blood plasma.

*In order to obtain water diuresis in an anesthetized animal with its abdomen opened and kidneys exposed for micropuncture, it is necessary to induce diabetes insipidus by electrolytic lesions in the brain that interrupt the supraopticohypophysial tract. Such lesions prevent the release of ADH in response to anesthesia and trauma.

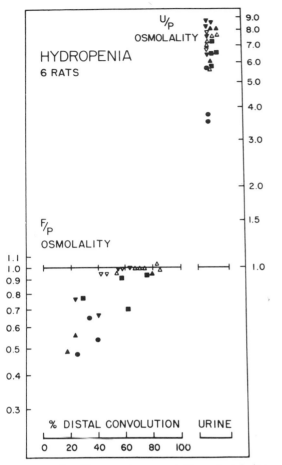

Fig. 7—7.—Change in osmolality of tubular urine in the distal nephron of the hydropenic rat. Hypotonic urine becomes isotonic by the middle of the distal segment. Concentration of the urine occurs in the collecting ducts. (From Gottschalk, C. W.: Physiologist 4:35, 1961.)

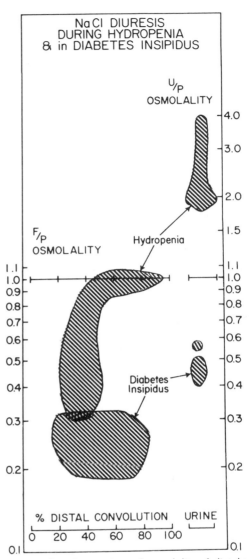

Fig. 7—8.—Comparison of osmolality of distal tubular urine in hydropenia and in diabetes insipidus in the rat. (From Gottschalk, C. W.: Physiologist 4:35, 1961.)

oped in the loop of Henle is maintained throughout the remainder of the nephron, whereas in the latter the urine becomes isotonic by the midpoint of the distal segment. The administration of ADH to rats with diabetes insipidus increases the permeability of the distal convolution to water and results in a rapid increase in osmolality of distal tubular fluid to an F/P ratio of 1.0† It likewise induces the formation of urine hypertonic to

———
†Recent micropuncture studies in hydropenic dogs have shown that distal tubule fluid does not reach osmotic equilibrium in late distal convolutions of this species (71). In the dog, ADH apparently acts only in the collecting ducts.

plasma in the collecting ducts. Therefore, ADH increases the water permeability of both distal tubules and collecting ducts.

The water permeability of isolated skin (68) and of isolated urinary bladder of the toad (69) is greatly enhanced by treatment with ADH. Permeability to small molecules (e.g., urea) is also enhanced; and this lends credence to the operational view that the hormones dilates pores having dimensions of the order of those of water and urea molecules (2 – 4 Å in diameter). Water permeability in the distal convoluted tubule during antidiuresis, estimated from the speed of osmotic equilibration across the tubular wall is only 7.6×10^{-8} ml/cm² × sec × cm H₂O, which is about 40% of the water permeability of proximal tubules (40). However, Ullrich (48) found a striking decline in permeability during water diuresis, the minimum permeability coefficient being less than one tenth of the antidiuretic value. Jaenike (70) showed that the permeability of the collecting ducts of the mammalian kidney to urea is also enhanced by ADH, presumably by an increase in pore diameter. It is probable that, in the absence of ADH (water diuresis), pores in the epithelium of distal tubules and collecting ducts are so small as to restrict severely the diffusion of water as well as urea. The continued active transport of ions and the restricted flow of water maintains the hypotonicity initially established in the loops of Henle. In the presence of ADH (hydropenia), the pores in the epithelium of distal tubules and collecting ducts enlarge. Water flows out of the distal convolutions to equalize the osmotic activity of the tubular fluid and of the cortical blood plasma. In collecting ducts, the movement of water continues and equalizes the osmotic activity of the final urine and that of the hypertonic medullary interstitium. The function of the loop of Henle in the establishment of medullary hypertonicity will be considered below.

Ion Transport in Distal Tubules and Collecting Ducts

Sodium. – Net reabsorption of sodium in distal convoluted tubules amounts to about 10 – 15% of the filtered load and proceeds against large sodium concentration gradients. In antidiuresis, early distal tubular fluid contains sodium at a concentration of about 60 mEq/L, indicating that more salt than water must have been reabsorbed along Henle's loop. There is a sustained decline in sodium concentration along the remaining portion of the distal tubule, to an approximate mean value of 30 mEq/L. Lower values have been found during osmotic diuresis (13, 42). The transtubular sodium concentration gradients at the end of the distal convolution may be in excess of 130 mEq/L, and the electrical gradient may reach 120 mV. This indicates that, compared to proximal tubules, either a stronger ion pump or a lower degree of ion and water permeability characterizes the distal tubular epithelium. In stop-flow microperfusions of distal tubules of rat kidneys, sodium and water reabsorption from isotonic NaCl solutions injected into the lumen was shown to be about one fourth of that in proximal tubules (72). Thus, it is fair to say that distal tubular sodium reabsorption is an active process, involving net movement of small amounts against a high electrochemical potential gradient.

The development of distal transtubular sodium concentration gradients is influenced by the amount of urea in fluid coming from the ascending limb of Henle's loop. During antidiuresis, an inverse relationship exists between the urea and sodium concentrations of distal tubular fluid samples. In states of sodium chloride diuresis, the amount as well as the concentration of urea found in early distal fluid is significantly reduced (73). This is probably due to the fact that, at increased rates of volume flow in the nephron, there is little recirculation of urea from collecting ducts to loops of Henle. Simultaneously, the sodium concentration fails to decline along the distal convolution (74). The presence of urea, a solute less permeable than water, seems to be prerequisite to the development of a sodium concentration gradient in the nondiuretic animal across the late distal tubule.

It is well recognized that the rate of sodium reabsorption along distal tubules is influenced by hormones. Most important in this respect is the action of mineralocorticoids, which will be discussed in more detail in another section of this chapter. However, other humoral factors may also affect the rate of distal tubular sodium transport.

Evidence derived from stop-flow analysis in dogs suggests that angiotensin II may act as an inhibitor of distal tubular sodium reabsorption (75). This hormone has also been implicated by Tobian *et al.* (76) as a likely regulator of distal tubular salt transport. Sodium reabsorption increased when the arterial perfusion pressure fell; therefore the suggestion was made that different levels of perfusion pressure are sensed by the juxtaglomerular apparatus. In the case of underdistention of the renal arterial tree, a lowering of secretion of angiotensin was thought to eliminate the inhibitory action of the hormone on distal tubular sodium reabsorption.

CHLORIDE. — Micropuncture studies on rats indicate that, under most experimental conditions, chloride is in electrochemical equilibrium across the distal tubular wall (42). This is borne out by the range of average transtubular chloride concentration ratios of 0.2 to 0.6 and the usually encountered late distal tubular potential (77) of about 50 mV (lumen negative). Kashgarian *et al.* (12) reached the same conclusion on the basis of stop-flow microperfusions of distal tubules of nondiuretic rat kidneys. There is, however, some evidence strongly suggesting that chloride can be actively transported by distal tubular epithelium. Rector and Clapp (78) measured the electrochemical potential gradient of chloride across distal tubular epithelium in normal and sodium-depleted rats, both groups being infused with sodium sulfate. Rats depleted of sodium chloride and infused with sodium sulfate form urine that is essentially chloride-free.

The chloride concentration of fluid collected from distal convoluted tubules by micropuncture may be as low as 0.1 mEq/L. At a plasma chloride concentration of 100 mEq/L, the ratio of plasma chloride to tubular fluid chloride may thus be as high as 10^3. At 38° C, the Nernst equation predicts that the transtubular potential difference would have to be 186 mV to explain passive reabsorption of this degree down an electrical gradient. Although Solomon (77) and Rector and Clapp (78) have observed higher transtubular potential differences in the distal than in the proximal segment of the rat kidney, the maximum has been about 120 mV. It is, therefore, evident that active chloride transport must be invoked to explain tubular fluid chloride concentrations below 1 mEq/L. Only under the abnormal circumstances outlined above is it possible to demonstrate active reabsorption. To what extent active chloride transport operates under normal conditions is undetermined; its nature is a mystery.

POTASSIUM. — Under normal conditions, the clearance of potassium is only 20% or so of the simultaneously determined rate of glomerular filtration. Accordingly, filtered potassium is largely reabsorbed. Some years ago, it was observed that in patients with chronic renal disease and markedly reduced rate of glomerular filtration the clearance of potassium approaches, and may occasionally exceed, the inulin clearance, suggesting tubular secretion. In 1948, Berliner, Mudge, Gilman and their respective associates (80) observed the net secretion of potassium in the normal dog. The secretion of potassium is enhanced by loading the animal with potassium salts, by alkalizing the urine and by loading with salts of nonreabsorbable or poorly reabsorbed anions, such as ferrocyanide and sulfate. Net secretion is also rendered more apparent if the rate of glomerular filtration is reduced by partial obstruction of the aorta above the origins of the renal arteries.

An interesting phenomenon is that of conditioning of potassium secretion by repeated loading with potassium salts. If a normal dog is given 5–10 Gm of potassium chloride orally each day for a week and then given an infusion containing the salt, the rate of secretion of potassium is greatly enhanced in comparison with that observed in an animal not so conditioned.

According to Berliner *et al.* (79, 80), virtually all the filtered potassium is reabsorbed proximally, and the excreted moiety, even under extreme conditions of reabsorption, is always added to tubular fluid in the distal segments of the nephron. Recent evidence obtained in micropuncture studies supports this view.

Figures 7–9 to 7–11 summarize the results of micropuncture studies on rats by Malnic *et al.* (22, 42). Rats kept on normal diet, rats kept on a potassium-deficient diet and rats subjected to procedures that enhance the rate of potassium excretion showed a similar pattern of proximal tubular potassium reabsorption. Despite variations in urinary K+ excretion rates from 3% to 150% of the filtered amount, net reabsorption of potassium in proximal tubules was relatively constant, at about four fifths of the quantity filtered.

Along the distal tubule, the potassium concentration rises as fluid passes through this nephron segment. Approximately 5–20% of the filtered load reaches the early part of the distal convolution, under control conditions as well as under conditions of potassium depletion or potassium loading. Only in rats in which a state of potassium deficiency is produced can the rise in potassium concentration be accounted for by distal tubular reabsorption of water. In all other conditions, overt net secretion of potassium takes place and accounts for at least 75% of urinary potassium.

It is possible that the low-potassium concentration and the small amounts of this ion (5–20% of the filtered load) that are detectable in the earliest portion of distal tubules

Fig. 7–9.—Potassium excretion along the nephron of rats on control diet. *Upper part*, tubular fluid/plasma (TF/P) concentration ratios as a function of tubular length. *Lower part*, potassium/inulin concentration ratios as a function of tubular length. (Data from Malnic, G., Klose, R. M., and Giebisch, G.: Am. J. Physiol. 206:674, 1964; figure from Giebisch, G., and Windhager, E. E.: Am. J. Med. 36:634, 1964.)

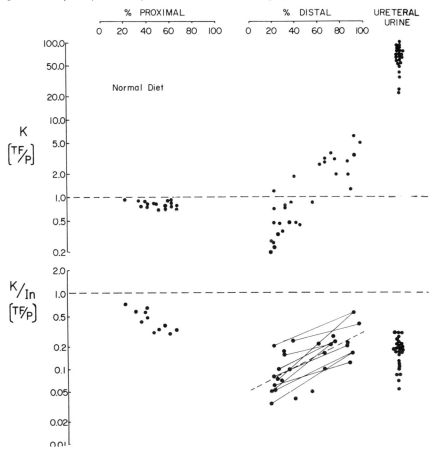

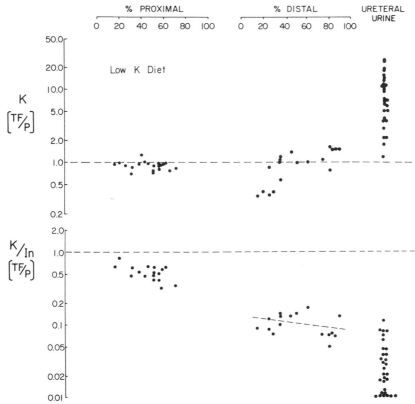

Fig. 7–10. — Potassium and potassium/inulin concentration ratios as function of tubular length in rats kept on low-potassium diet. Mean plasma K concentration was 1.99 mEq/L. (Data from Malnic, G., Klose, R. M., and Giebisch, G.: Am. J. Physiol. 206:674, 1964. Figure from Giebisch, G., and Windhager, E. E.: Am. J. Med. 36:634, 1964.)

accessible to micropuncture may not be the minimum escaping proximal reabsorption. Rather smaller amounts could be present in the first portion of the distal tubule. This suggestion follows from the fact that net secretion occurs over the entire length of the distal tubule where this segment is amenable to micropuncture. If this process includes the first fifth of the distal tubule, then the amount of potassium entering the macula densa portion of the nephron would be less than that found in the surface tubules and could conceivably be close to zero. Hence, the original hypothesis of Berliner (80) — that reabsorption of potassium in the proximal nephron is complete — is in accord with presently available micropuncture results.

In the collecting duct, significant net reabsorption has been observed under conditions of sodium or potassium depletion (22, 42, 81)

— situations characterized by low rates of potassium excretion. On the other hand, net secretion of potassium may also occur in the collecting duct during conditions of maximal rates of urinary excretion of potassium (82). Nonetheless, it would seem that, normally, most of the potassium appearing in the final urine is derived from distal tubular secretion and that little net transfer (probably reabsorptive in nature) takes place in the collecting duct.

Malnic and his associates (81, 83) have studied the net transfer of potassium by the distal tubule of rat kidneys in terms of the electrochemical driving forces, both under free-flow and stop-flow perfusion with isotonic raffinose solutions. Their results indicate that, even at the highest tubular K^+ secretion rates, the distal tubular potassium concentration is below the calculated equi-

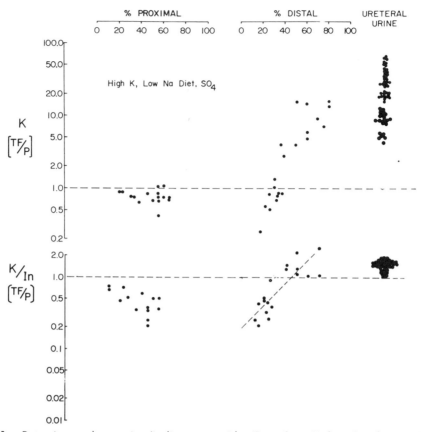

Fig. 7–11. — Potassium and potassium/inulin concentration ratios as function of tubular length in rats on high-potassium, low-sodium diet, receiving sodium sulfate and potassium chloride plus dichlorphena- mide. (Data from Malnic, G., Klose, R. M., and Gie- bisch, G.: Am. J. Physiol. 206:674, 1964. Figure from Giebisch, G., and Windhager, E. E.: Am. J. Med. 36: 634, 1964.)

librium value. To assume an active transport of potassium into the lumen is thus unneces- sary. Most important is the effect of changes in the distal transepithelial potential differ- ence on the distribution of potassium ions. Although an electrical driving force alone can explain the mechanism of secretion, it is necessary to postulate active reabsorptive movement of potassium, for, without such a transport, a state of electrochemical equilib- rium would be found, but this is not realized in stop-flow microperfusion experiments. Rather, what is present is a tubular potas- sium concentration lower than predicted on the basis of the magnitude of change in intra- luminal (negative) electrical potential. Such observations do not require the existence of a carrier-coupled secretory pump to explain

potassium movement into the lumen, in ex- change for reabsorbed sodium.

In the rat, neither the load nor the concen- tration of sodium reaching the distal convo- luted tubule is rate-limiting, if a 1:1 ex- change of sodium for potassium is taken to be the basis of potassium secretion (42). This is illustrated in Figure 7–12, which com- pares the fractions of filtered sodium and po- tassium remaining or appearing along the distal tubules. Considering the large differ- ence in the absolute amounts filtered, it is evident that the quantities of sodium reab- sorbed greatly exceed the amount of potassi- um secreted. However, potassium secretion can be reduced significantly, despite a more than adequate supply of sodium to distal tu- bules. This is illustrated by results obtained

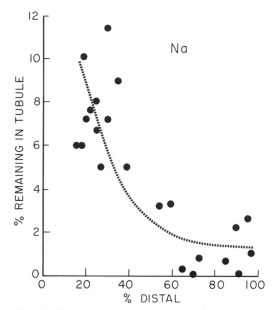

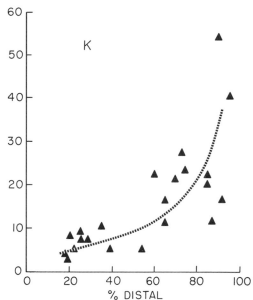

Fig. 7−12. − Fraction of filtered sodium and potassium remaining or appearing in tubular fluid as function of distal tubular length. (Data from Malnic, G., Klose, R. M., and Giebisch, G.: Am. J. Physiol. 206:674, 1964; and 211:529, 1966. Figure from Giebisch, G., and Windhager, E. E.: Am. J. Med. 36:634, 1964.)

in sodium-depleted rats with or without the administration of deoxycorticosterone acetate (DCA). In such animals, 4–6% of the filtered sodium enters the distal convoluted tubule. Ureteral urine is almost free of sodium ions, and the fractional excretion of potassium is about one fourth of the control value. Taking the mean values of sodium, potassium and inulin concentration ratios (tubular fluid/plasma) at the beginning and end of the distal tubule, it can be shown that, along the distal tubule, some 22 μEq of sodium are reabsorbed and about 1.2 μEq of potassium secreted (expressed per minute per kilogram rat). These results mean that the amount of sodium reabsorbed exceeds the quantity of potassium secreted by distal tubules by a factor of 20. In other words, potassium secretion has been compromised, as indicated by the low rate of potassium excretion, despite a more than adequate supply of sodium to the distal tubule. Neither could the sodium concentration in distal tubular fluid become rate-limiting for potassium secretion. This is borne out by the ob-

servation that, at least in the rat, the distal tubular epithelium cannot maintain a luminal sodium concentration below 10–20 mEq/L, even when an initially sodium-free raffinose solution is injected into the lumen. In every experimental condition studied, distal tubular sodium concentrations were found to exceed markedly the potassium concentration changes accompanying distal tubular potassium secretion.

SCHEMATIC REPRESENTATION OF DISTAL TUBULAR CELL

Figure 7–13 presents a model of a distal tubular cell. The lumen of distal tubules of rat kidneys is electrically negative by about 50 mV with respect to peritubular fluid (77, 84). Intracellular measurements of the electrical potential difference across the peritubular cell membrane gave values ranging between −70 and −90 mV. Hence, the potential drop across the luminal cell boundary amounts to some 20–40 mV.

The fact that the intracellular concentra-

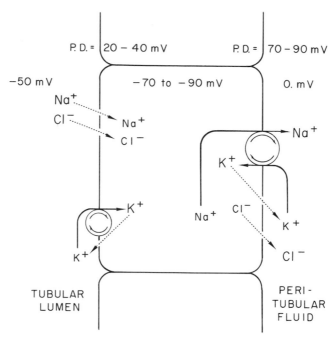

Fig. 7–13. — Schematic representation of ion transport in distal tubular cell.

tion of sodium is low and that the cell interior is electrically negative indicates that net reabsorption of sodium across the peritubular membrane occurs against an electrochemical gradient. Hence, sodium transport is active at this site. Furthermore, active uptake of potassium occurs at the peritubular cell border, because net movement of this ion takes place against a steep concentration gradient that outweighs the favorable electrical gradient. It is unknown to what extent the peritubular potassium pump is coupled stoichiometrically to active sodium extrusion.

At the luminal cell boundary, it is necessary to postulate active reabsorptive movement of potassium, as previously discussed (p. 120). Also, the possibility must be considered that transport of hydrogen ions involves a carrier mechanism, located at the luminal cell membrane.

Peritubular application of high potassium concentration results in reductions of the distal transepithelial potential (85). Accordingly, it is certain that the peritubular membrane acts as a barrier permeable to potassium ions. Although not tested directly, the over-all features of distal tubular chloride transfer make it likely that this cell border is also permeable to chloride.

Concerning the luminal membrane, studies by Giebisch et al. (85) suggest that the passive permeability to sodium and potassium are about equal and that the luminal potential difference is in part determined by the ratio of the sum of sodium and potassium concentrations in the luminal and cellular fluid compartments. This view is supported by the following observations: (1) Replacement of sodium and potassium by the poorly permeant cation choline reduces the transepithelial potential; the contribution of both sodium and potassium to diffusion potentials across the luminal membrane is thereby reduced. (2) For any given chloride concentration, both sodium and potassium are equally effective in maintaining a certain transepithelial potential difference. (3) The absolute magnitude of the distal transepithelial potential shows a significant correlation to the sum of quite variable combinations of sodium and potassium concentrations in tubular fluid.

The sum of sodium and potassium concentrations is relatively constant along the distal tubule, and, similarly, the transtubular potential difference shows no measurable change. These results strongly support the view that the luminal cell membrane is characterized by approximately equal permeabilities to sodium and potassium ions.

The mode of chloride transfer from tubular lumen into distal tubular cells has been less thoroughly analyzed than cationic transfer. As a simplifying assumption, it may be assumed that the permeability of the luminal membrane to chloride is of the same order of magnitude as that to sodium and potassium. Quantitative considerations (85), taking into account pertinent concentration gradients and assuming equal permeabilities for sodium and potassium, are in reasonable agreement with this thesis.

REGULATION OF POTASSIUM EXCRETION

Renal excretion of potassium ions is influenced by changes in sodium reabsorption and the acid-base status of the body. In general, the ratio of sodium and potassium excretion changes concordantly. With the notable exception of acidosis with simultaneous diuresis, metabolic or respiratory acidosis diminishes K excretion, and alkalosis leads to enhanced loss of potassium ions in the urine.

Enhanced tubular secretion of K ions in response to increased sodium excretion can best be explained by the fact that distal tubular K concentrations are equal in free flow and stop flow of fluid through the distal convolution. Because the concentration of potassium is independent of flow rate, the amount of sodium—i.e., the product of flow rate and concentration—leaving the tubule must vary in proportion to flow, other factors remaining constant. The kaliuresis observed during saline loading and in other diuretic conditions is, at least in part, explained by this diffusion limitation of distal tubular K secretion (86).

Although a 1:1 Na-K exchange by the distal tubule has been ruled out, some indirect coupling occurs. This dependence of K secretion on delivery of sodium to the distal nephron is probably due to electrical coupling (86). The more sodium ions that diffuse across the luminal membrane into the cell, the higher will be the distal transepithelial potential difference. It is the reabsorption of sodium that, in the last analysis, is responsible for the electronegativity of the tubular fluid and thus is responsible for maintaining an electrochemical driving force for K ions to enter the tubular lumen. The same argument holds for K secretion in the collecting duct. However, in this terminal tubular segment, active secretion of K ions has been demonstrated by Grantham *et al.* (87). Hence, a direct carrier-mediated exchange of K for Na could conceivably explain why potassium secretion falls drastically when collecting duct fluid is nearly sodium-free in states of dietary sodium deprivation or severe reductions in glomerular filtration rate.

The relationship between acid-base balance and K secretion has been examined in detail by Malnic *et al.* (86, 88), who measured the in situ pH, potassium and inulin concentrations of distal tubular fluid in a variety of conditions. Distal tubular bicarbonate reabsorption varied directly with bicarbonate concentration in the distal lumen. Assuming that hydrogen ion secretion is the primary cause of bicarbonate reabsorption, it appears that hydrogen ion secretion depends mainly on the amount of bicarbonate reaching the distal tubule. Therefore, contrary to expectation, in acidosis, an increase in distal hydrogen ion secretion does not occur (88) and, in alkalosis, hydrogen ion secretion is high. Potassium ion secretion, however, is depressed by acidosis and enhanced by alkalosis. The long-held view that cellular H^+ and K^+ ions compete for a common secretory pump of limited transport capacity is not supported by these findings. It is more likely that the effect of acid-base shifts on K secretion is due to a direct effect of intracellular pH changes on the peritubular K pump. Intracellular acidosis would diminish the rate of active K uptake by the cell. The intracellular K concentration will then be reduced and the driving force for passive diffusion of K ions into the lumen diminished. Intracellular alkalosis would have the opposite effect. The excretion of potassium is generally related to the concentration of potassium in plasma only in that plasma K reflects the concentration in the distal tubule cells; it is the latter that primarily determines potassium ion secretion.

EFFECT OF MINERALOCORTICOIDS ON TUBULAR ION TRANSFER

Using micropuncture technics, Hierholzer *et al.* (89, 90) demonstrated that mineralocorticoids affect sodium movement in both proximal and distal tubules. Thus, in adrenalectomized rats, net reabsorption of sodium from isotonic saline droplets injected into proximal tubules was found to be markedly diminished when compared with controls. Reabsorption could be restored, however, to normal after a latent period of 30–60 minutes by application of aldosterone. It was also observed that fractional sodium and fluid reabsorption was reduced in proximal tubules of adrenalectomized rats in which physiologic rates of flow were sustained with a perfusion pump. However, GFR was reduced, and estimates of proximal tubular transit time in nonperfused tubules showed that filtered fluid remained much longer in contact with the reabsorbing epithelium in adrenalectomized than in intact rats. Therefore, normal or even higher values of fractional reabsorption of salt and water are obtained for proximal tubules of adrenalectomized rats.

In the distal tubule, defects in the ability to establish limiting concentration gradients for sodium, as well as in the rate of net transport of sodium, have been found in adrenalectomized rats (89). Under conditions of free flow, distal tubular sodium concentrations were found to be higher than in normal animals—an effect that could be reversed by administration of aldosterone. There was also a reduction in distal tubular potassium concentrations in stop-flow microperfusions. On the basis of these experiments, Hierholzer and his associates (90) concluded that mineralocorticoids normally affect sodium transport in both proximal and distal tubules. However, the typical ionic abnormalities of adrenalectomized animals result primarily from distal tubular defects of sodium reabsorption and potassium secretion.

Mechanisms for Urine Concentration and Dilution

The ability to form concentrated urine has long been associated with the presence of loops of Henle interposed between proximal and distal segments of renal tubules. Crane (91) first observed that only mammals and birds can form urine hypertonic to plasma and that only these two classes possess loops of Henle. Much earlier, Peter (92) had noted, in studying a variety of mammalian species, that the greater the length of Henle's loop, the greater is the concentrating power of the kidney—an observation confirmed and extended by Sperber (93) and, more recently, by O'Dell and Schmidt-Nielsen (94). Such observations led to the view that ADH stimulates the active reabsorption of water by, and the formation of hypertonic urine in, the loops of Henle (95).

The results of early micropuncture studies on the rat (4) shattered this hypothesis, for if it were true, fluid collected from the distal tubules should be as hypertonic as ureteral urine. Actually, as pointed out above, distal tubular urine is either hypotonic or isotonic, never hypertonic. The site of final concentration of urine, therefore, had to be the collecting ducts; the mechanism of concentration was most simply envisioned as the active reabsorption of water. The loops of Henle were now believed to play only a minor role, namely, that of insuring osmotic equality of tubular fluid and blood prior to final elaboration of the urine in the distal tubules and final concentration of the urine in the collecting ducts.

ACTIVE TRANSPORT OF WATER VERSUS ACTIVE TRANSPORT OF IONS

The formation of concentrated urine by active reabsorption of water would be metabolically wasteful; the active reabsorption of ions and osmotic equilibration of water would be less demanding. For example, the reabsorption of 1 ml of isotonic saline solution by a mechanism that actively pumps sodium and permits the osmotic equilibration of water would require roughly 10^{20} successive combinations and dissociations of sodium with carrier. Reabsorption by a mechanism that actively pumps water and permits passive diffusion of sodium would require 300 times this number of successive combinations and dissociations of water and carrier. This derives from the fact that isotonic saline is 0.15 M with respect to sodium but 55.5 M with respect to water. According to Brodsky *et al.* (96), the energy required for concentrating the urine by the active transport of water is greatly in excess of that available to the kidney.

COUNTERCURRENT MULTIPLICATION OF CONCENTRATION

HYPOTHESIS. — The hypothesis of countercurrent multiplication of concentration was first developed in 1942 by Kuhn (99) to account for urinary concentration based on the hairpin configuration of the loops of Henle: a descending limb lying in close approximation to an ascending limb, with fluid flow in opposite directions in the two limbs. If the tubular epithelium were able to establish a small osmolar concentration difference between the fluid contents of the two limbs at each level along the course of the loop, this "single effect" could be greatly multiplied along the loop by countercurrent flow. An over-all effect — i.e., a high osmolar concentration difference — could be established between

the level of inflow and outflow (corticomedullary junction) and the point of reversal of flow (the bend of the loop at the tip of the papilla).

Kuhn described several possible mechanisms by which such an osmolar concentration difference could be developed. Subsequent work has shown that the pumping of salt out of the ascending limb of the loop of Henle into the medullary interstitium is the significant element of the process. The medullary interstitium becomes increasingly hypertonic from the corticomedullary junction to the tip of the papilla. The collecting ducts serve as osmotic exchangers, giving up water to the hypertonic medullary interstitium in their course from the cortex to the apexes of the renal papillae. The osmolar concentration of the urine in the collecting ducts becomes equal to that of the papillary interstitium. According to this concept, which has gained wide acceptance (6, 97, 98), the urine is concentrated by the pumping of ions in the loops of Henle and by the osmotic diffusion of water in the collecting ducts. No active pumping of water occurs.

PRINCIPLE OF COUNTERCURRENT MULTIPLICATION. — This principle is illustrated in Figure 7 – 14, in which concentration is portrayed as a series of discontinuous steps. In step *1*, the loop is filled with fluid containing 300 mOsm/L of sodium chloride. Let us assume that each segment of the ascending limb of the loop can establish a limiting gradient of 200 mOsm/L between its contents and that of the descending limb by active transport of chloride and passive diffusion of sodium ions.* This single effect is illustrated in step *2*. The fluid is now shifted along the tubule in step *3* by introducing more fluid having a concentration of 300 mOsm/L and by ejecting an equal volume of fluid having a concentration of 200 mOsm/L. The "single effect" is again developed in step *4*, the concentration difference at each point amount-

---

*This assumption is based on the fact that the osmotic concentration of the tubular fluid collected from the first part of the distal convolution is about 200 mOsm/L less than that of cortex and systemic blood.

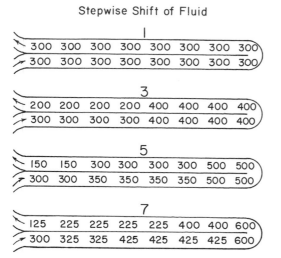

Stepwise Shift of Fluid

| 1 |
| 300 300 300 300 300 300 300 300 |
| 300 300 300 300 300 300 300 300 |

| 3 |
| 200 200 200 200 400 400 400 400 |
| 300 300 300 300 400 400 400 400 |

| 5 |
| 150 150 300 300 300 300 500 500 |
| 300 300 350 350 350 350 500 500 |

| 7 |
| 125 225 225 225 225 400 400 600 |
| 300 325 325 425 425 425 425 600 |

Development of "Single Effect"

| 2 |
| 200 200 200 200 200 200 200 200 |
| 400 400 400 400 400 400 400 400 |

| 4 |
| 150 150 150 150 300 300 300 300 |
| 350 350 350 350 500 500 500 500 |

| 6 |
| 125 125 225 225 225 225 400 400 |
| 325 325 425 425 425 425 600 600 |

| 8 |
| 112 175 175 225 225 313 313 500 |
| 312 375 375 425 425 513 513 700 |

Fig. 7–14.—The principle of countercurrent multiplication of concentration, based on the assumption that at any level along the loop of Henle a gradient of 200 mOsm/L can be established between ascending and descending limbs by active transport of ions.

ing to 200 mOsm/L. Steps *5, 6, 7* and *8* continue the process. By step *8,* a longitudinal gradient of 400 mOsm/L—i.e., a gradient significantly greater than the single effect of 200 mOsm/L—has developed. Continuation of these processes further increases the gradient. It should be noted that during the development of a gradient the outflowing fluid is hypotonic to the inflowing fluid and that the sodium chloride abstracted from the outflowing fluid is sequestered and progressively concentrated in the fluid contained in the loop, reaching its greatest concentration at the point of reversal of flow.

Fluid flow need not be discontinuous, as illustrated in Figure 7 – 14. Continuous flow, similar to that in the kidney, could result in the development of a like concentration gradient. Furthermore, the descending and ascending limbs of the loop need not be in apposition; in the kidney, they are separated by a small volume of interstitial fluid. There is, however, one condition that must be met both in the model and in the kidney: the ascending limb of the loop must be impermeable to water. Were it not, the transport of salt between the two limbs would be accompanied by the diffusion of an osmotically equivalent amount of water, and no concentration

gradient could be developed. Impermeability of the ascending limb to water is inherent in the premise that a concentration gradient of 200 mOsm/L can be established between the two limbs of the loop.

No useful osmotic work can be obtained from the system illustrated in Figure 7 – 14. An osmotic equilibrating device must be added, and, as noted at the beginning of this section, the collecting duct plays such a role. Its operation is described in the following paragraphs.

OPERATION OF COUNTERCURRENT MULTIPLICATION

The operation of countercurrent multiplication of concentration in the formation of hypertonic urine is illustrated in Figure 7 – 15. Isotonic fluid from the proximal tubule enters the descending limb of the loop of Henle. From the corresponding level of the ascending limb, chloride is actively extruded into the interstitium, reducing concentration in the ascending limb and increasing concentration in the interstitium. The concentration of sodium in the descending limb increases progressively as fluid flows toward the tip of the loop. This increase in

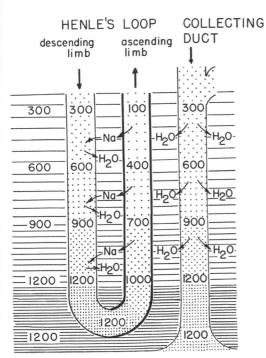

HENLE'S LOOP   COLLECTING
                                   DUCT
descending   ascending
  limb   limb

Fig. 7–15.—The operation of countercurrent multiplication of concentration in the formation of hypertonic urine. Recent evidence indicates that chloride is actively transported by the ascending limb of Henle's loop (64). (Adapted from Pitts, R. F.: *The Physiological Basis of Diuretic Therapy* [Springfield, Ill.: Charles C Thomas, Publisher, 1959].)

ing ADH, the permeability of collecting ducts to water is high. Isotonic fluid, entering the collecting ducts from the distal tubule, gives up water to the hypertonic interstitium. The final urine attains an osmolar concentration equal to that of the interstitium.

EXPERIMENTAL EVIDENCE FOR COUNTERCURRENT MULTIPLICATION.—In 1951, Wirz *et al.* (99) first presented experimental evidence for the countercurrent multiplication of concentration. Kidneys of thirsting rats were frozen in situ, removed, sectioned in a cold room and thawed gradually on a microscopic stage. The fluid contents of the cortical tubules were observed to melt at the same temperature as arterial blood plasma.

Fig. 7–16.—Osmolarity of tissue slices from the cortex and from the outer zone (O.Z.) and the inner zone (I.Z.) of the medulla of the kidney of the rat. Cortical slices are isosmotic with plasma. Those from the tip of the papilla are maximally hypertonic and are designed as having 100% of the observed osmotic concentration. (From Ullrich, K. J.; Kramer, K., and Boylan, J. W.: Prog. Cardiovas. Dis. 3:395, 1961.)

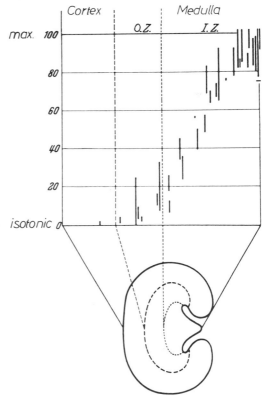

concentration results from the passive diffusion of water out of the descending limb into the interstitium and the passive diffusion of sodium from the interstitium into the descending limb. Which process is the more significant is not known. The concentration of salt in the ascending limb progressively decreases as fluid flows toward the cortex and the tubular urine becomes hypotonic before entering the distal tubule. In Figure 7–15, impermeability of the ascending limb to water is indicated by its heavily outlined wall. The descending limb is freely permeable to water and at least relatively permeable to sodium.

The collecting ducts serve as osmotic exchangers, which permit the equilibration of the final urine with the hypertonic interstitium of medulla and papilla. In hydropenia, i.e., in the presence of a high titer of circulat-

Hence, proximal tubular fluid is isotonic with systemic blood. The fluid contents of the tubules* in the outer medulla, inner medulla and papilla melted at progressively lower temperatures. Hence, these tubules contain fluid of increasing hypertonicity. Wirz's results are summarized in Figure 7 – 16.

Confirmatory results were obtained by Ullrich *et al.* (101), who showed that slices from cortex and outer and inner medulla of thirsting dogs must be immersed in progressively more hypertonic solutions to prevent swelling and gain in weight. Ullrich and Jarausch (102) subsequently showed that the increase in osmolar concentration of tubular cells from papillae, in comparison with those from cortex and outer medulla, was largely the consequence of increased concentrations

Fig. 7–17.—Concentration of urea, sodium and chloride in slices of cortex and of outer and inner zones of the medulla in hydropenic dogs. (Adapted from Ullrich, K. J., Kramer, K., and Boylan, J. W.: Prog. Cardiovas. Dis. 3:395, 1961.)

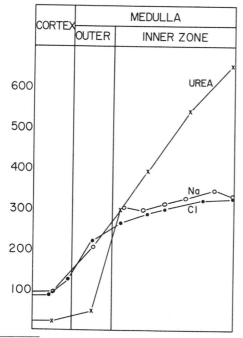

of sodium and chloride ions and urea (Fig. 7 – 17).

Evidence of Jamison *et al.* (103) indicates that even the thin limbs of Henle's loop act as countercurrent multipliers. When fluid samples collected from ascending limbs were compared with those from an adjacent descending limb, the osmolality was found to be lower by about 100 mOsm (Fig. 7 – 18). When the sodium concentrations of fluid from neighboring limbs were compared, the difference in sodium concentration accounted for about 90% of the difference in osmolality. These results support the view that transport of chloride and sodium out of ascending limbs across a relatively water-impermeable barrier provides the active step of countercurrent multiplication.

Additional evidence favoring countercurrent multiplication has been considered earlier (see Figs. 7 – 7 and 7 – 8). The fluid that enters the loops of Henle from the proximal tubules is isotonic, whereas that which leaves the loops of Henle to enter the distal tubules is hypotonic.

These several lines of evidence demonstrate that an osmolar gradient is developed along the loops of Henle between the cortex and the papilla. They suggest that the gradient is established by the pumping of salt out of the ascending limbs of the loops of Henle – a process that results in hypotonicity of fluid entering the distal tubules.

Hilger *et al.* (104) have catheterized collecting ducts of rats by introducing filamentous polyethylene tubes into the orifices of the ducts of Bellini at the tip of the papilla. They have shown, by comparing the inulin concentrations in samples collected high in the collecting tubules with those in samples collected near the orifices, that water is reabsorbed as fluid flows along the ducts. Furthermore, additional sodium is reabsorbed in the collecting ducts – some in exchange for hydrogen, ammonia and potassium, some in association with chloride. Figure 7 – 19 illustrates the fact that, in hydropenic animals in which the titer of ADH is high, fluids collected by micropuncture of loops of Henle, of

---

*Theoretically, the fluid contents of the ascending limbs of Henle's loops should melt at higher temperatures than those of descending limbs and collecting ducts at all levels of the medulla and papilla, for they are less hypertonic. Wirz *et al.* did not observe such differences, but Bray (100) has noted them.

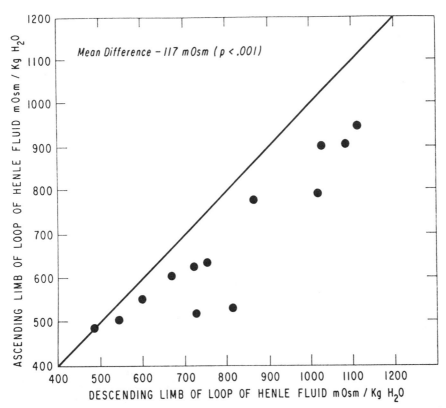

Fig. 7—18.—Comparison of osmolalities of fluid from ascending limbs and adjacent descending limbs of loops of Henle. (From Jamison, R. L., Ben- nett, C. M., and Berliner, R. W.: Am. J. Physiol. 212: 357, 1967.)

vasa recta and of collecting ducts near the tip of the papilla are essentially in osmotic equilibrium.* These two lines of evidence indicate that water is reabsorbed osmotically in the collecting ducts and that the final urine attains an osmolar concentration equal to that of the hypertonic papillary interstitium.† Figure 7–19 also shows that, in diabetes insipidus, urine from the collecting ducts is hypotonic, whereas blood in the vasa recta and fluid in the loops of Henle are equally, although modestly, hypertonic—a finding to which we shall return in considering the mechanism of dilution of the urine.

———

*Urine flow and osmolar concentration of the urine were varied by infusion of hypertonic mannitol at different rates.

†The osmolar concentration of blood in the vasa recta must be the same as that of papillary interstitial fluid, for osmotic equilibrium is rapidly established across capillary walls.

ADDITIONAL SIGNIFICANT FEATURES. — By now the discerning student may have some doubts as to whether the countercurrent multiplication mechanism as presented above will work. Indeed, it cannot work. The salt that is pumped out of the ascending limbs of the loops of Henle and reabsorbed from the collecting ducts cannot accumulate without limit in the medullary and papillary interstitium. The same is true of the water that diffuses out of the descending limbs of Henle's loops and the collecting ducts. Once a steady-state osmolar gradient is established along Henle's loop, both sodium and water must be removed, by the blood perfusing the medulla, as rapidly as they are reabsorbed. Because proportionally more salt than water is reabsorbed, the blood leaving the medulla must be modestly hypertonic. This follows from the fact that isotonic fluid enters the

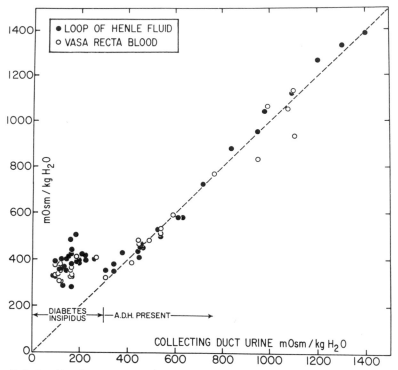

Fig. 7–19. — Relationships between osmolar concentration of fluid from loops of Henle, blood from vasa recta and urine from collecting ducts obtained by micropuncture at comparable levels near the tip of the papilla of rats. (From Gottschalk, C. W.: Physiologist 4:35, 1961.)

loop of Henle and hypotonic fluid leaves to enter the distal tubules. The fluid carried away from the medulla by the blood must, therefore, be hypertonic.* Removal of hypertonic fluid in the blood leaving the medulla is not the problem; rather, the problem is that of preventing the dissipation of the medullary osmotic gradient by the removal of fluid containing excessive amounts of osmotically active solutes. Two factors are significant in this respect: (1) the medullary blood flow is low and constitutes only a small fraction of total renal blood flow (105); and (2) the vasa recta behave as countercurrent exchangers, preventing excessive loss of osmotically active solutes from the medulla.

---

*The blood leaving the kidney in the renal vein must be hypotonic when the final urine is hypertonic, although blood flow is so high, relative to urine flow, that the fact could never be demonstrated experimentally.

COUNTERCURRENT EXCHANGE

PRINCIPLE. — The principle of countercurrent exchange is illustrated in Figure 7–20. The physical principles are illustrated in A and B; the application to conservation of medullary hyperosmolality is illustrated in C (106).

Consider the tube shown in A, through which water flows at a constant rate of 10 ml/min. A source of heat supplies 100 cal/min. If the fluid entering the system has a temperature of 30° C, that leaving the system must have a temperature of 40° C. If the tube is bent upon itself, as shown in B, insulated to prevent heat loss to the outside, but so arranged as to permit free exchange of heat between entering and emergent streams, certain features of operation will change. If the rate of fluid flow, the temperature of the entering stream and the rate of addition of heat are the same, the temperature of the emer-

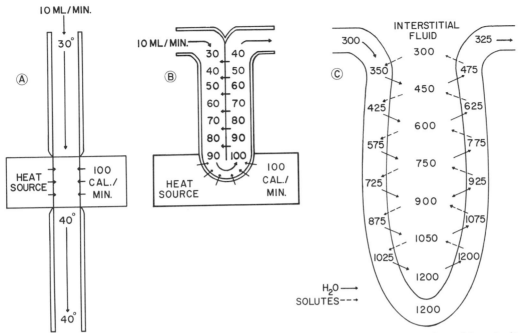

Fig. 7–20. — The principle of countercureent exchange. **A** and **B**, thermal models. **C**, operation of countercurrent exchange across the vasa recta to reduce the rate of dissipation of the osmolar gradient between cortex and medulla. (Adapted from Berliner, R. W.; Levinsky, N. G.; Davidson, D. G., and Eden, M.: Am. J. Med. 24:730, 1958.)

gent stream will be the same. However, the temperature at the heat source will be much higher in the countercurrent system, for heat will be transferred from emergent to entering streams. If the function of the fluid stream is considered to be that of cooling the heat source, then system *A* is much more effective than system *B*. Or, taking the opposite point of view, the countercurrent system in *B* has reduced the effective flow to a small fraction of the true flow.

The capillary shown in *C* illustrates the operation of the countercurrent vascular loop in terms of its effect in preserving the osmotic gradient in the renal medulla. Blood enters the loop at a concentration of 300 mOsm/L. As the capillary dips into the medullary and papillary interstitium, water diffuses out from, and osmotically active particles diffuse into, the blood. As blood traverses the loop and ascends, osmotically active particles diffuse out from, and water diffuses into, the blood. Water tends to short-circuit

the loop, passing more or less directly across the top of the loop. Red cells and plasma proteins are more concentrated at the tip of the loop, owing to this short-circuiting of water (6). The loop operates to reduce the effective blood flow with respect to the dissipation of the interstitial osmotic gradient.

COUNTERCURRENT MULTIPLICATION VERSUS COUNTERCURRENT EXCHANGE

Both these processes are dependent on the hairpin-loop configuration of ascending and descending limbs of medullary conduits. Countercurrent multiplication of concentration demands net active transport of solute from the ascending limbs of Henle's loops into the medullary interstitium. It alone can establish and maintain a gradient of osmolar concentration between the cortex and the tip of the papilla. Countercurrent exchange, in contrast, is a passive process and depends on diffusion of solutes and water in both directions across the permeable walls of the vasa recta. It plays no role in establishing an osmolar gradient. Indeed, it can only dissipate a gradient if that gradient is not actively maintained. However, countercurrent exchange reduces the rate of dissipation and therefore reduces the rate at which the countercurrent multiplier must pump sodium to maintain any given gradient.

ROLE OF DIETARY PROTEIN IN URINE CONCENTRATION

The ability of the kidney to concentrate the urine has long been used as a simple and informative test of renal function. The patient is maintained for 24 hours on a high-protein dry diet, and fluids are prohibited. If renal function is normal, the osmolar concentration of the urine will be some $4-5$ times that of the blood plasma. If protein intake is restricted before the test, the ability to eliminate hypertonic urine is reduced, whereas the ingestion of urea restores concentrating ability. A number of studies have shown that urea can be excreted in increased amounts without obligating the excretion of increased volumes of water.

Other than water and the blood gases, urea is the most diffusible substance in the body. Although in certain species there is evidence that urea may be reabsorbed actively (107), in most mammals passive diffusion down a concentration gradient will adequately explain the behavior of this solute. We shall assume only passive diffusion. Table $7-2$ summarizes data of Gottschalk (6), derived from micropuncture studies, which illustrate the relative amounts of urea that diffuse between tubular fluid and plasma at various sites within the nephron of the rat. In the late proximal tubule (i.e., in the most distal portion accessible to puncture), the urea F/P ratio is 1.5. At any point within the nephron the F/P ratio for urea divided by the F/P ratio for inulin is a measure of the amount of urea present relative to the amount filtered. Multiplying by 100 gives the percentage of

TABLE 7–2.— AVERAGE RATIOS OF TUBULAR FLUID TO PLASMA FOR INULIN AND UREA IN THE KIDNEY OF THE RAT*

	LATE PROXIMAL	DISTAL First Third	DISTAL Last Third	URETERAL URINE
F_{in}/P_{in}	3.0	6.9	14.9	690
F_u/P_u	1.5	7.7	10.5	90
$\dfrac{F_u/P_u}{F_{in}/P_{in}} \cdot 100$	50%	110%	70%	13%

*From Gottschalk, C. W.: Physiologist 4:35, 1961.

filtered urea remaining in the tubule. In the late proximal tubule, 50% of the filtered urea remains within the tubule; 50% has diffused into the peritubular capillaries of the cortex. The concentration gradient down which diffusion occurs has been established by the reabsorption of ions and water. The F/P ratio for inulin is 3.0, indicating that two thirds of the filtered fluid has been reabsorbed.

The fluid that has traversed the loops of Henle, although further reduced in volume (to 1/6.9th of the filtered volume), now contains as much urea as, or possibly more than, the original filtrate (110%). As Ullrich and Jarausch have shown (see Fig. $7-17$), the urea concentration of the medullary and papillary interstitium is high, providing the gradient down which urea diffuses into the loops of Henle. A modest fraction of the urea diffuses out of the distal tubule: 70% of the filtered moiety enters the collecting ducts. A major fraction is reabsorbed here, for only 13% is excreted in the urine. Because inulin is concentrated from an F/P ratio of 14.9 in the fluid entering the collecting ducts to an F/P ratio of 690 in that leaving as urine, a gradient is established to cause the diffusion of urea from the collecting ducts into the medullary and papillary interstitium.

It is evident that urea circulates from collecting ducts to medullary and papillary interstitium, to loops of Henle, to distal tubules and back to collecting ducts. Because the collecting ducts are relatively permeable to urea and because this solute is nearly as concentrated in the interstitial fluid of the medulla and papilla as it is in the urine, urea exerts only a small force in restraining the reabsorption of water. In essence, urea contributes little to the physiologically effective osmotic pressure of the urine. The kidney can concentrate other excretory products almost as though urea were not present.

OTHER FACTORS AFFECTING URINE CONCENTRATION

In his early studies, Kuhn enumerated the major factors that limit the degree to which the urine can be concentrated by countercurrent multiplication. Hypertonicity of the medullary and papillary interstitium, and therefore of the urine, is directly related to (1) the total quantity of salt pumped out of the ascending limbs of Henle's loops per unit time, (2) the magnitude of the gradient against which it is pumped and (3) the length of the countercurrent multiplier loop. Hypertonicity of interstitium and urine is inversely related to (1) the linear velocity of flow through the loops of Henle and (2) the cross-sectional area of the loops.

As mentioned earlier, animals in which all nephrons have long loops of small diameter (*Psammomys*, sand rat, deserts of northern Africa) form urine most hypertonic to plasma. Animals in which a majority of loops are short and of large diameter (beaver, man) concentrate the urine less. Concentration is favored by the delivery of a relatively small volume of fluid from the proximal tubules into the loops of Henle, provided the volume is large enough to deliver an adequate quantity of salt to the pumps of the loops. In osmotic diuresis, in which the volume of fluid reabsorbed by the proximal tubules is reduced, the linear velocity of flow through, and perhaps the diameter of, the loops of Henle are increased; medullary and papillary hypertonicity is reduced.

Two other factors must be considered:

1. An increase in medullary and papillary blood flow reduces tissue hypertonicity by washing out osmotically active solutes. Blood flow may well be increased in both water diuresis and osmotic diuresis; hence, tissue hypertonicity is reduced. In antidi-

uresis, ADH reduces medullary blood flow.

2. As noted earlier, ADH increases the permeability of the collecting ducts to water and to urea, permitting the attainment of more nearly perfect diffusion equilibrium. ADH may also stimulate the salt pumps of the ascending limbs of the loops of Henle, increasing both rate of transport and the gradient against which chloride can be extruded (95).

DILUTION OF URINE

The mechanism of dilution of the urine has been less adequately described than that of concentration, because of the difficulty of obtaining water diuresis in anesthetized and surgically manipulated animals. However, the essential features are known. As was shown in Figure 7–8, hypotonic fluid entering the distal tubules of hydrated rats with diabetes insipidus remains hypotonic during its passage along the distal tubules and collecting ducts. Both segments are relatively impermeable to water in the absence of circulating ADH; thus, osmotic equilibrium is not attained, as it is in hydropenia. The fact that the tubular fluid is hypotonic as it leaves the loops of Henle indicates that the pumps in the ascending limbs continue to operate in water diuresis and maintain at least some degree of medullary and papillary hypertonicity. This concept has been verified directly by studies of tissue osmolarity in water diuresis (100, 102) and indirectly by the observation that urine formed by one kidney during partial constriction of its renal artery may be hypertonic at a time when that formed by the opposite (control) kidney is hypotonic. Reduction of the rate of glomerular filtration and slowing of the flow of fluid along the collecting ducts on the side of arterial compression permits osmotic equilibration of urine and hypertonic medullary and papillary interstitium, even though the tubule is relatively impermeable to water (108).

The degree of hypertonicity of the medullary and papillary interstitium is less in hydrated than in dehydrated animals. In part, this may result from reduction in the rate of salt reabsorption and decrease in the NaCl gradient across the ascending limbs of Henle's loops. A reduction in hypertonicity of the interstitium may also result from increased medullary and papillary blood flow. ADH is believed to reduce blood perfusion of medulla and papilla.

Summary

Each day, 160 L of water is filtered through the glomeruli of normal man. Each liter contains 300 mOsm of solute, consisting largely of sodium, chloride and bicarbonate ions. As the filtrate flows along the proximal convoluted tubules, sodium is actively extruded into the interstitium of the cortex. Chloride follows sodium passively, and water is reabsorbed by osmosis. The ions and water deposited in the interstitium are rapidly carried away by blood perfusing the cortical capillaries. Although the volume of the tubular fluid is sharply reduced to perhaps 20% of that of the filtrate at the ends of the thick descending limbs of Henle's loops, the osmolar concentration remains unchanged at 300 mOsm/L. These facts are illustrated in Figure 7–21.

As the tubular fluid progresses down the

Fig. 7–21. — Summary of passive and active exchanges of water and ions in the nephron in the course of elaboration of hypertonic urine. Concentrations of tubular urine and peritubular fluid are given in milliosmoles per liter; large, boxed numerals are estimated percentages of glomerular filtrate remaining within the tubule at each level. Recent evidence indicates that chloride is actively transported by ascending limbs of Henle's loop (64).

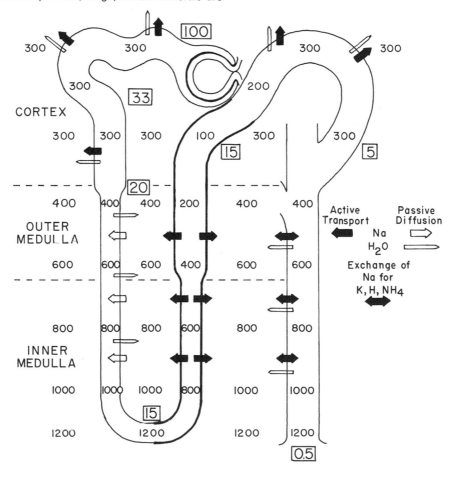

thin descending limbs of Henle's loops, water diffuses out into the hypertonic interstitium of the medulla and papilla and sodium diffuses in. Volume decreases and osmotic pressure increases progressively to the bends of the loops. In the ascending limbs of Henle's loops, chloride is extruded into the interstitium. Because the ascending limbs are impermeable to water, the osmolar concentration of the tubular fluid is reduced. At each level, a gradient of about 200 mOsm/L is established between tubular contents and hypertonic interstitium. Indeed, it is this capacity of the tubular epithelium to establish a modest osmolar gradient at each level that accounts for the much more significant gradient of 300:1,200 mOsm/L developed along the length of the loops. This process is termed "countercurrent multiplication of concentration."

The fluid that enters the distal convoluted tubules is hypotonic to the surrounding cortical interstitial fluid. Its volume is perhaps 15% of that of the glomerular filtrate. In hydropenia, in which the titer of circulating ADH is high, the epithelium of the distal tubules and collecting ducts is freely permeable to water. The tubular fluid becomes isotonic with cortical interstitial fluid by the middle of the distal segment. The continued extrusion of chloride and sodium and the passive osmotic diffusion of water continue in the distal tubule, reducing volume to a small proportion of that of the filtrate as fluid enters the collecting duct. This fluid, initially isosmotic, becomes progressively concentrated as it flows along the collecting duct and gives up water to the hypertonic medullary and papillary interstitium. The final urine, entering the renal pelvis, is essentially as concentrated as the interstitial tissue of the tips of the papillae.

The water, which diffuses out of the descending limbs of Henle's loops and out of the collecting ducts, and the salt, which is pumped out of the ascending limbs of Henle's loops, are removed by blood perfusing the vasa recta of the medulla and papilla. These vessels serve as countercurrent exchangers to reduce excessive loss of osmotically active solutes from the medulla and papilla.

In water diuresis, in which the titer of circulating ADH is low, the epithelium of the distal tubules and collecting ducts is impermeable to water. The hypotonicity of the tubular urine leaving the loops of Henle is maintained throughout the remainder of the nephron and is increased by the continued active extrusion of ions. The final urine is dilute and its volume large.

REFERENCES

1. Smith, H. W.: The Evolution of the Kidney, in *Lectures on the Kidney* (Porter Lectures, Series IX) (Lawrence: University of Kansas Press, 1943).
2. Smith, H. W.: *From Fish to Philosopher* (Boston: Little, Brown & Company, 1953).
3. Walker, A. M., Hudson, C. L., Findley, T., Jr., and Richards, A. N.: The total molecular concentration and the chloride concentration of fluid from different segments of the renal tubule of amphibia, Am. J. Physiol. 118:121, 1937.
4. Walker, A. M., Bott, P. A., Oliver, J., and MacDowell, M. C.: The collection and analysis of fluid from single nephrons of the mammalian kidney, Am. J. Physiol. 134:580, 1941.
5. Clapp, J., Watson, J., and Berliner, R. W.: Osmolality, bicarbonate concentration, and H_2O reabsorption in proximal tubule of the dog nephron, Am. J. Physiol. 205:273, 1963.
6. Gottschalk, C. W.: Micropuncture studies of tubular function in the mammalian kidney, Physiologist 4:35, 1961.
7. Gottschalk, C. W., and Mylle, M.: Micropuncture study of the mammalian urinary concentrating mechanism: Evidence for the countercurrent hypothesis, Am. J. Physiol. 196:927, 1959.
8. Wesson, L. G., and Anslow, W. P.: Excretion of sodium and water during osmotic diuresis in the dog, Am. J. Physiol. 153:465, 1948.
9. Shipp, J. C., Hanenson, I. B., Windhager, E. E., Schatzmann, H. J., Whittembury, G., Yoshimura, H., and Solomon, A. K.: Single proximal tubules of the *Necturus* kidney: Methods for micropuncture and microperfusion, Am. J. Physiol. 195:563, 1958.
10. Windhager, E. E., Whittembury, G., Oken, D. E., Schatzmann, H. J., and Solomon, A.

K.: Single proximal tubules of the *Necturus* kidney: III. Dependence of water movements on NaCl concentration, Am. J. Physiol. 197:313, 1959.

11. Giebisch, G., Klose, R. M., Malnic, G., Sullivan, W. J., and Windhager, E. E.: Sodium movement across single perfused proximal tubules of rat kidneys, J. Gen. Physiol. 47: 1175, 1964.

12. Kashgarian, M., Stöckle, H., Gottschalk, C. W., and Ullrich, K.: Transtubular electrochemical potentials of sodium and chloride in proximal and distal renal tubules of rats during antidiuresis and water diuresis (diabetes insipidus), Arch. ges. Physiol. 277:89, 1963.

13. Windhager, E. E., and Giebisch, G.: Micropuncture study of renal tubular transfer of sodium chloride in the rat, Am. J. Physiol. 200:581, 1961.

14. Ullrich, K. J., Schmidt-Nielsen, B., O'Dell, R., Pehling, G., Gottschalk, C. W., Lassiter, W., and Mylle, M.: Micropuncture study of composition of proximal and distal tubular fluid in rat kidney, Am. J. Physiol. 204:527, 1963.

15. Giebisch, G.: The contribution of measurement of electrical phenomena to our knowledge of renal electrolyte transport, Prog. Cardiovas. Dis. 3:463, 1961.

16. Giebisch, G.: Electrical potential measurements on single nephrons of *Necturus*, J. Cell. & Comp. Physiol. 51:221, 1958.

17. Spring, K. R., and Paganelli, C. V.: Sodium flux in *Necturus* proximal tubule under voltage clamp, J. Gen. Physiol. 60:181, 1972.

18. Boulpaep, E. L., and Seely, J. F.: Electrophysiology of proximal and distal tubules in the autoperfused dog kidney, Am. J. Physiol. 221:1084, 1971.

19. Burg, M. B., and Orloff, J.: Electrical potential differences across proximal convoluted tubules, Am. J. Physiol. 219:1714, 1970.

20. Lutz, M. D., Cardinal, J., and Burg, M. B.: Electrical resistance of the renal proximal tubule, Am. J. Physiol. 225:729, 1973.

21. Bloomer, H. A., Rector, R. C., Jr., and Seldin, D. W.: The mechanism of potassium reabsorption in the proximal tubule of the rat, J. Clin. Invest. 42:277, 1963.

22. Malnic, G., Klose, R. M., and Giebisch, G.: Micropuncture study of renal potassium excretion in the rat, Am. J. Physiol. 206: 674, 1964.

23. Giebisch, G., and Windhager, E. E.: Measurements of chloride movement across single proximal tubules of *Necturus* kidney, Am. J. Physiol. 204:387, 1963.

24. Boulpaep, E. L.: Ion Permeability of the

Peritubular and Luminal Membrane of the Renal Tubular Cell, in Krück, F. (ed.): *Transport and Funktion intracellulärer Elektrolyte: Symposion in Schüren* (Berlin: Urban and Schwarzenberg, 1967), pp. 98–105.

25. Ussing, H. H., and Windhager, E. E.: Nature of shunt-path and active sodium transport path through frog epithelium, Acta physiol. scandinav. 61:484, 1964.

26. Koefoed-Johnsen, U., and Ussing, H. H.: The nature of the frog skin potential, Acta physiol. scandinav. 42:298, 1958.

27. Windhager, E. E., Boulpaep, E. L., and Giebisch, G.: Electrophysiological Studies on Single Nephrons, in Schreiner, G. E. (ed.): *Proceedings of the 3rd International Congress on Nephrology, Washington, D.C., 1966* (Basel: Karges, 1967), Vol. 1, pp. 35–47.

28. Farquhar, M. G., and Palade, G. E.: Junctional complexes in various epithelia, J. Cell. Biol. 17:375, 1962.

29. Tisher, C. C., and Yarger, W. E.: Lanthanum permeability of the tight junction (zonula occludens) in the renal tubule of the rat, Kidney Internat. 3:238, 1973.

30. Diamond, J. M., and Tormey, J. McD.: Studies on the structural basis of water transport across epithelial membranes, Fed. Proc. 25:1458, 1966.

31. Whittembury, G.: Sodium extrusion and potassium uptake in guinea pig kidney cortex slices, J. Gen. Physiol. 48:699, 1965.

32. Lassen, N. A., Munck, O., and Thaysen, J. H.: Oxygen consumption and sodium reabsorption in the kidney, Acta physiol. scandinav. 51:371, 1961.

33. Deetjen, P., and Kramer, K.: Sodium reabsorption and oxygen consumption by the kidneys, Klin. Wchnschr. 38:680, 1960.

34. Fujimoto, M., Nash, F. D., and Kessler, R. H.: Effects of cyanide, Q_0 and dinitrophenol on renal sodium reabsorption and oxygen consumption, Am. J. Physiol. 206:1327, 1964.

35. Skou, J. C.: The influence of some cations on adenosinetriphosphatase from peripheral nerves, Biochim. et biophys. acta 23:394, 1957.

36. Gottschalk, C. W.: Renal tubular function: Lessons from micropuncture, Harvey Lect. 58:99, 1962–63.

37. Smith, H. W.: The excretion of water, Bull. New York Acad. Med. 23:177, 1947.

38. Lewy, J. E., and Windhager, E. E.: Peritubular control of proximal tubular fluid reabsorption in the rat kidney, Am. J. Physiol. 214:943, 1968.

39. Arrizurieta-Muchnik, E. E., Lassiter, W. E., Lipham, E. M., and Gottschalk, C. W.: Micropuncture study of glomerulo-tubular balance in the rat kidney, Nephron 418, 1969.

40. Landwehr, D. M., Schnermann, J., Klose, R. M., and Giebisch, G.: Effect of reduction in filtration rate on renal tubular sodium and water reabsorption, Am. J. Physiol. 215: 687, 1968.

41. Rodicio, J., Herrera-Acosta, J., Sellman, J. C., Rector, R. C., Jr., and Seldin, D. W.: Studies on glomerulotubular balance during aortic constriction, ureteral obstruction and venous occlusion in hydropenic and saline-loaded rats, Nephron 6:437, 1969.

42. Giebisch, G., and Windhager, E. E.: Renal transfer of sodium, chloride and potassium, Am. J. Med. 36:634, 1964.

43. Spitzer, A., and Windhager, E. E.: Effect of peritubular oncotic pressure changes on proximal tubular fluid reabsorption, Am. J. Physiol. 218:1188, 1970.

44. Brenner, B. M., and Troy, J. L.: Postglomerular vascular protein concentration: Evidence for a causal role in governing fluid reabsorption and glomerulo-tubular balance by the renal proximal tubule, J. Clin. Invest. 50:336, 1971.

45. Green, R., Windhager, E. E., and Giebisch, G.: Effects of transepithelial protein oncotic pressure difference on proximal tubular fluid movement in the rat, Am. J. Physiol. (accepted for publication).

46. Brenner, B. M., Falchuk, K. H., Keimowitz, R. I., and Berliner, R. W.: The relationship between peritubular capillary protein concentration and fluid reabsorption by the renal proximal tubule, J. Clin. Invest. 48: 1519, 1969.

47. Falchuk, K. H., Brenner, B. M., Tadokoro, M., and Berliner, R. W.: Oncotic and hydrostatic pressures in peritubular capillaries and fluid reabsorption by proximal tubule, Am. J. Physiol. 220:1427, 1971.

48. Ullrich, K., Rumrich, G., and Fuchs, G.: Wasserpermeabilität und transtubulärer Wasserfluss corticaler Nephronabschnitte bei verschiedenen Diuresezuständen, Arch. ges. Physiol. 280:99, 1964.

49. Curran, P. F., and MacIntosh, J. R.: A model system for biological water transport, Nature, London 193:347, 1962.

50. Boulpaep, E. L.: Permeability changes of the proximal tubule of *Necturus* during saline loading, Am. J. Physiol. 222:517, 1972.

51. Lorentz, W. B., Jr., Lassiter, W. E., and Gottschalk, C. W.: Renal tubular permeability during increased intrarenal pressure, J. Clin. Invest. 51:484, 1972.

52. Bank, N., Yarger, W. E., and Aynedijian, H. S.: A microperfusion study of sucrose movement across the rat proximal tubule during renal vein constriction, J. Clin. Invest. 50:294, 1971.

53. Imai, M., and Kokko, J. P.: Effect of peritubular protein concentration on reabsorption of sodium and water in isolated perfused proximal tubules, J. Clin. Invest. 51:314, 1972.

54. Grantham, J. J., Qualizza, P. B., and Welling, L. W.: Influence of serum proteins on net fluid reabsorption of isolated proximal tubules, Kidney Internat. 2:66, 1972.

55. De Wardener, H. H., Mills, I. H., Clapham, W. F., and Hayter, C. J.: Studies on the efferent mechanism of the sodium diuresis which follows the administration of intravenous saline in the dog, Clin. Sc. 21:249, 1961.

56. Cortney, M. A., Mylle, M., Lassiter, W. E., and Gottschalk, C. W.: Renal tubular transport of water, solute, and PAH in rats loaded with isotonic saline, Am. J. Physiol. 209:1199, 1965.

57. Landwehr, D. M., Klose, R. M., and Giebisch, G.: Renal tubular sodium and water reabsorption in the isotonic sodium chloride-loaded rat, Am. J. Physiol. 212:1327, 1967.

58. Dirks, J. H., Cirksena, W. J., and Berliner, R. W.: Effect of saline infusion on sodium reabsorption by the proximal tubule of the dog, J. Clin. Invest. 44:1160, 1965.

59. Johnston, C. I., and Davis, J. O.: Evidence from cross circulation studies for a humoral mechanism in the natriuresis of saline loading, Proc. Soc. Exper. Biol. & Med. 121: 1058, 1966.

60. Brenner, B. M., Troy, J. L., Daugharty, T. M., and MacInnes, R.: Quantitative importance of changes in postglomerular colloid osmotic pressure in mediating glomerulotubular balance in the rat, J. Clin. Invest. 52: 190, 1973.

61. Buckalew, V. M., Jr., Martinez, F. J., and Green, W. E.: The effect of dialysates and ultrafiltrates of plasma of saline-loaded dogs on toad bladder sodium transport, J. Clin. Invest. 49:926, 1970.

62. Hoshiko, T., Swanson, R. E., and Visscher, M. B.: Excretion of Na^{22} and K^{42} by the perfused bullfrog kidney and the effect of some poisons, Am. J. Physiol. 184:542, 1956.

63. Anagnostopoulos, T., Kinney, M., and Windhager, E. E.: Salt and water reabsorption by short loops of Henle during renal vein constriction, Am. J. Physiol. 200:1060, 1971.

64. Burg, M. B., and Green, N.: Function of the thick ascending limb of Henle's loop, Am. J. Physiol. 224:659, 1973.

65. Burg, M. B., and Grantham, J. J.: Ion Movements in Renal Tubules, in Bitter, E. E. (ed.): *Membranes and Ion Transport* (London: John Wiley & Sons, Ltd., 1971), Vol. 3, p. 77.

66. Kokko, J. P.: Membrane characteristics governing salt and water in the loop of Henle, Fed. Proc. 33:25, 1974.

67. Wirz, H.: Der osmotische Druck in den corticalen Tubuli der Rattenniere, Helvet. physiol. et pharmacol. acta 14:353, 1956.

68. Andersen, B., and Ussing, H. H.: Solvent drag on nonelectrolytes during osmotic flow through isolated toad skin and its response to antidiuretic hormone, Acta physiol. scandinav. 39:228, 1957.

69. Hays, R. M., and Leaf, A.: The problem of clinical vasopressin resistance: in vitro studies, Ann. Int. Med. 54:700, 1961.

70. Jaenike, J. R.: The influence of vasopressin on the permeability of the mammalian collecting duct to urea, J. Clin. Invest. 40:144, 1961.

71. Clapp, J. R., and Robinson, R. I.: Osmolality of Distal Tubular Fluid in the Dog, in Schreiner, G. E. (ed.): *Proceedings of the 3rd International Congress on Nephrology, Washington, D.C., 1966* (Basel: Karger, 1967), Vol. I., p. 171.

72. Gertz, K. H.: Transtubuläre Natriumchloridflüsse und Permeabilität für Nichtelektrolyte im proximalen und distalen Konvolut der Rattenniere, Arch. ges. Physiol. 276:336, 1963.

73. Lassiter, W. E., Gottschalk, C. W., and Mylle, M.: Micropuncture study of net transtubular movement of water and urea in rat kidney during saline diuresis, Am. J. Physiol. 206:669, 1964.

74. Giebisch, G., Klose, R. M., and Windhager, E. E.: Micropuncture study of hypertonic sodium chloride loading in the rat, Am. J. Physiol. 206:687, 1964.

75. Vander, A. J.: Inhibition of distal sodium reabsorption by angiotensin II, Am. J. Physiol. 205:133, 1963.

76. Tobian, L., Coffee, K., Ferreira, D., and Meuili, J.: The effect of renal perfusion pressure on the net transport of sodium out of distal tubular urine as studied with the stop-flow technique, J. Clin. Invest. 43:118, 1964.

77. Solomon, S.: Transtubular potential differences of rat kidney, J. Cell. & Comp. Physiol. 49:351, 1957.

78. Rector, F. C., Jr., and Clapp, J. R.: Evidence for active chloride reabsorption in the distal tubule of the rat, J. Clin Invest. 41:101, 1962.

79. Berliner, R. W., Kennedy, T. J., Jr., and Orloff, J.: Factors affecting transport of potassium and hydrogen ions by renal tubules, Arch. internat. pharmacodyn. 97:299, 1954.

80. Berliner, R. W.: Renal mechanism for potassium excretion. Harvey Lect. 55:141, 1959–60.

81. Malnic, G., Klose, R. M., and Giebisch, G.: Micropuncture study of distal tubular potassium and sodium transport in rat nephron, Am. J. Physiol. 211:529, 1966.

82. Hierholzer, K.: Secretion of potassium and acidification in collecting ducts of mammalian kidney, Am. J. Physiol. 201:318, 1961.

83. Malnic, G., Klose, R. M., and Giebisch, G.: Microperfusion study of distal tubular potassium and sodium transfer in rat kidney, Am. J. Physiol. 211:548, 1966.

84. Windhager, E. E., and Giebisch, G.: Electrophysiology of the nephron, Physiol. Rev. 45:214, 1965.

85. Giebisch, G., Malnic, G., Klose, R. M., and Windhager, E. E.: Effect of ionic substitutions on distal potential differences in rat kidney, Am. J. Physiol. 211:560, 1966.

86. Giebisch, G.: Renal Potassium Excretion, in Rouiller, C., and Muller, A. F. (eds.): *The Kidney* (New York: Academic Press, Inc., 1971), Vol. 3, p. 329.

87. Grantham, J. J., Burg, M., and Orloff, J.: The nature of transtubular Na and K transport in isolated rabbit renal collecting tubules, J. Clin. Invest. 49:1815, 1970.

88. Malnic, G., Mello Aires, J., and Giebisch, G.: Potassium transport across renal distal tubules during acid-base disturbances, Am. J. Physiol. 221:1192, 1971.

89. Hierholzer, K., Wiederholt, M., Holzgreve, J., Giebisch, G., Klose, R. M., and Windhager, E. E.: Micropuncture study of renal transtubular concentration gradients of sodium and potassium in adrenalectomized rats, Arch. ges. Physiol. 285:193, 1965.

90. Hierholzer, K., Wiederholt, M., and Stolte, H.: Hemmung der Natriumresorption im proximalen und distalen Konvolut adrenalektomierter Ratten, Arch. ges. Physiol. 291:43, 1966.

91. Crane, M. M.: Observations of the function of the frog's kidney, Am. J. Physiol. 81:232, 1927.

92. Peter, C.: *Untersechungen über Bau und Entwicklung der Niere* (Jena: Fischer, 1909).

93. Sperber, I.: Studies on the mammalian kidney, Zool. Birdrag Uppsala 22:249, 1944.

94. O'Dell, R., and Schmidt-Nielsen, B.: Concentrating ability and kidney structure, Fed. Proc. 19:366, 1960.

95. Burgess, W. W., Harvey, A. M., and Marshall, E. K., Jr.: The site of antidiuretic activity of pituitary extract, J. Pharmacol. & Exper. Therap. 49:237, 1933.

96. Brodsky, W. A., Rehm, W. S., Dennis, W. H., and Miller, D. G.: Thermodynamic analysis of the intracellular osmotic gradient hypothesis of active water transport, Science 121:302, 1955.

97. Winters, R. A., and Davies, R. E.: The role of countercurrent mechanisms in urine concentration, Ann. Int. Med. 54:810, 1961.

98. Ullrich, K. J., Kramer, K., and Boylan, J. W.: Present knowledge of the countercurrent system in the mammalian kidney, Prog. Cardiovas. Dis. 3:395, 1961.

99. Wirz, H., Hargitay, B., and Kuhn, W.: Lokalisation des Konzentrierungsprozesses in der Niere durch direkte Kryoskopie, Helvet. physiol. et pharmacol. acta 9:196, 1951.

100. Bray, G. A.: Freezing point depression of rat kidney slices during water diuresis and antidiuresis, Am. J. Physiol. 199:915, 1960.

101. Ullrich, K. J., Drenckhahn, F. O., and Jarausch, K. H.: Untersuchungen zum Problem der Harnkonzentrierung und Verdünnung: Über das osmotische Verhalten von Nierenzellen und die begleitende Elektrolytanhäufung im Nierengewebe bei verschiedenen Diuresezuständen, Arch. ges. Physiol. 261: 62, 1955.

102. Ullrich, K. J., and Jarausch, K. H.: Untersuchungen zum Problem der Harnkonzentrierung und Verdünnung: Über die Verteilung der Elektrolyte. Harnstoff. Aminosäuren und exogenem Kreatinin in Rinde und Mark bei verschiedenen Diuresezuständen, Arch, ges. Physiol. 262:537, 1956.

103. Jamison, R. L., Bennett, C. M., and Berliner, R. W.: Countercurrent multiplication by the thin loops of Henle, Am. J. Physiol. 212:357, 1967.

104. Hilger, H. H., Klümper, J. D., and Ullrich, K. J.: Wasserrückresorption und Ionentransport durch die Sammerlrohrzellen der Säugetierniere, Arch. ges. Physiol. 267:218, 1958.

105. Kramer, K., Thurau, K., and Deetjen, P.: Hämodynamik des Nierenmarkes, Arch. ges. Physiol. 270:251, 1960.

106. Berliner, R. W., Levinsky, N. G., Davidson, D. G., and Eden, M.: Dilution and concentration of the urine and action of antidiuretic hormone, Am. J. Med. 24:730, 1958.

107. Schmidt-Nielsen, B.: Urea excretion in mammals, Physiol. Rev. 38:139, 1958.

108. Berliner, R. W., and Davidson, D. G.: Production of hypertonic urine in the absence of pituitary antidiuretic hormone, J. Clin. Invest. 36:1416, 1957.

8

Tubular Secretion

TUBULAR SECRETION resembles tubular reabsorption in many respects; the major difference is in the orientation of transport. Tubular secretory mechanisms transport materials from peritubular fluid to tubular lumen; tubular reabsorptive mechanisms transport materials in the reverse direction. Active tubular secretion, like active reabsorption, implies transport against an electrochemical gradient and therefore demands a continuous supply of energy. There are, in fact, three types of secretory mechanisms analogous to the three types of reabsorptive mechanisms described in preceding chapters: (1) active secretory mechanisms that exhibit an absolute limitation of transport capacity—i.e., Tm-limited mechanisms; (2) active secretory mechanisms that exhibit gradient-time limitation of transport capacity; and (3) passive secretory mechanisms, which involve diffusion of materials down gradients of concentration or of electrical potential.

Active Secretion by
Tm-Limited Mechanisms

GENERAL CHARACTERISTICS

Only three secretory mechanisms that exhibit an absolute limitation of transport capacity are presently known. One mechanism secretes a heterogeneous group of compounds, of which many, but not all, are carboxylic or sulfonic acids, including phe-

nol red, hippurate, p-aminohippurate (PAH), penicillin, chlorothiazide, a variety of glucuronides and sulfuric acid esters, various acetylated sulfonamides and a group of urologic contrast agents, such as Diodrast, Uroselectan, Topax, Neo-Iopax and Skiodan. Creatinine may also be secreted by this mechanism, although recent evidence favors the view that it is secreted by the strong base transport system. A second mechanism secretes a group of strong organic bases, including guanidine, thiamine, choline, histamine, tetraethylammonium, piperidine, tolazoline (Darstine), mepiperphenidol (Priscoline) and hexamethonium. A third mechanism secretes ethylenediaminetetraacetate (EDTA) and possibly other, as yet unidentified, substances. The existence of only three Tm-limited secretory mechanisms contrasts sharply with the existence of many, more or less independent, Tm-limited reabsorptive mechanisms.

Many of the substances secreted by these mechanisms are foreign to the body. Furthermore, all of them are eliminated by glomerular filtration; and the quantities secreted into the urine are, in some instances, of minor significance (e.g., creatinine in man). One wonders why these mechanisms exist and what useful purposes they serve. Undoubtedly, the mechanism that secretes PAH, phenol red, penicillin, etc., was not evolved to rid the body of these foreign substances. Hippurate, glucuronides and even phenol esters, all of which are normal excretory products, are relatively nontoxic. Perhaps the mechanism was evolved to secrete some unknown substance that, because of high toxicity, must be maintained in very low concentration in the body fluids. Other substances, in consequence of structural similarities, are also transported by the mechanism.

Although these three secretory mechanisms are present in most vertebrate orders so far studied, they are not identical in all. In the course of evolution, variations on a general theme have appeared.

QUANTIFICATION

Any substance secreted by the renal tubules is also filtered through the glomeruli. Accordingly, the rate of excretion is the sum of the rate of filtration and the rate of tubular secretion. Conversely, the rate of secretion (T_x) equals the rate of excretion ($U_x \cdot V$) minus the rate of filtration ($P_x \cdot C_{in}$):

$$T_x = U_x \cdot V - P_x \cdot C_{in}$$

Many, but not all, substances secreted are partly bound to plasma proteins and, consequently, are incompletely filterable through glomerular capillaries. For a substance bound to protein, the rate of filtration is the product of that fraction of the substance present in plasma that is freely filterable, $P \cdot F \cdot W$, and the rate of glomerular filtration, C_{in}, F being the ratio of the concentration in the ultrafiltrate (P_f) to that in whole plasma (P), or P_f/P. Properly, one should relate P_f to P_w, the latter being the concentration in milligrams per milliliter of plasma water. To convert P_f/P to P_f/P_w, one must multiply F by W, the latter being the fraction of the plasma that is water — normally 0.93 – 0.94. The formula* for calculating secretion of substances partly bound to protein is, therefore,

$$T_x = U_x \cdot V - P_x \cdot F \cdot W \cdot C_{in}$$

---

*If the substance is filtered, reabsorbed and in part secreted, exact quantification of rate of secretion is impossible. One can only calculate net secretion or net reabsorption. However, in some instances it is possible to block either reabsorption or secretion with a transport inhibitor and gain some idea of the true magnitude of the two processes.

Protein binding of secreted substances varies widely: phenol red is about 80% bound, 20% free; PAH is 10 – 20% bound, 80 – 90% free.

SECRETION OF ORGANIC ACIDS

SECRETORY MECHANISM TRANSPORTING ORGANIC ACIDS. — The general characteristics of the secretory mechanism that transports phenol red, Diodrast, PAH and various other compounds are illustrated in Figure 8 – 1, which relates rate of filtration, secretion and total excretion to plasma concentration of PAH. To perform such a titration of the secretory system in man, inulin is infused at a rate sufficient to maintain a constant plasma concentration between 15 and 20 mg/100 ml. PAH is infused at a slowly increasing rate to elevate plasma concentration gradually from 1 to 100 mg/100 ml. Urine and plasma samples, collected at frequent intervals, are analyzed for inulin and PAH; and the appropriate calculations of clearance and rates of filtration, excretion and secretion are performed, using the formula given in the preceding paragraph.

At plasma concentrations of 1 – 6+ mg/100 ml of free unbound PAH,† rates of excretion, secretion and filtration increase in proportion to the increase in plasma level. Above 10 mg/100 ml, secretion of PAH becomes constant and independent of plasma concentration. The maximum rate of secretory transport of PAH averages 80 mg/min per 1.73 m² of surface area, in normal man. It is evident from Figure 8 – 1 that, if plasma concentration is less than 60 mg/100 ml, tubular secretion accounts for the major fraction of urinary PAH, whereas, if plasma concentration exceeds 60 mg/100 ml, filtration accounts for the major fraction. If plasma concentration is less than 10 mg/100 ml, more than 80% of the PAH excreted is secreted by the renal tubules.

KINETICS OF SECRETORY TRANSPORT OF

---

†The rate of filtration of a substance partly bound to plasma protein is a linear function of the concentration of the free unbound moiety in plasma, not necessarily of total concentration, unless the free fraction is constant and is independent of plasma concentration.

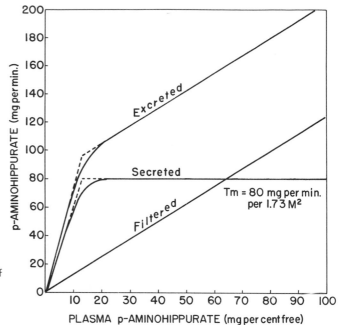

Fig. 8—1. — Rates of filtration, secretion and excretion of p-aminohippurate as functions of plasma concentration in man.

PAH. — The kinetics of the secretory transport of PAH can be described in the same terms used in describing the reabsorptive transport of glucose (1, 2). A substance, B, present in the cell membrane or perhaps within the cell in a fixed and limited amount, combines with PAH to form a complex $(PAH) \cdot B$. The dissociation of this complex is the rate-limiting step in tubular transport:

$$(PAH) + B \leftrightarrows (PAH) \cdot B \rightarrow B + (PAH)$$

One must assume that the affinity of PAH for substance B is high and that the rate of attainment of equilibrium in the reaction $(PAH) + B \rightleftarrows (PAH) \cdot B$ is rapid in comparison with the rate of breakdown of $(PAH) \cdot B$. When sufficient PAH is presented to the secretory cells in the peritubular blood stream to convert all of B into the complex $(PAH) \cdot B$, the secretory system is saturated and the rate of secretion is determined by the rate of breakdown of the complex. If less than saturation quantities of PAH are presented to the tubules — i.e., if plasma concentration is less than 4–6 mg/100 ml — the affinity of PAH for the carrier component is sufficiently high to remove essentially all of the PAH from the blood in one circulation through the peritubular capillaries. We shall return to this point in a discussion of the measurement of renal plasma flow and renal blood flow, in Chapter 9.

COMPETITION IN TUBULAR TRANSPORT. — The competition in tubular transport finds ready explanation in this kinetic scheme. In man, Tm values for phenol red, Diodrast-iodine* and PAH average 36, 57, and 80 mg/min per 1.73 m² of surface area, respectively. If the secretory mechanism is saturated with phenol red, the infusion of PAH, Diodrast or any of the other substances transported by this mechanism reduces the secretion of phenol red. Thus, these latter substances compete for the common carrier, displace phenol red and reduce its secretion. Because PAH and Diodrast have a greater affinity for the carrier than has phenol red, they readily inhibit secretion of the dye. However, competition obeys the mass law; and, if the concentration of phenol red is increased sufficiently, this can depress the secretion of PAH and Diodrast.

---

*Because Diodrast in plasma and urine is determined iodometrically, it is customary to express quantities and concentrations in terms of iodine.

Karl Beyer and his associates (3) suggested during World War II that competitive inhibition could be used to conserve penicillin. At this time, penicillin was expensive, in very short supply and nearly unobtainable for civilian use. Administered in high dosage, it is rapidly excreted in the urine and wasted. From its high rate of excretion, Beyer inferred that penicillin is secreted. He observed that, if PAH and penicillin are infused simultaneously, the secretion of penicillin is blocked and high plasma penicillin levels are sustained for prolonged periods of time. This observation led to the synthesis of two compounds, carinamide and probenecid, that depress the transport of penicillin and related compounds. According to Beyer, carinamide and probenecid become tangled in the secretory machinery, forming stable, slowly dissociating complexes with the cell carrier. Although they are themselves only slowly secreted under normal conditions, they effectively block the transport of other compounds. A different explanation has been given by Weiner, Washington and Mudge, namely, that probenecid and carinamide are rapidly secreted but are passively reabsorbed from acid or neutral urine. Both probenecid and carinamide are weak acids. Their dissociation is depressed in acid urine, and they exist largely as unionized compounds to which the tubular epithelium is permeable. In alkaline urine, both compounds exist as dissociated salts to which the tubular epithelium is impermeable. Accordingly, their clearances are high in alkaline urine and exceed the rate of glomerular filtration. The blocking of penicillin secretion with PAH, probenecid or carinamide is not done today, largely because the antibiotic is readily available and inexpensive and the need for conservation of limited supplies no longer exists.

BIOCHEMICAL PROCESSES OF TUBULAR SECRETION. — These processes are somewhat better understood than are those of tubular reabsorption, because of the development of in vitro methods of study. Years ago, Taggart and Forster (4) observed that renal tubules of marine teleosts, such as the flounder, when teased apart and immersed in a balanced salt solution containing minute amounts of phenol red, concentrate the dye in the tubular lumen many hundred-fold. The flounder tubule preparation, observed under the microscope, is ideal for the qualitative study of the effects of inhibitors and accelerators of phenol red transport. Subsequently it was observed that slices of the renal cortex of a number of laboratory mammals accumulate Diodrast, PAH, etc., in relatively high concentration from a dilute bathing medium. Transport can be expressed in quantitative terms of slice/medium ratios attained within a given period of time. It is probable that most of the material accumulated in a slice is concentrated within tubular cells, not within the tubular lumen. Nevertheless, observations of the action of inhibitors and accelerators of transport and of competition made on slices of cortex correlate well with those made on the intact kidney. Accordingly, the in vitro slice preparation is very useful, even though the secretory system is incomplete.

Relatively low concentrations of azide, cyanide, and arsenite, as well as cold and anaerobiosis, block the uptake of phenol red, PAH and Diodrast by teased tubules or slices of renal cortex. All interfere with the oxidative processes that serve as sources of energy to turn the secretory machinery. Dinitrophenol (DNP), which uncouples oxidation and phosphorylation, also depresses the uptake of secreted materials. Furthermore, the administration of DNP to intact animals (dogs) reduces Tm_{PAH} to one third or less of

$$\begin{array}{l} \text{OXYGEN} + \\ \text{SUBSTRATE} \end{array} \xrightarrow{\text{(Cyclophorase system)}} CO_2 + H_2O$$

$$AMP \longrightarrow ATP$$
$$PP + AMP \rightarrow \begin{array}{l} \text{ENERGY TO TURN} \\ \text{SECRETORY MACHINERY} \end{array}$$

its control value without affecting tubular reabsorption of either glucose or amino acids. Therefore, phosphate bond energy is more or less specifically and obligatorily involved in tubular secretory transport (5).

The mitochondria of renal tubular cells contain an enzyme complex (cyclophorase system) capable of catalyzing all reactions of the citric acid cycle and incorporating inorganic phosphate into adenosine triphosphate (ATP). The gross elements of the provision of energy to the secretory system are illustrated in the above diagram. The addition of certain metabolic intermediates to the medium enhances the uptake of secreted materials by kidney slices; these intermediates are pyruvate, lactate and, especially, acetate. Other intermediates, including succinate, α-ketoglutarate, fumarate, glycine, alanine, glutamate and fatty acids of intermediate length, depress uptake by slices and isolated tubules. In dogs, the infusion of sodium acetate increases Tm_{PAH} promptly by as much as 50–100%.

An interesting phenomenon is evident in the dog and cat but absent in man: *self-depression of secretory transport*. If the plasma concentration of PAH is raised to extremely high levels in the determination of Tm in the dog and cat, secretory transport progressively declines and may cease entirely.* If acetate is now infused, Tm is restored to normal values or may even attain supernormal values. Apparently, the availability of acetate is a limiting factor in the rate of turning of the citric acid cycle and thus in the rate of provision of phosphate bond energy to the secretory mechanism. Unfortunately, details as to the nature of the cellular carrier and the manner of cycling energy into the system are unknown. Certainly, secreted materials are not themselves phosphorylated; nor, as was once believed, do they couple with coenzyme A in the course of transport. Neither

are all of the compounds transported by this "organic acid" secretory system actually organic acid anions. Therefore, ionic reactions are probably not involved in transport (5). According to Hoeber (6), secretion depends on the presence within the molecule of a polar hydrophilic group and a nonpolar organophilic group. The suggestion has been made that this structure is necessary for orientation of the molecule within the membrane prior to attachment to the carrier.

STEPS IN TRANSPORT OF PAH. — Earlier it was stated that, although the basic "organic acid" transport mechanism exists in the renal tubules of most vertebrate species studied, variations on a general theme have appeared in the course of evolution. In the tubule of the flounder, the transport of phenol red involves at least two active steps. Uptake of phenol red from the medium is separate from and independent of secretion into the tubular lumen (7). Ordinarily, transport across the cell is so rapid that one sees no staining of the cytoplasm. Certainly, dye is not concentrated in the cell in granules or vacuoles before ejection into the tubular lumen. The two-step nature of the process can be demonstrated in the following manner: If flounder tubules are placed in a balanced salt solution containing Na^+, K^+, Ca^{++}, Mg^{++}, Cl^-, HCO_3^- and $HPO_4^=$ ions, phenol red is rapidly concentrated in the tubular lumen; none is visible in the cell. If K^+ and Ca^{++} ions are omitted from the medium, no dye is secreted into the lumen, and none is visible in the cell; i.e., the transport mechanism is completely blocked. If K^+ ions are now added, dye is rapidly taken up by cells, staining them diffusely and intensely red. No dye appears in the lumen. If Ca^{++} and K^+ ions are added, the dye is immediately ejected into the lumen, and transport continues without evidence of concentration within the cell. Apparently, two mechanisms exist in the flounder tubule capable of concentrating phenol red: one located in the peritubular membrane, the other in the luminal membrane. Under normal conditions, the peritubular mechanism is the one that limits overall transport of phenol red. The luminal

---

*The mechanism of self-depression of Tm is unknown, as is also that of the depression of transport induced by the group of metabolites listed above. However, both phenomena are consequences of reduced production of phosphate bond energy, of uncoupling of energy supply and secretory machinery, or of competition for the common transport mechanism.

mechanism ejects dye into the tubular urine at such a rapid rate that it never accumulates in the cytoplasm.

There is evidence that, in the rabbit, only a single concentrating step is involved in the transport of PAH (8). This compound diffuses down a concentration gradient from blood capillary to interstitial fluid and into the tubular cell, where it is segregated in some undefined intracellular compartment at essentially the same concentration as in the peritubular fluid. Within a second intracellular compartment, PAH is actively accumulated in high concentration. From this compartment, it diffuses down a second concentration gradient into the tubular urine. Evidence for this concept is indirect, and it may or may not describe the transport of PAH accurately.

OTHER METHODS FOR STUDYING SECRETORY TRANSPORT.—Still other methods for studying secretory transport have been devised, as follows: Mesonephric tubules, isolated from embryonic chicks, can be grown in tissue culture. Fragments of these tubules seal their ends, become cysts and secrete phenol red into their lumens (9). The cells become modestly stained in the process; however, the concentration of dye in the lumen of a cyst is far higher— some 20–30 times that in the medium. Furthermore, only cysts formed of proximal tubules secrete phenol red; those of distal tubules do not. When dye is injected into the lumen of a tubular cyst, the cells take up little or none. Accordingly, the apical aspect of the cell must be effectively impermeable to phenol red. If a cyst forms so that one wall is supplied by the glass of a cover slip, dye is secreted. However, isolated cells or those at the ends of a tubular fragment take up no dye. Loosening of the cells, one from another, by omission of Ca^{++} ions from the culture medium stops secretion. Chambers (10) remarked, "There seems to be a significant relation between the constrained shape of cells and their functional polarity." Obviously, we are far from a true understanding of secretion.

Blood is supplied to the kidney of the adult chicken from two sources: the aorta and the veins draining the legs and pelvis. The aortic supply first perfuses the glomeruli and then the peritubular capillaries, as in the mammal. The venous portal supply enters the peritubular capillary plexes directly. If a solution containing PAH and inulin is infused into the saphenous vein of one leg and if urine is collected separately from the two kidneys by catheters introduced into the cloacal ureteral orifices, it will be observed that inulin is excreted at equal rates by the two kidneys. whereas PAH is largely eliminated by the kidney on the side infused. The reason is obvious: inulin passes through the peritubular capillary network, enters the systemic circulation and is filtered at equal rates by the glomeruli of both kidneys; but PAH is largely extracted from the peritubular capillaries and secreted into the tubular urine on the side infused, so that little enters the systemic circulation and, therefore, little reaches the opposite kidney.

SITE OF SECRETORY MECHANISM FOR PAH, PHENOL RED, ETC.—The secretory mechanism for PAH, phenol red, etc., is localized in and restricted to the proximal tubule. Marine fish, which have only a single renal tubular segment, homologous with the proximal tubule of higher forms, secrete the several substances transported by the organic acid secretory mechanism. Secretion of phenol red can be observed under the microscope only in the living blood-perfused proximal tubules of the frog and *Necturus*. In cultures of cysts of the mesonephros of the chick embryo, only those derived from the proximal segment secrete phenol red into their lumens. Finally, stop-flow studies definitely establish the proximal site of secretion of PAH in the dog (see Figure 6–10, p. 91).

SECRETORY CLEARANCE.—The clearance of PAH, phenol red, etc., is very high at low plasma concentrations and decreases with increasing plasma concentration to approach the inulin clearance asymptotically. The general relationships are described in Figure 8–2, in which the clearance of PAH is related to plasma concentration. An explanation of this curvilinear relationship requires reference to Figure 8–1. Over a range of

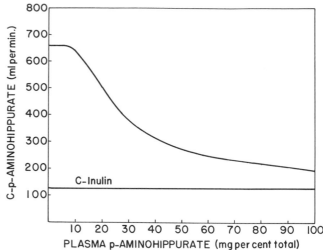

Fig. 8–2.—Clearance of p-aminohippurate as a function of plasma concentration in man.

1–8 mg/100 ml of plasma, PAH clearance is constant and equal to 660 ml/min. From Figure 8–1, it is evident that, over this range, the rate of excretion, $U_{PAH} \cdot V$, varies in direct proportion to the plasma concentration, P_{PAH}. Therefore, the total clearance, $U_{PAH} \cdot V/P_{PAH}$, is constant. Total clearance is equal to the glomerular clearance plus the tubular clearance. Glomerular clearance is equal to the rate of filtration of PAH divided by the plasma concentration, and it remains constant at all plasma levels. Over a range of 1–8 mg/100 ml, the tubular clearance likewise remains constant, because the rate of tubular secretion increases in exact proportion to the plasma level. However, at plasma concentrations in excess of 10 mg/100 ml, the secretory mechanism becomes saturated. Because the rate of secretion remains constant with increasing plasma concentration, tubular clearance progressively decreases. The sums of a constant glomerular clearance and a declining tubular clearance account for the curvilinear decrease in total clearance evident in Figure 8–2. At plasma concentrations sufficient to saturate the secretory mechanism, the following relationship holds:

At a plasma concentration of 60 mg/100 ml of PAH,

$$\frac{U_{PAH} \cdot V}{C_{PAH}} = \frac{125 \text{ ml/min} \cdot 0.6 \text{ mg/ml} \cdot 0.9}{0.6 \text{ mg/ml}} + \frac{80 \text{ mg/min}}{0.6 \text{ mg/ml}}$$

$$C_{PAH} = 113 \text{ ml/min} + 133 \text{ ml/min} = 246 \text{ ml/min}$$

As plasma concentration is further increased, the ratio Tm_{PAH}/P_{PAH} progressively declines, to reach zero at infinitely high plasma concentrations. One might expect $C_{in} \cdot P_{PAH} \cdot F \cdot W/P_{PAH}$ to remain constant at 113 ml/min at all plasma levels. Therefore, the asymptote that C_{PAH} would approach at infinitely high plasma levels would be $C_{in} \cdot 0.9$; i.e., 90% of filtration rate. Obviously, the experiment has never been performed and never will be; but, if plasma concentration could be raised to infinity, the fraction of the PAH bound to plasma protein would approach zero and the clearance of PAH would become equal to the clearance of inulin.

TUBULAR SECRETION OF CREATININE IN MAN.—In man, the tubular secretion of creatinine is apparently effected by the same mechanism as that which transports Diodrast, PAH, etc. The creatinine/inulin clearance ratio in normal man averages 1.4 at

$$\underset{\text{Total clearance}}{\frac{U_{PAH} \cdot V}{P_{PAH}}} = \underset{\text{Glomerular clearance}}{\frac{C_{in} \cdot P_{PAH} \cdot F \cdot W}{P_{PAH}}} + \underset{\text{Tubular clearance}}{\frac{Tm_{PAH}}{P_{PAH}}}$$

low plasma concentrations of creatinine—a fact that indicates definite, although slight, renal tubular secretion (11). Tm creatinine is small: on average, 16 mg/min. As the plasma creatinine level is elevated, the clearance ratio decreases, in line with the behavior of compounds actively secreted by Tm-limited mechanisms. The clearance ratio is immediately depressed to 1.0 by the administration of large amounts of Diodrast, PAH or carinamide (12). Tubular secretion of creatinine in the rat is also suppressed by PAH and Diodrast.

For many years, the renal tubules of the dog, sheep and seal have been considered to be qualitatively different from those of the rat, ape and man, in that the former are unable to secrete creatinine. Evidence of Swanson et al. (13) and O'Connell et al. (14) suggests that the differences may be quantitative rather than qualitative. The creatinine and inulin clearances of the dog are the same, within limits of experimental error, under conventional free-flow conditions. However, in stop-flow experiments the proximal U/P ratios for creatinine exceed those for inulin. By slowing or stopping flow and filtration, one exaggerates the contribution of creatinine secretion to final urine composition. Although this observation renders the creatinine U/P ratio suspect as a measure of water reabsorption in stop-flow experiments, the minute contribution of secretion to the creatinine clearance in conventional experiments does not introduce a significant error in its use as a measure of glomerular filtration.

Recent evidence of Selkurt, referred to earlier, suggests that the secretion of creatinine in the squirrel monkey involves the organic base secretory mechanism to be described subsequently. Transport by this mechanism seems logical in view of the fact that creatinine is a base. Perhaps the apparent competition of substances secreted by the organic acid mechanism with creatinine is of a nonspecific character and thus may not indicate true competition for a common transport mechanism.

TUBULAR SECRETION OF UREA IN THE BULLFROG.—The tubular secretion of urea in the bullfrog is a function of the organic acid secretory mechanism. Forster (15) showed that urea secretion is completely blocked by DNP and probenecid and depressed significantly by the infusion of PAH. Again, it is unknown why the secretory mechanism transports urea in the bullfrog but not in its amphibian relative *Necturus*. Furthermore, no evidence for urea secretion exists in higher vertebrate species that actively transport phenol red, PAH, etc. However, it may be that urea is secreted in these species, but in amounts so small and so outweighed by reabsorption that experimental demonstration is impossible. It is evident that the secretory mechanism, although basically the same, is not identical in all species. Evolutionary modifications occur sporadically throughout the animal kingdom.

Owen, Robinson, Schmidt-Nielsen and Shrauger (16–18) observed that arginase is present in varying amounts in the kidneys of a number of vertebrate species—which suggests that urea may be formed in the kidney by reactions of the Krebs-Henseleit cycle and secreted into the urine passively. This view is strengthened by the fact that urea is produced in homogenates of kidneys of frogs and mammals from existing substrate and that urea is produced in increased amounts by the kidneys of frogs and chickens in vivo when arginine is administered parenterally. However, at normal plasma levels of arginine, no significant amount of urea is produced in the kidney, and the weight of evidence is against the view that the reactions of the Krebs-Henseleit cycle are in any way involved in the net transport of urea across the renal tubules of the frog.

FUNCTIONAL MEASUREMENT OF TUBULAR MASS.—Tm_{PAH} (80 mg/min), $Tm_{Diodrast}$ (57 mg of iodine per minute) and $Tm_{phenol\ red}$ (36 mg/min) are used as measures of functional tubular mass (more specifically, as measures of proximal tubular mass) in the assessment of renal function in man. Because of the ease and precision of analysis, Tm_{PAH} is the measurement of choice. Although numerically different, the functional significance of Tm_{PAH} is the same as that of $Tm_{glucose}$. In chronic renal disease, both diminish in rough proportion to tubular destruction and replacement fibrosis. In acute renal disease, the correlation is less evident, for Tm values are depressed not only by loss of secretory and reabsorptive tissue but also by biochemical sickness of intact cells. The nature of these relationships will be considered in Chapter 13, on renal disease.

SECRETION OF STRONG ORGANIC BASES

A group of normal constituents of plasma and urine, and certain synthetic compounds as well, all of which are strong organic bases, are secreted by a single transport mechanism. Fourteen such compounds are listed in Table 8 – 1; half of them occur naturally, and the remainder are foreign synthetic materials. Some are amines; others are quaternary ammonium compounds (19).

SECRETORY MECHANISM TRANSPORTING STRONG ORGANIC BASES. — The general characteristics of this mechanism are much like those described for the mechanism that secretes organic acids. In 1947, Rennick *et al.* (20) observed that tetraethylammonium (TEA) is rapidly excreted by the kidney of the dog. TEA/creatinine clearance ratios varied between 2.0 and 2.5 at low plasma levels. As the plasma concentration of TEA increased, the clearance ratio declined. Tm_{TEA} amounts to 1 – 1.4 mg/min per square meter of surface area in the dog.

It has been impossible to establish whether or not most of the other strong bases exhibit Tm limitation of transport. When administered in the large quantities needed to saturate the transport mechanism, they give rise to profound pharmacologic responses, which render suspect any conclusion concerning the existence of a Tm. Because of these pharmacologic responses, much of the work on secretion has been performed on mammalian renal cortical slices or in experiments in which the bases have been infused

TABLE 8-1.—STRONG ORGANIC BASES SECRETED BY MAMMAL AND BIRD TUBULE*

NATURALLY OCCURRING COMPOUNDS	FOREIGN SYNTHETIC COMPOUNDS
Guanidine	Tetraethylammonium (TEA)
Methylguanidine	Tetramethylammonium (TMA)
Piperidine	Tetrabutylammonium (TBA)
N^1-methylnicotinamide (NMN)	Trimethyloctylammonium
Thiamine	Mepiperphenidol (Darstine)
Choline	Tolazoline (Priscoline)
Histamine	Hexamethonium

*From Peters, L.: Pharmacol. Rev. 12:1, 1960.

into the renal portal system of the chicken.

COMPETITION FOR A SINGLE TRANSPORT MECHANISM. — Such a competition has been demonstrated in studies of the effect of one base on the accumulation of others in tissue slices (19). The uptake of TEA by the slices has been inhibited by the addition, to the medium, of tolazoline, piperidine, guanidine and methylguanidine. Similarly, the uptake of N^1-methylnicotinamide (NMN) has been inhibited by the addition of tolazoline, mepiperphenidol, choline, guanidine and methylguanidine. Sperber (21) showed that many of these bases interfere with the excretion of others when infused into the renal portal system of chickens. Finally, Kandel and Peters (22) observed the depression of NMN secretion by the infusion of mepiperphenidol in the dog and the reverse depression of mepiperphenidol secretion by the infusion of NMN. NMN also competes with TEA for secretion in the chicken.

A cyanine dye, no. 863, suppresses the secretion of strong organic bases by the kidney of the intact dog and chicken and reduces the uptake of these bases by renal cortical slices (19). Inhibition is long-lasting; the dye is accumulated in tubular cells in high concentration; and excretion is extremely slow, continuing over a period of some 96 hours. The parallelism of the effect of cyanine no. 863 on the strong base secretory mechanism and that of probenecid

(Benemid) and carinamide on the organic acid secretory mechanism is evident. Cyanine gets tangled in the secretory machinery and, because of its extremely high affinity for the carrier, blocks the secretion of other strong bases.

Competition for secretion among strong bases has the same explanation as competition among strong acids: the existence of a limited amount of a carrier component with which the transported materials combine. A strong base of high affinity for the carrier displaces other strong bases of lower affinity. Similarly, one presented in large amounts displaces others, even though its affinity may be somewhat less, because secretory competition obeys the mass law. In studies on the chicken kidney, the order of decreasing affinity for the secretory transport mechanism is mepiperphenidol, tetrabutylammonium (TBA), trimethyloctylammonium, tolazoline, tetraethylammonium (TEA), tetramethylammonium (TMA), N^1-methylnicotinamide (NMN) and choline. In the dog kidney, the order of decreasing affinity is Darstine, tolazoline, TEA, choline, methylguanidine and guanidine.

SPECIFICITY OF TRANSPORT MECHANISM FOR STRONG BASES. — The specificity of the transport mechanism for strong bases is well established. Abundant evidence shows that none of the members of the organic acid group of compounds competes with or depresses the secretion of strong bases. Conversely, none of the strong bases competes with or depresses the secretion of organic acids. These findings hold whether the test system is the intact kidney of the dog (or chicken) or slices of mammalian renal cortex. Although the two secretory mechanisms have a number of properties in common, they are biochemically and functionally independent (19).

METABOLIC REQUIREMENTS OF STRONG-BASE SECRETION. — The metabolic requirements of strong base secretion are less well defined than are those of organic acid secretion. A continuous supply of oxidative energy is necessary for the transport of ma-

terials by both systems. Furthermore, both depend on phosphate bond energy, because transport by both mechanisms is depressed by DNP in the intact dog kidney and in renal cortical slices. In the intact kidney of the dog, DNP has no effect on simultaneously measured glucose or amino acid transport. Therefore, the effect of the inhibitor is specifically related to depression of secretory transport, not to alteration of cell permeability or to loss of integrity of cell structure.

The effects of the addition of acetate, pyruvate and lactate on the uptake of strong bases is not especially prominent. Malonate and fluoroacetate, which suppress secretion of PAH in vivo, have no effect on TEA transport. One may tentatively conclude that the energy for TEA transport, and presumably for transport of other strong bases, comes from oxidative mechanisms not obligatorily dependent on the citric acid cycle.

SECRETORY CARRIER OF STRONG BASES. — That the secretory carrier of strong bases may be a phospholipid is suggested by the fact that cyanine dyes and transportable strong bases bind to the phospholipid fraction of homogenates of rabbit kidney. The fraction most active in the binding of strong bases is the cephalin fraction made up of phosphatidylserine, phosphatidylethanolamine and phosphatidylinositol. Because these components have a negative charge, owing to their phosphate groups, they may be able to bind cationic strong bases reversibly in the course of transport. The fact that cell membranes contain phospholipids tempts one to place carrier molecules either at the peritubular border or the luminal border (19).

SITE OF SECRETION OF STRONG BASES. — Like that of organic acids, the site of secretion of strong bases is the proximal tubule. This is indicated not only by the fact that these compounds are secreted by the kidneys of marine fish, which have only a proximal tubule, but also by stop-flow studies in the dog, carried out by Rennick (20). The region that secretes TEA in the dog is coextensive with that which secretes PAH.

EDTA Secretory Mechanism

Foreman *et al.* (23) in 1953 first observed that the anion ethylenediaminetetraacetate (EDTA), administered parenterally to rats as the calcium chelate, is rapidly excreted in the urine: some 95–98% is eliminated in 6 hours. They inferred that its excretion involved both glomerular filtration and tubular secretion. Heller and Vostal (24) subsequently noted that the clearance of EDTA in the rat is comparable to that of Diodrast and is some 4 times that of inulin. The secretion of EDTA is unaffected by the simultaneous administration of PAH, Diodrast or probenecid. Neither is it affected by the administration of quinine. Thus the secretory system appears to be different from those for organic acids and bases. Secretion is not affected by changes in pH of the urine; therefore it is not dependent on mechanisms that involve non-ionic diffusion. Furthermore, in the chicken, EDTA is eliminated solely by glomerular filtration. The bird kidney lacks the ability to secrete EDTA, whereas it secretes organic acids and bases copiously. Relatively little is known of the properties and energy requirements of the EDTA secretory mechanism or of other substances secreted by it.

Active Secretion by Gradient-Time-Limited Mechanisms

Hydrogen ions are transported from tubular cells into tubular fluid along the entire length of the nephron against an electrochemical gradient. Thus, transport is active. However, the gradient, against which transport occurs, differs in the several segments of the nephron. The proximal tubule can establish a hydrogen ion gradient no greater than 0.4 pH unit between blood and tubular fluid, whereas the collecting duct can establish a gradient as high as 3 pH units. The proximal tubule is specialized to secrete large numbers of hydrogen ions against a small gradient, whereas the collecting duct is specialized to transport small numbers of hydrogen ions against a high gradient. In severe acidosis, the kidney can produce urine no more acid than pH 4.4; therefore it is obvious that the maximum hydrogen ion gradient the collecting duct can establish is approximately 1,000:1. Large quantities of hydrogen ions are secreted by the renal tubules if the intracellular concentration is high and if the transtubular gradient is maintained at a low value by the presence in the urine of large quantities of buffer of favorable pK. If the intracellular concentration is low, relatively few hydrogen ions are secreted.

Formerly, it was thought that hydrogen ions and potassium ions are secreted by a common mechanism and that the relatively more abundant intracellular ion could displace the relatively less abundant ion from the transport mechanism. Thus, in hyperkalemia, potassium ions were thought to displace hydrogen ions from the transport mechanism, restricting their excretion and resulting in acidosis. Conversely, in hypokalemia, hydrogen ions were thought to displace potassium ions from the transport mechanism, resulting in alkalosis. This view is no longer tenable; for, as shown by Giebisch *et al.* (27), the secretion of potassium is passive and is determined by the transtubular potential gradient that exists across the distal tubule and the collecting duct. However, reciprocal variations in excretion of hydrogen ions and potassium ions just described are real, although the basis for their interactions must be reinterpreted. In hyperkalemia, the potassium concentration within tubular cells is high, and the hydrogen ion concentration is relatively low. Few hydrogen ions are actively secreted; much potassium is passively secreted down the transtubular potential gradient. In hypokalemia, the concentration of potassium ions within tubular cells is relatively low and that of hydrogen ions is higher than normal. Accordingly, hydrogen ions are copiously secreted, whereas potassium ions are conserved. The secretion of hydrogen ions is described in detail in Chapter 11.

Passive Tubular Secretion

Passive tubular secretion, like passive tubular reabsorption, implies transfer of material down an electrochemical gradient. No energy is expended directly in moving the transported substance, although energy is required for the establishment of the gradient down which passive diffusion occurs. The secretion of weak bases and the secretion of weak acids illustrate passive transport down gradients of concentration of the undissociated, lipid-soluble, permeant molecular species. The secretion of potassium illustrates passive transport of a readily permeating ion down a gradient of transtubular potential.

DIFFUSION TRAPPING OF WEAK BASES

The rate of excretion of a number of weak bases, including quinine, quinacrine, procaine, chloroquine, neutral red and ammonia, is greatly augmented if the urine is acidified by the administration of ammonium chloride. If the urine is alkalized, either by the infusion of sodium bicarbonate or by the administration of acetazolamide, the rates of excretion of weak bases are reduced. Changing the pH of the urine from 8 to 5 may alter the clearances of these substances from low values, indicative of marked reabsorption, to very high values, indicative of tubular secretion (25, 26).

The pK values of these weak bases vary over a range of 6.85–9.35. Therefore, at the pH of blood plasma they exist as equilibrium mixtures of the charged cationic species and the uncharged free base; the lower the pK, the greater is the proportion of uncharged free base. The lipid solubility of the free base is much greater than that of the cationic form. Therefore, the free base penetrates cell membranes much more readily than does the ionic species.

In acid urine, weak bases also exist as equilibrium mixtures of ionized and union-ized forms, but the equilibrium is shifted in favor of the cationic form; i.e., free base binds hydrogen ion to form cation. Accordingly, free base diffuses from peritubular fluid at pH 7.4 through tubular cells and into urine of pH 5, where hydrogen ions are bound to convert the diffusible base into nonpenetrating cation. A gradient of concentration down which the free base can diffuse is maintained as long as the urine is more acid than the blood. If the urine is alkalized, and especially if urine pH is about 8, the gradient for diffusion is reversed, and the weak base delivered into the tubules in the glomerular filtrate is reabsorbed passively by diffusion into peritubular fluid.

Passive secretion of weak bases is best described as diffusion trapping; i.e., diffusion of the free base through tubular cells and trapping of the ionic species within the tubular urine. For diffusion to continue, energy must be supplied—not to move the weak base but to maintain the hydrogen ion gradient between peritubular fluid and tubular urine. If the pH of the urine is low, the gradient of the free base is high and the rate of diffusion is little affected by urine flow. If the pH of the urine is only slightly below that of the blood, the rate of diffusion becomes dependent on urine flow. The higher the flow, the greater is the diffusion of free base, merely because the free base is continually removed in the urine and fresh filtrate is supplied—filtrate into which further diffusion can occur.

An alternative view is that weak bases are actively secreted in the proximal tubule by the same mechanism that transports strong bases (19, 27). If the urine becomes alkaline in the distal portions of the nephron, the ratio of free base to cationic base alters in favor of the free base. Back diffusion of the free base occurs, leading to net reabsorption. However, if the urine becomes acid, rather than alkaline, in the distal portions of the nephron, the ratio of free base to cationic base alters in favor of the cationic base. No back diffusion occurs, and net secretion, established in the proximal tubule, is maintained. The passive secretion of the weak base, ammonia, will be further considered in Chapter 11, on the renal regulation of acid-base balance.

DIFFUSION TRAPPING OF WEAK ACIDS

Theoretically, a weak acid, present in part in undissociated form in blood plasma of pH 7.4, can diffuse into alkaline urine, dissociate hydrogen ion and be converted into nondiffusible anion. Because the urine, as it leaves the renal tubules, is never more alkaline than pH 8.2, the maximum concentration gradient of undissociated weak acid between plasma and alkaline urine is less than 10:1. Accordingly, diffusion processes are less likely to be important in the secretion of weak acids than in that of weak bases.

In fact, only two weak acids—salicylic acid and phenobarbital—have been shown to be excreted by a diffusion-trapping secretory mechanism. The clearance of salicylate in acid urine is less than the inulin clearance, indicating reabsorption. When the urine is alkalized by the administration of sodium bicarbonate or acetazolamide or by hyperventilation, the clearance of salicylate exceeds the inulin clearance, indicating tubular secretion. The phenobarbital clearance varies in a similar manner with change in urine pH. The administration of sodium bicarbonate is, therefore, of value in the treatment of patients with salicylate and phenobarbital intoxication. However, both drugs can be more rapidly removed from the body by dialysis with the artificial kidney (see treatment of uremia).

Weiner and Mudge (28) proposed that weak acids are secreted in the proximal tubule by the organic acid secretory mechanism and are passively reabsorbed by nonionic diffusion in more distal portions of the nephron when the urine is acidified. Such a view is not incompatible with passive secretion of at least minor proportions; for, if the tubule is sufficiently permeable to the undissociated species to permit passive back diffusion, it would no doubt permit passive diffusion into the tubule in a secretory direction as well, if an appreciable amount of undissociated acid exists in plasma.

PASSIVE SECRETION OF POTASSIUM

Under normal conditions, the clearance of potassium is only 20% or so of the simultaneously determined rate of glomerular filtration. Accordingly, filtered potassium is largely reabsorbed. Some years ago, it was observed that, in patients with chronic renal disease and markedly reduced rates of glomerular filtration, the clearance of potassium approaches, and may occasionally exceed, the inulin clearance; this suggests tubular secretion. In 1948, Berliner, Mudge, Gilman and their respective associates observed the net secretion of potassium in the normal dog. The secretion of potassium is enhanced by loading the animal with potassium salts, by alkalizing the urine and by loading with salts of nonreabsorbable or poorly reabsorbed anions, such as ferrocyanide and sulfate. Net secretion is also rendered more apparent if the rate of glomerular filtration is reduced by partial obstruction of the aorta above the origins of the renal arteries.

An interesting phenomenon is that of conditioning of potassium secretion by repeated loading with potassium salts. If a normal dog is given 5–10 Gm of potassium chloride orally each day for a week and then given an infusion containing the salt, the rate of secretion of potassium is greatly enhanced in comparison with that observed in an animal not so conditioned. Renal conditioning of potassium secretion, acute loading with potassium salts and the infusion of poorly reabsorbed anions (including excess bicarbonate) all operate to increase potassium secretion, either by raising the potassium concentration within tubular cells or by enhancing the transtubular potential gradient across distal tubules and collecting ducts.

SITES OF POTASSIUM TRANSPORT. — According to Giebisch et al. (27), filtered potassium is actively reabsorbed against a small concentration gradient as urine flows through proximal tubules. A gradient of 0.8:1 is maintained throughout the proximal segment between tubular fluid and plasma. About five sixths of the filtrate is reabsorbed by the time the fluid leaves the proximal tubule; therefore it is obvious that the bulk of the filtered load of potassium is reabsorbed in this segment, as was postulated earlier by Davidson *et al.* (29). Most of the potassium excreted in the urine is added by passive secretion as the urine flows through distal tubules and collecting ducts. The quantity of potassium added at these sites is determined largely by the intracellular concentration of potassium and by the transtubular potential gradient. If body stores of potassium, including those of tubular cells, are depleted, active reabsorption continues throughout the distal nephron, and minimal quantities are excreted in the urine.

Tubular Structure

Renal tubular cells are amazingly complicated bits of biochemical machinery enclosing a number of semi-independent reabsorptive and secretory mechanisms plus the several metabolic systems required to power them. Recent electron-microscopic studies have revealed an equally amazing complexity of cytologic structure (30). Unfortunately, our understanding of both structure and function is too inadequate to permit the formulation of any but the simplest correlations between the two. The following structural features appear, to a physiologist, to have the most evident correlation with function.

The luminal and basal surfaces of both proximal and distal tubular cells are tremendously increased by a complicated series of evaginations and invaginations of the plasma membrane. Figures 8–3 and 8–4 illustrate the dense population of the luminal surface with cylindrical evaginations called microvilli—the "brush border" of the light microscopists. These processes are 1 μ in length by 700 Å in diameter. They are covered by a plasma membrane about 50 Å thick. In fixed material, the lumen of the tubule is collapsed and the microvilli are clumped (some $215/\mu^2$), although in the living distended tubule they no doubt float freely in the tubular urine. Tiny coiled invaginations of the luminal membrane at the bases of the microvilli penetrate into the soma of proximal cells. Some of these microducts connect with cytoplasmic vacuoles. Microvilli and microducts are most numerous in the convoluted portions of the proximal tubule. They diminish in number in the descending thick limb of the loop of Henle and are present only in rudimentary form in the remainder of the nephron. The microvilli greatly increase the luminal surface of proximal cells, facilitating diffusion of materials into the cell from the tubular fluid. The microducts may be significant in the secretory activities of proximal cells.

The bases of the cuboidal cells making up both the proximal and the distal tubule project laterally along the basement membrane, much as buttress roots of a tree project from the base of the trunk. These projections extend under adjacent cells, infolding the basilar surface to form cytoplasmic lamellae. Not only do these lamellar infoldings greatly increase the basilar surface of the cells; they also lock adjacent cells together to form a tight tube. Mitochondria are lined within the channels formed by the multiple infoldings of the basilar plasma membrane, accounting for the striation described by light microscopists. The close association of mitochondria and basilar plasma membrane may well be significant for the transfer of energy to membrane carriers concerned with the extrusion of materials from, and the active concentration of materials within, tubular cells.

The apical borders of adjacent tubular cells are sealed by terminal bars, which, again, may be a specialization to form a tight tube. The sealing of chinks between cells insures the passage of materials across the limiting plasma membrane and prevents leakage between cells.

Finally, the delicate structure of the peritubular capillaries, consisting of a very thin

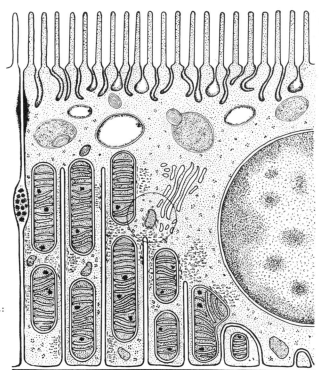

Fig. 8–3. — Schematic representation of the structure of a proximal tubular cell as revealed by electron microscopy. (From Rhodin, J.: Thesis, Karolinska Institute, Stockholm, 1954.)

fenestrated endothelial layer and a thin basement membrane, is such as to permit the ready transfer of water and solutes between tubular cells and blood stream. Although cytoplasmic organelles are numerous in all portions of the nephron, there is little evidence on which one can base inferences as to their function.

Summary

Three types of secretory mechanisms are involved in the transport of materials from peritubular fluid to tubular lumen: Tm-limited mechanisms, gradient-time-limited mechanisms and passive secretory mechanisms. Both Tm-limited and gradient-time-limited mechanisms are active and demand a continuous supply of energy to move the transported materials from blood to urine. Passive secretion occurs by diffusion down a gradient of concentration or of electrical potential. Although no energy is directly used in the movement of the transported material, maintenance of the hydrogen ion or potential gradient, down which diffusion occurs, requires the expenditure of energy.

Three Tm-limited mechanisms secrete a variety of organic compounds. One mechanism secretes a group of substances; many, but not all, of these are organic acids (phenol red, penicillin, PAH, Diodrast, etc.). The other secretes a group of strong organic bases (histamine, guanidinc, NMN, etc.). The substances secreted by either of these two mechanisms compete with each other for their common transport system. However, no cross-competition occurs between members of the two groups. Accordingly, the two mechanisms are discrete. Although these two secretory mechanisms are present throughout all vertebrate orders, minor evolutionary modifications have occurred sporadically to alter secretory transport of specific compounds. Creatinine is secreted in significant amounts by man but not by the dog. Urea is secreted by the frog but not by *Necturus*. The organic acid and organic base secretory mechanisms are localized in the proximal tubule. A third active secretory

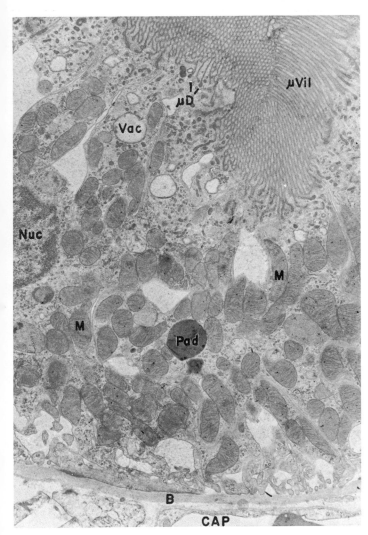

Fig. 8—4. — Electron micrograph of a proximal tubular cell of the rat, illustrating microvilli (μVil), microducts (μD), vacuole (Vac), nucleus (Nuc), protein absorption droplet (Pad), mitochondrion (M), basement membrane (B) and peritubular capillary (CAP). (Illustration prepared by Marilyn G. Farquhar.)

mechanism transports EDTA. Although little is known of the characteristics of this mechanism, it seems to be distinct from those transporting organic acids and bases.

Hydrogen ions are transported by an active mechanism, which exhibits gradient and perhaps time limitation of transport capacity. This mechanism is present throughout the length of the nephron but is differently specialized in its several parts. In the proximal tubule, the mechanism is specialized to transport large quantities of hydrogen ions against a small concentration gradient. In the collecting duct, the mechanism is specialized to transport small quantities of hydrogen ions against a large gradient.

A series of weak bases and at least two weak acids are passively secreted by a mechanism of diffusion trapping. Renal tubules are permeable to the undissociated weak base and the undissociated weak acid and are impermeable to the cationic and anionic forms, respectively. Accordingly, undissociated weak bases diffuse into acid urine, where they bind hydrogen ions to become cations to which the tubules are impermeable. As long as the urine is more acidic than the blood, a gradient will exist in favor of the diffusion of undissociated base from peritubular fluid to tubular lumen. Conversely, undissociated weak acids diffuse into alkaline urine, where they dissociate hydrogen ions to become anions to which the tubules are impermeable. As long as the urine is more alkaline than the blood, a gradient favoring the diffusion of undissociated acid from peritubular fluid to tubular urine will exist. Accordingly, the clearance of weak bases (ammonia, quinine, quinacrine, etc.) is greater in acidic than in alkaline urine, whereas the clearance of weak acids, such as salicylic and phenobarbital, is greater in alkaline than in acidic urine. Passive secretion of weak bases and of weak acids occurs in all regions of the tubule but is most evident in those in which the highest hydrogen ion gradients are established; i.e., its terminal portions.

The secretion of potassium ions is passive and occurs down a gradient of potential established by the active reabsorption of sodium ions. Normally, only 10–20% of the filtered load of potassium is excreted; the remainder is reabsorbed. However, when potassium salts or the sodium salts of poorly absorbed anions are administered, the potassium excreted may exceed the filtered load. The bulk of the excreted potassium is added to the tubular urine in the distal tubules and collecting ducts.

REFERENCES

1. Shannon, J. A.: Renal tubular excretion, Physiol. Rev. 19:63, 1939.
2. Beyer, K. H.: Functional characteristics of renal transport mechanisms, Pharm. Rev. 2:227, 1950.
3. Beyer, K. H., Peters, L., Woodward, R., and Verwey, W. F.: The enhancement of the physiological economy of penicillin in dogs by the simultaneous administration of para-amino-hippuric acid, J. Pharmacol. & Exper. Therap. 82:310, 1944.
4. Taggart, J. V., and Forster, R. P.: Renal tubular transport: Effects of 2,4-dinitrophenol and related compounds on phenol red transport in the isolated tubules of the flounder, Am. J. Physiol. 161:167, 1950.
5. Taggart, J. V.: Mechanisms of renal tubular transport, Am. J. Med. 24:774, 1958.
6. Hoeber, R.: *Physical Chemistry of Cells and Tissues* (Philadelphia: Blakiston Company, 1945).
7. Puck, T. T., Wasserman, K., and Fishman, A.: Some effects of inorganic ions on the active transport of phenol red by isolated kidney tubules of the flounder, J. Cell. & Comp. Physiol. 40:73, 1952.
8. Foulkes, E. C., and Miller, B. F.: Steps in p-aminohippurate transport by kidney slices, Am. J. Physiol. 196:86, 1959.
9. Chamber, R., and Kempton, R. T.: Indications of function of the chick mesonephros in tissue culture with phenol red, J. Cell. & Comp. Physiol. 3:131, 1933.
10. Chambers, R.: The relation of extraneous coats to the organization and permeability of cellular membranes, Cold Spring Harbor Symp. Quant. Biol. 8:144, 1950.
11. Shannon, J. A.: The renal excretion of creatinine in man, J. Clin. Invest. 14:403, 1935.
12. Crawford, B.: Depression of exogenous creatinine/inulin or thiosulfate clearance ratios in man by Diodrast and p-aminohippuric acid, J. Clin. Invest. 27:171, 1948.
13. Swanson, R. E., and Hakins, A. A.: Stop-flow analysis of creatinine excretion in the dog, Am. J. Physiol. 203:980, 1962.
14. O'Connell, J. M. B., Romeo, J. A., and Mudge, G. H.: Renal tubular secretion of creatinine in the dog, Am. J. Physiol. 203:985, 1962.
15. Forster, R. P.: Active cellular transport of urea by the frog renal tubules, Am. J. Physiol. 179:372, 1954.
16. Owen, E. E., and Robinson, R. R.: Urea production and excretion by chicken kidney, Am. J. Physiol. 206:1321, 1964.
17. Robinson, R. R., and Schmidt-Nielsen, B.: Distribution of arginase within kidneys of several vertebrate species, J. Cell. & Comp. Physiol. 62:147, 1963.
18. Schmidt-Nielsen, B., and Shrauger, C. R.: Handling of urea and related compounds by the renal tubules of the frog, Am. J. Physiol. 205:483, 1963.
19. Peters, L.: Renal tubular excretion of organic bases, Pharmacol. Rev. 12:1, 1960.
20. Rennick, B. R., Moe, G. K., Lyons, R. H., Hoobler, S. W., and Neligh, R.: Absorption and renal excretion of the tetraethylammonium ion, J. Pharmacol. & Exper. Therap. 91:210, 1947.
21. Sperber, I.: Competitive inhibition and specificity of renal tubular transport mechanisms, Arch. internat. pharmacodyn. 97:221, 1954.
22. Kandel, A., and Peters, L.: Observations concerning the renal tubular transport characteristics of three quaternary bases in dogs, J. Pharmacol. & Exper. Therap. 119:550, 1957.
23. Foreman, H., Vier, M., and Magee, M.: The

metabolism of C^{14}-labeled ethylenediamine-tetraacetic acid in the rat, J. Biol. Chem. 203:1045, 1953.

24. Heller, J., and Vostal, J.: Renal excretion of calcium-disodium ethylenediaminetetraacetic acid, Experientia 20:99, 1964.

25. Orloff, J., and Berliner, R.: The mechanism of excretion of ammonia in the dog, J. Clin. Invest. 35:223, 1956.

26. Milne, M. D., Scribner, B. H., and Crawford, M. A.: Non-ionic diffusion and the excretion of weak acids and bases, Am. J. Med. 24:709, 1958.

27. Giebisch, G., Klose, R. M., and Malnic, G.

H.: Renal tubular potassium transport, Proc. 3rd Internat. Congr. Nephrology. Washington, D. C., 1966, 1967.

28. Weiner, I. M., and Mudge, G. H.: Renal tubular mechanisms for excretion of organic acids and bases, Am. J. Med. 36:743, 1964.

29. Davidson, D. G., Levinsky, N. G., and Berliner, R. W.: Maintenance of potassium excretion despite reduction of glomerular filtration during sodium diuresis, J. Clin. Invest. 37:548, 1958.

30. Rhodin, J.: Electron microscopy of the kidney, Am. J. Med. 24:661, 1958.

Renal Circulation

Measurement of Renal Blood Flow

As WAS POINTED OUT in the preceding chapter, the clearance of PAH is very high and is independent of plasma concentration over a range of from 1 to 6 or 8 mg/100 ml. Both facts suggest that within this range the clearance of PAH may be limited by, and be a measure of, renal plasma flow. The PAH clearance in normal man at low plasma levels averages 660 ml/min per 1.73 m² of surface area. If the hematocrit is 45%, renal blood flow must be no less than $660 \cdot 1/(1-0.45)$, or 1,200 ml/min. Because the resting cardiac output of normal man is 5–6 L/min, the kidneys must receive one fourth to one fifth of the blood ejected by the heart each minute. That the kidneys should receive significantly more would be difficult even for a dedicated renal physiologist to concede. In fact, all evidence suggests that the apparent or

minimum effective renal blood flow measured by the plasma clearance of PAH and hematocrit represents some 90% of total blood flow through the kidneys of normal man. Indeed, Smith (1) maintained that it measures the true rate of blood perfusion of excretory tissue; the remaining 10% perfuses capsule, pelvis and perinephric fat (i.e., non-excretory tissues).

FICK PRINCIPLE

PAH CLEARANCE FOR MEASURING MINIMUM EFFECTIVE RENAL PLASMA FLOW. — The use of the PAH clearance in measuring minimum effective renal plasma flow is an extension of the well-known Fick principle used in measuring cardiac output. In this latter role, the following equation applies:

$$\text{Cardiac output} = \frac{\dot{Q}_{02}}{A_{02} - V_{02}}$$

where $\dot{Q}_{0_2}$ represents the milliliters of oxygen consumed by the person each minute and A_{0_2} and V_{0_2} represent, respectively, the oxygen contents of 1 ml of arterial blood and of 1 ml of mixed venous blood. If the oxygen consumption at rest is 240 ml/min and the arterial and mixed venous oxygen contents are 0.2 ml and 0.16 ml, respectively, per milliliter of blood, then

$$\text{Cardiac output} = \frac{240 \text{ ml/min.}}{0.20 \text{ ml/ml} - 0.16 \text{ ml/ml}} = \frac{240}{0.04} = 6,000 \text{ ml/min}$$

In a similar vein, one can use the Fick principle in the measurement of renal plasma flow (RPF), as follows:

$$\text{RPF} = \frac{U_X \cdot V}{RA_X - RV_X}$$

where $U_x \cdot V$ represents the rate of excretion of a substance in milligrams per minute and RA_x and RV_x represent, respectively,

158

renal arterial and renal venous plasma concentrations of x in terms of milligrams per milliliter. The A-V difference is the amount of x removed from each ml of plasma as it perfuses the kidney. Dividing the A-V difference into rate of excretion yields the volume of plasma that must perfuse the kidney each minute to supply the quantity of x excreted.

With the Fick procedure, one may use any substance for the measurement of renal plasma flow, so long as it is excreted in the urine and is not used by or manufactured in the kidney. The mechanism of excretion is of no significance—whether filtered, secreted or partly reabsorbed. If a normal subject excretes 6.6 mg of urea nitrogen per minute and if arterial and renal venous concentrations are 0.1 and 0.09 mg of urea nitrogen per milliliter of plasma, then

$$\text{RPF} = \frac{6.6 \text{ mg/min}}{0.1 \text{ mg/ml} - 0.09 \text{ mg/ml}} = \frac{6.60}{0.01} = 660 \text{ ml/min}$$

From renal plasma flow and hematocrit, renal blood flow (RBF) is calculated as follows:

$$\text{RBF} = \text{RPF}\left(\frac{1}{1 - \text{Hct.}}\right)$$

Strictly speaking, the simple Fick formula is incorrect, because it neglects the fact that the renal venous outflow is less than the renal arterial inflow by the volume of urine flow. The error is small if urine flow is low and if extraction of the substance by the kidney is high. A formula that corrects this error has been devised by Wolf:

$$\text{RPF} = \frac{(U_X - RV_X) \cdot V}{(RA_X - RV_X)}$$

The difficulty in using the Fick method for the measurement of renal plasma flow is that of obtaining renal venous plasma. In the dog, one kidney can be explanted subcutaneously in the flank and a skin tube constructed around the renal vein. Renal venous blood can then be obtained by venipuncture with minimum disturbance to the animal. Arterial blood can, of course, be obtained by puncture of any peripheral artery, for its com-

position is the same throughout the body. Obviously, such heroic methods are inapplicable in man. However, it is possible to introduce a radiopaque cardiac catheter into a peripheral vein, maneuver it into the inferior vena cava and then direct it into a renal vein under fluoroscopic observation. In the author's experience with dogs, the procedure is by no means as difficult as it sounds. However, the technic is demanding and is unsuited for routine clinical studies.

BASIS FOR USE OF PAH CLEARANCE.—The basis for the use of the PAH clearance is the following: Let us assume for the moment that all of the PAH is removed from the blood in one passage through the kidney. If extraction is complete, the renal venous concentration is zero and the Fick formula reduces to the clearance formula

$$\text{RPF} = \frac{U_{\text{PAH}} \cdot V}{A_{\text{PAH}} - 0}$$

Because peripheral tissues extract no PAH from blood, one may use venous blood drawn from a superficial vein in the performance of a PAH clearance test. Arterial puncture is unnecessary.

PAH EXTRACTION.—The extraction of PAH in one passage through the kidney of normal man is, on an average, only 90% complete (1). Therefore, the true renal plasma flow exceeds the PAH clearance by about 10%. Although the PAH clearance is a reasonable approximation of true renal plasma flow in the normal human kidney, by no means does it have the same significance in the diseased kidney. The percentage of extraction (E), calculated by the equation

$$E_{\text{PAH}} = \frac{RA_{\text{PAH}} - RV_{\text{PAH}}}{RA_{\text{PAH}}} \cdot 100$$

progressively declines with damage to the renal parenchyma (see Chapter 13, on renal disease). Therefore, in renal disease, if one wishes a true measure of renal plasma flow, percentage of extraction must be determined and the clearance of PAH appropriately corrected. In the dog, the extraction of PAH is appreciably less nearly complete than in man, averaging 75–80%.

Not only the blood that perfuses the capsule, perirenal fat and pelvis but also that which perfuses the medulla and papilla contributes to reduced extraction. PAH is secreted only by proximal tubules; therefore, blood perfusing the medulla and papilla (i.e., that flowing in the vasa recta) has only that fraction of its PAH extracted that is removed by filtration (about one fifth in man).* Blood flow in the vasa recta is relatively low; nevertheless, it is probably equal to or greater than blood flow to inert renal tissues. The PAH clearance, therefore, represents more nearly cortical plasma flow than minimum effective plasma flow to the kidney as a whole.

DIODRAST CLEARANCE.—The Diodrast clearance at low plasma levels is equal to, and has the same functional significance as, the PAH clearance; therefore, both can be considered to represent minimum effective cortical plasma flow. Diodrast was used extensively in early studies, but, owing to difficulties of chemical analysis, it has now been entirely displaced by PAH and by ^{131}I-Diodrast. The latter is easily quantified by scintillation counting. The chemical analysis of PAH is relatively easy and remarkably precise.

NECESSITY FOR STEADY STATE.—The use of clearance methods for measurement of renal blood flow demands maintenance of a steady state during the period of measurement, which is usually 10–20 minutes. Plasma concentration of the test material, percentage of extraction, plasma flow and urine flow must all be constant during the test period. If any parameter varies, the flow measurement is in error in some degree. Accordingly, clearance methods are unreliable for measurement of flow transients, and physical instruments such as the bubble flowmeter, thermostromuhr or electromagnetic flowme-

ter must be used. Unfortunately, these instruments must be inserted into or placed around the renal artery; so they have not been used in studies on man. Furthermore, in order to use clearance methods, an adequate urine flow must be maintained, and this makes it impossible to use them under conditions of anuria. Despite these restrictions, most of our knowledge of the renal circulation has been derived from clearance studies. The phenol red clearance was actually the first to be used as an approximation of renal plasma flow, but, because of grossly incomplete extraction, it is no longer so used (1).

FILTRATION FRACTION.—If one measures simultaneously the clearance of inulin and the clearance of PAH at low plasma PAH concentrations, one may calculate the fraction of plasma that is filtered through the glomeruli:

$$\text{Filtration fraction} = \frac{C_{\text{in}}}{C_{\text{PAH}}} = \frac{125 \text{ ml/min}}{660 \text{ ml/min}} = 0.19$$

The filtration fraction in normal man is 16–20%; in the dog, 20–30%.

RENAL ISCHEMIA AND HYPEREMIA.—If the renal plasma flow of a person at rest is significantly less than 660 ml/min per 1.73 m² of surface area, absolute renal ischemia exists. In chronic renal disease, the renal vasculature is reduced more or less in proportion to the reduction of tubular mass. Whether or not the remaining tubular tissue is ischemic or hyperemic can be determined by performing PAH clearance measurements —first at low plasma concentrations, to measure renal plasma flow, and then at high plasma concentrations, to measure Tm_{PAH}.* Normally, the ratio of C_{PAH} to Tm_{PAH} is 660 ml/min to 80 mg/min, or 8.3 ml of plasma per milligram of Tm_{PAH}. In chronic renal disease, Tm_{PAH} is reduced because of destruction of tubules and replacement fibrosis. If the plas-

---

*Some PAH may be extracted by the most distal parts of the proximal tubules in their course through the outer medulla; i.e., by the thick descending limbs of Henle's loops.

*In renal disease, extraction of PAH must be measured to obtain a valid estimate of renal plasma flow. Furthermore, C_{PAH} and Tm_{PAH} must be measured consecutively and the assumption made that the infusion of large amounts of PAH during Tm measurement has not altered renal plasma flow.

ma flow per milligram of residual Tm_{PAH} is less than 8.3 ml, the renal tissue still functional is relatively ischemic. If plasma flow is greater, the functional renal tissue is relatively hyperemic. Variations in perfusion of tubular tissue characteristic of renal diseases are considered in Chapter 13.

RENAL BLOOD FLOW AND OXYGEN CONSUMPTION. — High blood flow in relation to kidney weight (i.e., 1,200 ml/min per 300 Gm in man) is more an expression of the renal processes involved in regulating the composition of extracellular fluid than of excessive metabolic demands. As a consequence, the renal arterial-venous oxygen difference is low: 1.7 ml of oxygen per 100 ml of blood, in comparison with an arterial-venous oxygen difference of 4 – 6 ml of oxygen per 100 ml of blood for the body as a whole (1). However, the kidneys of man, which constitute less than 0.5% of the weight of the body, consume some 8% of the oxygen used at rest (i.e., 20 ml/min). Obviously, the metabolic cost of renal function is considerable.

A number of years ago, the renal oxygen consumption of the dog was observed to vary more or less in proportion to blood flow. Thus, the renal arterial-venous oxygen difference remains constant and is independent of blood flow (2). In contrast, the oxygen consumption of other organs tends to remain constant, and the arterial-venous oxygen difference varies inversely with blood flow.

Recent observations have shed some light on this anomalous behavior of the kidney (3, 4). The significant variable is not blood flow but glomerular filtration rate. A reduction in blood flow (e.g., in consequence of reduced arterial pressure) is accompanied by a reduction in glomerular filtration rate. A large proportion of the energy turnover of the kidney is concerned with the active reabsorption of sodium. If less sodium is filtered, less is reabsorbed, and oxygen consumption decreases. The energy cost of reabsorption averages 1 micromole (μmol) of oxygen for each 24 – 28 μmol of sodium. In the dog, the oxygen consumption of the normally functioning kidney is 4 – 6 μmol/Gm per minute. If renal arterial pressure is reduced to such a value that filtration ceases, oxygen consumption falls to 1 – 1.5 μmol/Gm per minute; i.e., to one fourth to one sixth of normal. Accordingly, the energy requirements of tubular reabsorption, obligated by the high rate of glomerular filtration, account for three fourths to five sixths of the energy turnover of the kidney. As Homer Smith has so aptly stated: "There is enough waste motion here to bankrupt any economic system other than a natural one, for Nature is the only artificer who does not need to count the cost by which she achieves her ends."*

Control of Renal Circulation

The renal circulation is subject to two types of regulation: (1) an extrinsic hormonal and nervous regulation and (2) an intrinsic or autonomous autoregulation.

PRESSURE GRADIENTS AND RESISTANCE TO FLOW

The pressure gradients and sites of major resistance to flow within the kidney are illustrated in Figure 9–1. These pressure gradients are based on measurements in the rat and may not be precisely representative of all forms. According to Brenner, whose observations are described on p. 42, the glomerular capillary pressure is approximately half the aortic pressure and is of the order of 50 mm Hg. The afferent vessels that supply the glomerular capillary tufts and the efferent vessels that drain the tufts have the characteristics of arterioles. Smooth muscle fibers, richly supplied with sympathetic nerve endings, wind spirally around their lumens, exerting a sphincter-like action to control diameter and resistance to flow. It is evident, from Figure 9–1, that the pressure gradient across the efferent arteriole is less than that across the afferent arteriole when

*Smith, H. W.: *Lectures on the Kidney,* Porter Lecture Series IX (Lawrence, Kansas: University of Kansas Extension Division, 1943).

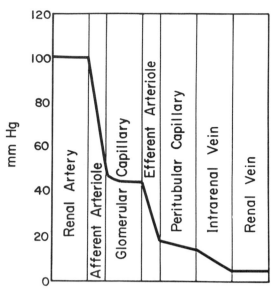

Fig. 9–1.—Pressure gradients in the renal circulation.

aortic pressure is normal. When aortic pressure increases, the afferent arteriole constricts further, to maintain constancy of glomerular capillary pressure. This reaction is independent of extrinsic nervous and hormonal control and therefore is termed "autoregulation." As a consequence of the reaction, the pressure drop across the afferent arteriole tends to exceed even more the drop across the efferent arteriole. In fact, under most conditions, the resistances of afferent and efferent arterioles are coordinated so as to maintain constancy of glomerular capillary pressure, and, therefore, constancy of filtration rate. The pressure within the peritubular capillary network is of the order of 15 mm Hg and is equal to the hydrostatic pressure within the renal tubules. The renal parenchyma is, therefore, under uniform and moderate positive pressure and is constrained by the inelastic capsule. The living blood-perfused kidney is firm to the touch. A third resistance, of small magnitude, is offered by the venous side of the peritubular capillary network. It may represent resistance imposed by compression of interlobar veins at the points where they leave the distended parenchyma and enter the loose areolar and adipose tissue of the renal sinus.

On the other hand, they, like the afferent and efferent arterioles, are innervated by sympathetic nerve fibers.

DISTRIBUTION OF FLOW WITHIN THE KIDNEY

The distribution of flow within the kidney is not uniform. This fact cannot be derived from clearance measurements of plasma flow, for at best such measurements yield over-all, rather than regional, flow rates. Several methods have been used to study the distribution of flow in the cortex, medulla and papilla of the dog. The first involves the fractional uptake of ^{42}K or ^{86}Rb (radioactive potassium or rubidium) by tissues in specific areas when one of these isotopes is administered by rapid intravenous injection. The animal is sacrificed immediately after the isotope is given, and the distribution of the isotope is measured in separated fragments of tissue. Under appropriate conditions, the rate of accumulation is proportional to blood flow. The second method involves the introduction of a microlight source into a given area, the placement of a photoelectric cell on the surface of the cortex or papilla, the injection of Evans blue into the renal artery and the recording of the dye-dilution curve. From measurements of local blood volume and mean transit time, flow rates can be calculated. Figure 9-2 illustrates the brisk entry and washout of dye in cortical vessels and the sluggish flow in medullary vessels (6). Flow in the cortex of the dog kidney is 4–5 ml/Gm per minute; in the medulla, 0.7 –1 ml/Gm per minute; and in the papilla, 0.2–0.25 ml/Gm per minute. Accordingly, of the total flow, only 1–2% perfuses the papilla, 8–10% the medulla and nearly 90% the cortex. Low blood perfusion of the medulla and papilla is of special significance in the operation of the countercurrent mechanism that concentrates the urine (see Chapter 7). In a third method, ^{85}Kr (radioactive krypton) dissolved in saline solution is rapidly injected into one renal artery of a dog through a chronically implanted catheter,

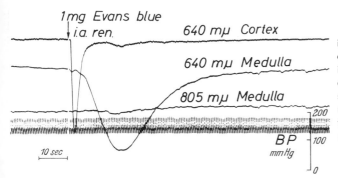

Fig. 9–2.—Dye-dilution curves inscribed by photocells monitoring cortex and medulla during the injection of Evans blue into the renal artery. Delayed appearance and sluggish disappearance of dye in the medulla are indicative of prolonged transit time and low blood perfusion rate. (Courtesy of K. Thurau.)

and the rate at which the radioactive material is washed out of the kidney is measured by a scintillation detector positioned externally over the lumbar region (7, 8). A typical wash-out curve is illustrated in Figure 9–3. Disappearance of radioactivity is a complex function of time and can be described as the sum

of several exponentials, each of which represents blood flow through a discrete region of the kidney. By graphic methods, the composite curve can be analyzed into its component exponentials. From the partition coefficient for krypton, the slope of each exponential, and the density of the tissue, blood

Fig. 9–3.—Typical ^{85}Kr disappearance curve (*heavy black curve*) following injection of the isotope into the renal artery. Graphic analysis of the resultant exponentials is shown by thinner lines: *I*, cortical

flow; *II*, outer medullary flow; *III*, inner medullary flow; and *IV*, perirenal and hilar fat flow. (Modified from Barger, A. C.: Ann. New York Acad. Sc. 139:276, 1966.)

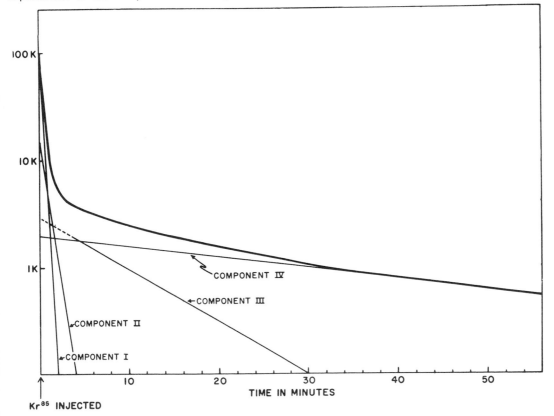

flow per gram of tissue can be calculated for some four differently perfused masses of renal tissue, as Figure 9–3 shows. By radio-autography, these tissue masses have been identified and flows assigned as follows: cortex, 4–5 ml/Gm per minute; outer medulla, 1.2–1.5 ml/Gm per minute; inner medulla (papilla), 0.12–0.20 ml/Gm per minute; and perirenal and hilar fat, 0.02 ml/Gm per minute.

Grossly, the latter two methods yield values of distribution of blood that agree reasonably well. However, all of these methods involve procedures that are traumatic. A fourth method, applicable in man, is based on the following arguments (9,10): In normal man, about 90% of the PAH contained in plasma perfusing the kidneys is extracted if concentration is low (1–2 mg/100 ml). If one assumes that PAH is extracted by the combined processes of filtration through glomeruli and secretion by the convoluted portions of proximal tubules, then only cortical structures participate in its removal from renal blood. If one further assumes that extraction from plasma perfusing the cortex is complete, then one may grossly divide the renal blood perfusate into two moieties: one completely cleared and representing cortical flow (90% of total) and one not cleared at all and representing medullary flow (10% of total). In essence, this is an extension of Homer Smith's view that the PAH clearance represents minimum effective renal plasma flow. In order to estimate flow distribution in this manner, both PAH clearance and true renal plasma flow must be measured, the latter by quantifying renal arterial-venous extraction of PAH as well as rate of excretion. Most investigators believe that too many assumptions are required for this method to yield meaningful results. At best, it can yield only a gross estimate of flow distribution.

Interest in the distribution of flow within the kidneys is related primarily to the operation of the countercurrent multiplier and exchange mechanisms described in Chapter 7. All methods that purport to describe distribution of flow agree in showing that med-ullary-papillary flow is low in comparison with cortical flow, which is essential to the maintenance of a gradient of osmolality from cortex to tip of papilla along Henle's loop. Slow flow in the vasa recta relative to that in cortical capillaries is a consequence of their much greater lengths, of the increased viscosity of their contained blood due to the shunting of water from descending to ascending limbs at the corticomedullary junction, and of the distribution of the flow from any single efferent arteriole of a juxtamedullary glomerulus among the many parallel channels that constitute the vasa recta.

EXTRINSIC CONTROL OF RENAL CIRCULATION

The vessels of the kidney are richly supplied with sympathetic nerve fibers derived from the fourth thoracic segment to the fourth lumbar segment. These fibers are distributed through the celiac and renal plexuses. All are vasoconstrictor; no evidence of innervation by vagal or sympathetic dilator fibers exists.

EMERGENCY FUNCTION OF THE RENAL NERVES. —According to Smith (1,11), the renal nerves of a normal person in a supine position, completely at rest physically and mentally and in an environment of neutral temperature, transmit few, if any, impulses; i.e., tonic vasoconstrictor activity is minimal or nonexistent. Let such a person sit up or stand up, or even read an exciting mystery story, and the situation changes: vasoconstrictor tone increases. If the stress is mild, renal blood flow may be minimally reduced, with no change in glomerular filtration rate. If the stress is more marked, blood flow decreases significantly, but filtration rate may remain constant. The filtration fraction accordingly increases. If a life-threatening situation arises, then both blood flow and filtration rate may be reduced profoundly— the former to a greater extent than the latter. In general, it may be stated that the renal blood flow is regulated to maintain relative stability of filtration rate. Regulation obviously must involve alterations of the caliber of afferent and efferent glomerular arterioles so as to maintain constancy of effective filtration pressure. If a grave emergency arises, both filtration rate and blood flow are sacrificed in defense of the blood perfusion of organs more immediately vital to existence; i.e., the heart and the brain.

Fright, pain, syncope, cold, severe exercise, deep anesthesia and hemorrhage constitute grave emergencies. Because renal blood flow normally amounts to 1,200 ml/min (i.e., one fifth or more of the resting output of the heart), reduction to 200 ml/min obviously provides an additional liter of blood each minute to perfuse active skeletal muscles or to compensate general circulatory inadequacy.

Figure 9–4 illustrates the response of the renal circulation of a subject who, during the course of an experiment, became alarmed about the significance of the clearance tests that were being performed (11). The Diodrast clearance (renal plasma flow) fell from 700 to less than 400 ml/min. Because the glomerular filtration rate changed but little, the filtration fraction increased. Although the situation was explained and the subject's apprehension was apparently dissipated, renal ischemia persisted for the remainder of the experiment.

Figure 9–5 describes the response of the renal circulation to change from the horizontal to the 80° head-up position on a tilt-table. Under these circumstances, blood pools in capillaries and veins below the level of the heart, and venous return and cardiac output decrease. Blood pressure is initially sus-

Fig. 9–4. — Psychogenic renal vasoconstriction induced by alarm. (Adapted from Smith, H. W.: Harvey Lect. 35:166, 1939–40.)

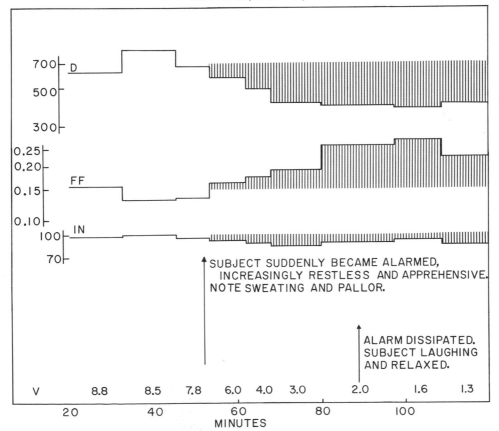

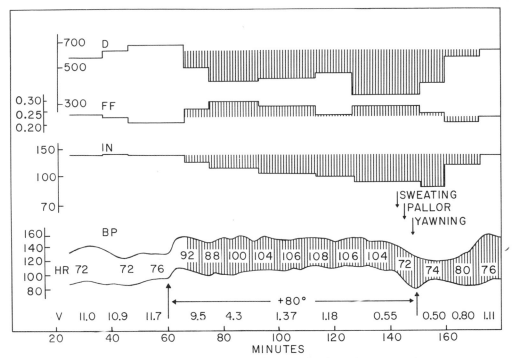

Fig. 9—5.—Renal ischemia induced by tilting a normal subject from the horizontal to the 80° head-up position. (Adapted from Smith, H. W.: Harvey Lect. 35:166, 1939—40.)

tained by vasoconstriction of skin and viscera, including the kidneys. The syncopal crisis was foreshadowed by an increase in heart rate, sweating, yawning and pallor. Syncope was precipitated by a fall in blood pressure and cerebral ischemia brought on by slowing of the heart and vasodilation of skeletal muscles. When the subject was returned to the horizontal position, normal circulatory relationships were promptly restored, and renal plasma flow returned to its control value. In this experiment, filtration rate fell significantly; i.e., afferent arteriolar constriction was greater than efferent by an amount sufficient to cause a reduction in filtration pressure despite an increase in mean arterial pressure.

EFFECTS OF HORMONES ON RENAL CIRCULATION.—Epinephrine and norepinephrine constrict renal vessels. Moderate doses (0.5 mg), administered intramuscularly, reduce renal blood flow as much as 50% but do not change filtration rate significantly. Because both hormones increase blood pressure, it is evident that they must constrict the afferent and efferent arterioles more or less equally. When administered in higher dosage, and especially when infused intravenously, epinephrine and norepinephrine cause a precipitous fall in renal blood flow and filtration rate. Under these circumstances, afferent arteriolar constriction must be greater than efferent. The two hormones also cause constriction of renal veins, resulting in an elevation in peritubular capillary, interstitial and intratubular pressures and swelling of the kidney. This paradoxical swelling of the kidney despite reduced blood flow was observed by Richards and Plant many years ago.

Vasopressin, better termed "antidiuretic hormone," when administered at physiologic rates induces marked oliguria but has no effect on total renal blood flow or filtration rate. In pharmacologic doses, the hormone raises blood pressure and reduces renal blood flow and filtration rate. The name "vasopressin" is a misnomer because the hormone probably is never liberated from the pituitary in amounts sufficient to raise blood pressure or to alter renal hemodynamics.

Serotonin, in pharmacologic doses, also constricts renal arterioles, reducing renal blood flow and filtration rate. Renin and angiotensin, in moderate doses, reduce renal blood flow without having any major effect on filtration rate. In high dosage, they reduce both blood flow and filtration rate.

EFFECTS OF ANESTHESIA ON RENAL CIRCULATION. — In unanesthetized animals, the blood flow and filtration rate of a denervated kidney and of a normally innervated kidney are equal. Under anesthesia, however, flow and filtration rate are slightly higher on the denervated side. Induction of anesthesia causes a moderate decrease in blood flow and filtration rate on the innervated side and no change on the denervated side. Sympathetic outflow to the kidney is obviously enhanced by anesthesia, which constitutes a stress, threat or emergency situation.

A presumed stimulation of sodium reabsorption by sympathetic impulses impinging on tubular cells has been described, on the basis of experiments in which one kidney of an anesthetized animal has been acutely denervated. Denervation results in a prompt, although moderate, increase in sodium excretion, which is almost always accompanied by increased renal blood flow and filtration rate. Excretion of a small proportion of an increased filtered load is a more probable explanation of the finding of enhanced sodium output than reduced reabsorption from withdrawal of impulses stimulating tubular reabsorption (12). No really valid evidence of nervous control of tubular reabsorptive or secretory function exists.

RENAL HYPEREMIA. — No neural mechanism of renal vasodilation, other than that of reduction of sympathetic vasoconstrictor outflow, is known. However, the kidneys of normal man, under conditions such that sympathetic tone is minimal, respond to intravenously administered pyrogens with a dramatic increase in blood flow. This pyrogenic reaction was first observed following the administration of inulin that had been contaminated with bacterial protein during preparation. Triple typhoid vaccine and other pyrogens produce a similar response. Typically, renal hyperemia has its onset about 70–90 minutes after the pyrogen is given; i.e., at about the time of the chill and beginning rise of temperature. The blood pressure increases at the same time, and the subject complains of nausea, back pain and headache. Renal blood flow increases by 50–100%, and hyperemia persists for 5 hours or more. Filtration rate is unchanged; hence filtration fraction decreases.

If one administers the antipyretic drug aminopyrine, prior to the pyrogen, no rise in blood pressure, no chill and no fever occur, and the subject experiences none of the malaise associated with a febrile reaction. Nevertheless, renal blood flow increases and filtration fraction decreases exactly as in the febrile state. Because blood flow increases while filtration rate remains unchanged, both afferent and efferent arterioles must be dilated. Because pyrogenic hyperemia has been observed in totally sympathectomized patients (i.e., those with kidneys denervated), a neural mechanism is not involved. It is probable that the pyrogen relaxes renal arterioles by a direct action on the smooth muscle of their walls.

AUTOREGULATION OF RENAL CIRCULATION

The vasculature of the kidney is subject to a type of control that, if not unique, is certainly far better developed than in any other organ. Figure 9–6 illustrates the fact that renal blood flow and glomerular filtration rate change but little as arterial pressure is varied over a range of 80–180 mm Hg. Because renal blood flow is relatively independent of arterial pressure in denervated and in isolated perfused kidneys, control must reside wholly within the kidney, must be independent of extrinsic nerves and blood-borne hormones, and, accordingly, is termed "auto-

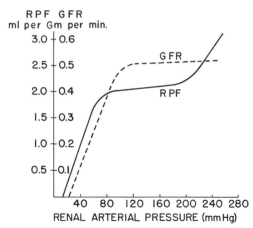

Fig. 9—6.—Autoregulation of glomerular filtration rate and renal plasma flow in the dog over a range of 8–180 mm Hg perfusion pressure. (Adapted from Ochwadt, B.: Prog. Cardiovas. Dis. 3:501, 1961.)

regulation." Autoregulation is organized to stabilize renal blood flow and filtration rate in the face of changes in renal arterial pressure. Sympathetic neural regulation is superimposed to permit the shunting of a portion of the renal blood to other organs while maintaining filtration rate as nearly stable as is possible.

The relation between blood flow (F), the pressure head that drives the blood from artery to vein (ΔP), and resistance (R) is given by the equation $F = k \cdot \Delta P / R$. If the resistance were to remain constant—i.e., if the caliber of the vessels were not to change—a 50% increase in pressure would cause a 50% increase in flow. In the perfused hind limb of the dog, a 50% increase in pressure actually causes a 60–70% increase in flow, because the elevated pressure stretches the vessels, increasing their diameter and reducing their resistance. A similar relationship holds in the kidney over a range of pressure from a yield pressure of about 14 mm Hg, required to initiate flow, to 70–80 mm Hg. However, within a range of 80–180 mm Hg, a 50% increase in pressure causes only a 6–8% increase in flow. Resistance, therefore, increases with increasing pressure. Because the glomerular filtration rate changes little over this mid-

range of pressure, the increase in resistance must be localized almost entirely in the afferent arterioles. Filtration decreases sharply with decreasing pressure below 100 mm Hg and ceases at pressures less than 55–60 mm Hg (13–15), resulting in anuria. Thurau (16) showed that only the cortical fraction of renal blood flow is subject to autoregulation; medullary blood flow varies directly with arterial pressure. However, inasmuch as medullary flow is only a minor fraction of total flow, the latter, like cortical flow, exhibits autoregulation.

AUTOREGULATION OF RENAL BLOOD FLOW AND GLOMERULAR FILTRATION RATE.—The mechanism of autoregulation of renal blood flow and glomerular filtration rate is one of great interest and of equally great controversy. In fact, some deny its existence in the normal kidney (17); but this view is difficult to reconcile with its obvious demonstration in unanesthetized animals (15). However, among the vast majority of investigators who do accept its existence, four concepts are held as to its origin: the cell separation hypothesis, the intrarenal pressure hypothesis, the myogenic hypothesis, and a group of hypotheses that involve the sensing of blood pressure, intratubular hydrostatic pressure, or tubular fluid composition by one or the other component of the juxtaglomerular apparatus, and the control of glomerular and tubular blood perfusion through the renin-angiotensin effector system. A symposium on autoregulation published in *Circulation Research*, in 1964, demonstrated the lack of a generally acceptable explanation of the phenomenon.

HYPOTHESIS OF CELL SEPARATION.—The cell separation hypothesis proposes that the increase in resistance to flow that occurs within the pressure range of autoregulation is brought about not by a change in the caliber of vessels but by an increase in the viscosity of blood (18,19). Blood flowing in the interlobular arteries exhibits axial streaming of cells; plasma flows more slowly, in a peripheral cuff next to the vessel walls. The afferent arterioles, branching at right angles from the interlobular arteries near their origins on the arciform arteries, receive plasma-rich blood; i.e., plasma-skimming occurs. Red cells become progressively more concentrated as blood flows toward the periphery, and viscosity increases. Afferent arterioles that branch off more distally are supplied with blood of increased hematocrit.

Skimming also occurs beyond the efferent arterioles: the plasma is directed into long, tortuous peritubular capillaries; the red cells flow into veins by short, direct shunts.* The higher the perfusion pressure, the greater is the skimming of plasma and the more marked is the increase in blood viscosity in the periphery. The viscosity of blood changes only a little, with small variations in hematocrit around the normal range of 45%. However, small variations in hematocrit cause an inordinate change in viscosity at hematocrits around 80%—a value presumably attained in the postglomerular red cell shunts of peripherally located glomeruli. The basic thesis is the following: an increase in pressure energy is expended in forming a fluid of greater viscosity; relatively little of the energy is expended in increasing flow.

If this view were correct, it would follow, as a corollary, that autoregulation must be impaired in anemia and nonexistent in kidneys perfused with cell-free fluid. Furthermore, the distribution of flow among the nephrons must be greatly altered with change in pressure. An increase in pressure should increase blood perfusion of juxtamedullary and deep cortical nephrons, while that of more superficial cortical nephrons should decrease. Total flow should increase only slightly. Although it is true that autoregulation is most effective in unanesthetized animals that are normal in all respects other than renal denervation, it is by no means absent in isolated kidneys perfused with oxygenated, cell-free dextran solutions. Fur-

---

*Evidence for preglomerular and postglomerular plasma-skimming is indirect and by no means conclusive.

thermore, such evidence as exists does not favor the view that distribution of flow to nephrons is greatly altered over the range of autoregulation. Thus, cell separation cannot adequately explain certain features of autoregulation. Whether or not it contributes to autoregulation, to any significant degree, is undetermined.

HYPOTHESIS OF INTRARENAL PRESSURE. — The intrarenal pressure hypothesis is based on the presumption that an increase in renal arterial pressure is accompanied by an increase in renal interstitial fluid pressure (20, 21). This latter pressure compresses the peritubular network of capillaries and the intrarenal veins, impeding flow and increasing resistance. The major evidence in favor of this thesis has been derived from the so-called needle-pressure measurements of interstitial fluid tension. A fine hypodermic needle, plunged into the renal parenchyma, registers an apparent interstitial pressure, which increases with increasing arterial pressure over the range of autoregulation. Just what such needle-pressure measurements mean is subject to debate. In all likelihood, small arteries are ruptured, and the recorded pressures are some undetermined average of interstitial and arterial values. In any event, they do not agree with micropuncture determinations of intratubular pressures, which change little with arterial pressure over the range of autoregulation (22). The author does not favor this intrarenal pressure explanation.

MYOGENIC HYPOTHESIS. — The myogenic hypothesis holds that the increase in renal resistance that accompanies an increase in perfusion pressure is effected by the contraction of smooth muscle in the walls of afferent arterioles. Many years ago, Bayliss observed that smooth muscle in the vessels of a number of organs responds to distention with an increase in contractile tone. However, the increase in tone is insufficient to prevent an increase in the diameter of the vessels and a decrease in resistance. It may well be that the response of the smooth muscle in renal afferent arterioles is qualitatively similar but quantitatively much greater. In renal vessels, the contraction of smooth muscle might be great enough to cause a reduction in diameter and an increase in resistance.

The major evidence in favor of the myogenic hypothesis of autoregulation is the fact that the phenomenon is abolished by the infusion into the renal artery of cyanide, procaine and papaverine in amounts sufficient to paralyze the contraction of smooth muscle. Furthermore, the time course of the autoregulatory response is in accord with a myogenic origin. Thus, a sudden increase in perfusion pressure causes an immediate marked increase in flow, lasting a few seconds, followed by an overcompensating reduction in flow and a readjustment to an intermediate value within about 30 seconds (23). This phasic response could well result from sluggish contraction of smooth muscle. When contraction is abolished by drugs, an increase in pressure causes an immediate increase in flow, and no subsequent readjustments occur; i.e., autoregulation is lost (Fig. 9–7).

JUXTAGLOMERULAR HYPOTHESES. — These hypotheses are myogenic in the sense that they implicate the smooth muscle of the arterioles as the means of control of renal vascular resistance; but they differ in that they assume that the tone of the arterioles is under the control of the renin-angiotensin system (described below). Thus, the degree of distention of afferent arterioles might influence the rate of liberation of renin from the granular cells of the polkissen and the rate of production and, therefore, the concentration of angiotensin in the environment of the micromuscular sphincters. Thurau (24) has recently implicated both elements of the juxtaglomerular apparatus: in his view, the macula densa of the distal tubule senses the concentration of sodium in tubular fluid and controls the liberation of renin by its associated polkissen.

An increase in glomerular capillary pressure presumably increases filtration rate. If reabsorption in the proximal tubule and the loop of Henle did not change instantaneously, one would expect the concentration of sodium in the distal tubular fluid to increase. This increase in sodium concentration, sensed by the macula densa, presumably increases the liberation of renin and formation of angiotensin in the afferent arteriole of the glomerulus attached to that specific tubule. Arteriolar contraction reduces filtration, reduces the delivery of sodium to the macula densa and restores conditions to normal. The major evidence in favor of this thesis is Thurau's observation that the reverse perfusion of a distal tubule toward the macula densa with solutions of high sodium content causes cessation of filtration in the associated glomerulus and collapse of the proximal tubule. If this mechanism is physiologically significant, it could play a role not only in autoregulation of blood flow and filtration but also in the maintenance of glomerular tubular balance. Which of the several juxtaglomerular mechanisms play significant roles is uncertain.

Fig. 9–7.—Evidence for the myogenic nature of autoregulation of renal blood flow. (Adapted from Thurau, K., and Kramer, K.: Arch. ges. Physiol. 269:77, 1959.)

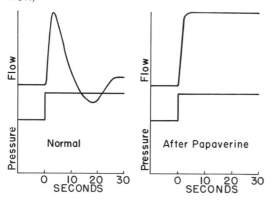

Renal Hormonal Factors in Blood Pressure Regulation

Ever since Richard Bright, in 1827, published his observations on the association of cardiac hypertrophy* with chronic renal disease, an understanding of the role of the kidney in the pathogenesis of hypertension has been sought. At present, there is evidence that the kidneys play at least two distinct roles: (1) under certain conditions they liberate an enzyme that reacts with a component of plasma to produce a pressor substance, which causes generalized arteriolar constriction, increased vascular resistance and elevated blood pressure; and (2) normal kidneys either destroy a circulating pressor factor or add to the blood a depressor factor.

Renin-Angiotensin System

Late in the last century, Tigerstedt and Bergman observed that the intravenous injection of a crude extract of kidney tissue causes a slowly developing and sustained increase in blood pressure. They called the active principle renin. Subsequently, it was shown that repeated injections of crude renin cause successively lessening pressor responses—a property termed "tachyphylaxis." It was later noted that purification of the active protein enhances its pressor activity when injected intravenously but reduces its capacity to constrict the vessels of the ear of a rabbit perfused with Ringer-Locke solution. However, the addition of plasma to the perfusate containing purified renin results in intense constriction of the vessels of the ear.

In the 1940s, Page and his colleagues (25) in the United States and Houssay, Braun-Menendez and their associates in Argentina showed that renin is a proteolytic enzyme and that it reacts with a plasma component to produce a nonprotein pressor substance, which the two groups of investigators called

---

*Cardiac hypertrophy occurs in response to the increased work load imposed on the heart by an increase in mean arterial pressure. Following the development of means of measuring systolic and diastolic blood pressures in man, it became evident that hypertension almost invariably occurs in chronic renal disease. Hypertension also occurs in the absence of significant renal disease and in the presence of essentially normal renal function. The role of the kidney in such benign essential hypertension is by no means clear.

"angiotonin" and "hypertensin," respectively. In the interest of Pan-American solidarity, this substance is now called angiotensin. More recent work has shown that the plasma substrate is an α_2-globulin and that the initial product of its lysis by renin is a nonpressor or weakly pressor decapeptide, angiotensin I. The decapeptide is converted into a highly active pressor octapeptide, angiotensin II, by a chloride-activated enzyme in plasma (26). When a small amount of angiotensin II is injected intravenously, blood pressure rises sharply and remains elevated for 5–10 minutes or so. In contrast, the injection of purified renin causes a slow rise in pressure, which is sustained at an elevated level for 40–60 minutes. The prolonged action of renin is due to the continued slow formation of angiotensin in the circulating blood plasma. Angiotensinase, which destroys the pressor octapeptide, is present in circulating blood plasma and in many organs, including kidney, intestine and liver. Angiotensin II is relatively heat-stable, water- and alcohol-soluble and dialyzable. Some five different renin substrates have been isolated from hog plasma and have been found to differ only in the carbohydrate moiety of the glycoprotein molecule. Renin acts to split a leucine-leucine bond linking amino acids 10 and 11 of the protein to form the decapeptide, angiotensin I. The converting enzyme removes histidine and leucine from the C-terminal of this peptide to form the active octapeptide, angiotensin II, which has the following structure:

Asp · Arg · Val · Tyr · Ile · His · Pro · Phe

Angiotensins of the hog and horse are identical; that of the cow differs in the amino acid in position 5, where valine rather than isoleucine is found (27). A series of angiotensin analogues have been synthesized, and the requirements for biologic activity have been defined. The structure of human angiotensin is unknown at present.

Experimental renal hypertension. — In 1934, Goldblatt *et al.* (28) first conclusively demonstrated that persistent hypertension can be induced in experimental animals by the partial ligation of a renal artery. In the dog, if only one artery is constricted, blood pressure rises, but after a few weeks it returns to normal. If both renal arteries are partly ligated or if one is constricted and the opposite kidney removed, hypertension is stable and persistent. In most other laboratory animals, including the rat, rabbit, goat and sheep, constriction of only one renal artery leads to persistent hypertension. If the constriction of the renal artery is excessive, extreme hypertension develops, renal function deteriorates rapidly, and the animal dies. Widespread necrotizing arteriolar lesions are observed along with retinal hemorrhages and papilledema—changes similar to those of malignant hypertension in man.

Subsequent to the work of Goldblatt, a variety of methods were developed to produce sustained hypertension; these included the tying of a figure-eight ligature around the two poles and body of the kidney and wrapping the kidney in silk or cellophane. This latter procedure stimulates a foreign-body reaction in the capsule of the kidney, which thickens tremendously and compresses the renal parenchyma in a thick, collagenous hull. Hypertension develops slowly and increases progressively. Surgical removal of portions of the kidney and tying off branches of the renal artery are less dependable methods of inducing hypertension.

Partial ligation of a renal artery, encapsulating the kidney or tying a figure-eight ligature around body and poles alters renal blood perfusion. What change in renal hemodynamics is significant is uncertain. Because hypertension can be induced by any of these procedures in animals with kidneys denervated, subjected to total sympathectomy or even with the spinal cord destroyed, it is evident that neural reflexes originating in the ischemic kidney are not obligatorily involved. Clamping of a renal artery results in an increased content of pressor material in renal venous blood when the circulation is re-established. Early workers presumed that

the pressor material was either renin or angiotensin, although methods of assay were nonspecific. Although many have demonstrated increased titers of pressor substances in peripheral blood in experimental renal hypertension, others have not. Accordingly, all investigators do not accept the renin-angiotensin origin of such hypertension The demonstration of pressor substances in peripheral blood in chronic renal disease and in benign essential hypertension has been even less uniformly successful—whether a reflection of lack of sensitivity of assay procedures or lack of causal relationship is uncertain. It may well be that cases of experimental, and especially human, renal and essential hypertension, all of which develop slowly in comparison with the rise in pressure produced by intravenous injections of pharmacologic doses of renin or angiotensin, are expressions of the effects of the continuous liberation of minute amounts of the active agent.

Early in the hypertensive phase, removal of the offending kidney returns blood pressure to normal. Later, nephrectomy may be less effective. Also, in long-established hypertension, most investigators have failed to demonstrate increased titers of pressor substances in the blood. These latter results have inclined some to the belief that a humoral mechanism of early hypertension is replaced by a neural one, in which the set point of the buffer regulatory reflexes is adjusted upward. However, in experimental chronic renal hypertension, the fact that the stimulation of production of antirenin antibodies by the injection of a foreign renin often significantly reduces blood pressure argues in favor of a humoral mechanism throughout (29). Needless to say, the matter is controversial. In the author's judgment, the evidence that the renin-angiotensin mechanism plays a major role in the genesis of the Goldblatt type of hypertension outweighs contrary evidence; but the evidence of its role in chronic renal disease and in benign essential hypertension in man is much less impressive.

The fact that, in the dog, compression of

one renal artery does not result in permanent hypertension and that, in other animals, the degree of hypertension is exaggerated by removing the normal kidney suggests an ability of normal renal tissue to destroy or excrete angiotensin. That destruction, and not excretion, is significant is indicated by the fact that ureterovenous anastomosis of the normal kidney does not impair its ability to moderate the hypertension. Very likely the kidney is a major site of destruction of angiotensin, probably owing to its content of angiotensinase. The sensitivity of an animal to intravenous administration of angiotensin is increased acutely by bilateral nephrectomy; again, this suggests that the kidneys may play a major role in the destruction of angiotensin.

JUXTAGLOMERULAR CELLS. — Juxtaglomerular cells, rather than tubular cells, probably produce renin and secrete it into the blood stream (30, 31). The smooth muscle of the media of the afferent arteriole gradually gives way to large, round or polygonal epithelioid cells as the vessel approaches the glomerulus. These cells pile up as an expanding and often asymmetrical cuff, which abuts the vascular pole of Bowman's capsule. They contain many granules, which stain brilliantly with fuchsin. The Hartrofts, some years ago, introduced the method of counting granules as a semiquantitative procedure for determining secretory activity.

This perivascular cuff of cells was named the polkissen ("polar cushion") by Zimmerman. Zimmerman also noted that a cytologically specialized loop of the distal convoluted tubule is applied closely to the polkissen. The cells of this loop are high-columnar rather than cuboidal, and the nuclei are large and prominent; accordingly, it was named the macula densa. Together, the polkissen and the macula densa constitute the juxtaglomerular apparatus. As commonly used, the term "juxtaglomerular cells" refers to the granular cells of the polkissen. Figure 9–8 illustrates the locus and appearance of the juxtaglomerular cells.

A variety of evidence suggests that renin is secreted by juxtaglomerular cells:

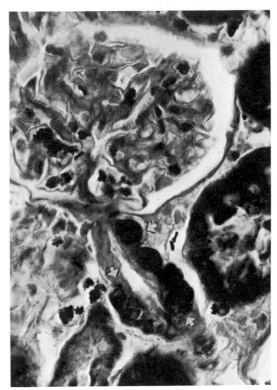

Fig. 9–8. — Juxtaglomerular cells (polkissen) in the afferent arteriole just ahead of its entry into Bowman's capsule. (From Tobian, L.: Ann. Int. Med. 52:395, 1960.)

1. In rats made hypertensive by the Goldblatt procedure, the kidney with artery constricted contains juxtaglomerular cells loaded with granules (high secretory activity). Juxtaglomerular cells of the opposite, normally perfused, kidney contain fewer granules than the kidneys of control rats (depressed secretory activity).

2. Isolated kidneys of rats perfused with blood under high pressure lose the granulation of the juxtaglomerular cells. Those perfused at low-normal pressure retain the granulation. These two observations suggest that a reduction in afferent arteriolar pressure by partial ligation of one renal artery stimulates secretion of renin by juxtaglomerular cells. The formation of angiotensin II in the circulating blood results in a compensatory increase in arterial pressure. In contrast, increased renal arterial pres-

sure reduces basal rate of secretion of renin.

3. High salt intake plus injection of deoxy-corticosterone causes hypertension accompanied by loss of granularity of juxtaglomerular cells. A sodium-free diet reduces blood pressure, as does adrenalectomy. Both procedures markedly increase the granularity of the juxtaglomerular cells.

4. Renin can be extracted from the renal cortex, which contains glomeruli, but not from the medulla or papilla, which are wholly tubular in composition. Isolation of glomeruli and their attached vessels by magnetic means after injection of iron particles has shown that the source of renin is either the glomeruli or their attached vessels.

5. The quantity of renin that can be extracted from kidneys correlates well with the granulation of juxtaglomerular cells.

6. Antibodies to rabbit renin, tagged with fluorescein, localize specifically in the granules of juxtaglomerular cells.

These several lines of evidence suggest that the polkissen is both a pressure-sensing and a hormone-secreting organ, that the granules in the juxtaglomerular cells represent the hormone, renin, and that compression of one renal artery in the Goldblatt procedure results in increased secretion of renin and compensatory elevation of arterial perfusion pressure. To what extent this system plays a role in autoregulation of glomerular filtration and renal blood flow and in maintenance of glomerular tubular balance has not been precisely defined.

However, angiotensin has been implicated in the normal control of arterial blood pressure in a variety of functional states. Furthermore, it is now apparent that angiotensin is a prime determinant of aldosterone secretion—which means that it indirectly promotes renal tubular conservation of sodium and expansion of extracellular volume (32, 33). Acting directly on renal tubules, angiotensin depresses reabsorption of sodium (34) and thus tends to counteract the indirect conservation of this ion mediated by aldosterone.

The varied functional roles of renin and angiotensin, outlined above, make it unlikely that a single factor governs activity of the system. Vander (35) reviewed, in detail, evidence suggesting that no fewer than four factors control the rate of renin release: change in intraluminal pressure of afferent arterioles; change in composition of tubular fluid at the macula densa; sympathetic nerve impulses; and catecholamines and other known and unknown humoral agents.

Following the demonstration by Goldblatt that constriction of a renal artery induces hypertension, renal ischemia was assumed to be the major determinant of renin release. Subsequently, it was shown that renal hypoxia and hypercapnia are not effective stimuli. Furthermore, a reduction in renal pulse pressure, per se, is not effective, although a reduction in mean renal arterial pressure, so small that no change in flow is apparent, induces release of renin. The thesis has therefore evolved that the granular cells of the polkissen are exquisitely sensitive to mean intraluminal pressure; i.e., are intrarenal baroreceptors. When pressure decreases, renin is released.

A second control is in some way exerted by the macula densa responding to the composition of early distal tubular fluid. Changes in osmolality and sodium concentration and in the quantity of sodium delivered per unit time have all been implicated as stimuli of the macula densa. By some unknown method of coupling, the macula densa controls liberation of renin by the granular cells of the polar pad. Support for these views derives from micropuncture and microperfusion studies and from responses to salt depletion, diuretics and salt loading.

Stimulation of renal nerves and the infusion of catecholamines into a renal artery cause the release of renin. This suggests that the system is subject to extrarenal reflex as well as intrarenal control. The suggestion is borne out by the observation that carotid occlusion stimulates renin release. It is uncertain whether nerve impulses act directly on granular cells to liberate renin or induce renin release indirectly by constricting afferent arterioles, thus reducing both intraluminal pressure at the polkissen and the rate of glomerular filtration. The latter might result in a change in composition of tubular fluid at the site of the macula densa.

The release of renin is subject to a negative feedback type of control; i.e., an increase in circulating angiotensin reduces the liberation of renin, even when arterial pressure is kept constant. Vasopressin similarly inhibits release of renin. In contrast, aldosterone and a number of other hormones do not significantly affect renin release. Evidence from studies on salt depletion suggests that hormones other than aldosterone may regulate proximal sodium reabsorption. These hormones might influence renin release by altering composition of the urine at the macula densa site.

RENIN-ANGIOTENSIN SYSTEM AND HUMAN HYPERTENSION.—The role played by the renin-angiotensin system in human hypertension is highly controversial. There are instances of human hypertension in which constriction of one renal artery by an arteriosclerotic plaque, by compression or by kinking has been demonstrated angiographically. Plastic repair of the artery or removal of the damaged kidney has occasionally resulted in dramatic and complete cure of hypertension. Such instances constitute a small fraction of the total number of cases of human hypertension. Opinions vary concerning the origin of hypertension in chronic bilateral renal diseases and in essential hypertension. If the renin-angiotensin system is significant, it is no doubt a consequence of structural narrowing of afferent arterioles and therefore is not amenable to surgical treatment. The student should keep an open mind as to the genesis of human hypertension; conclusive evidence regarding its cause is not available.

RENOPRIVAL HYPERTENSION

Bilateral nephrectomy causes hypertension in animals maintained in good condition by careful dietary control and by repeated hemodialysis with an artificial kidney. Following nephrectomy, blood pressure progressively increases over a period of 10 days or so. At autopsy, nephrectomized animals exhibit arteriolar changes similar to those seen in malignant hypertension induced by excessive constriction of the renal arteries.

If the ureters are ligated or implanted into the small bowel or vena cava—procedures that result in uremia of a degree equivalent to that induced by bilateral nephrectomy—hypertension is of brief duration, if it occurs at all. Hemodialysis does not increase the incidence of hypertension (36).

Renoprival hypertension occurs without expansion of volume and in the presence of normal composition of extracellular fluid. Its mechanism is obviously different from that induced by renal artery constriction. The hypertension is unrelated to failure of excretion of pressor substances, because neither ureteral ligation nor diversion of urine into the blood stream elevates the blood pressure. Normal renal tissue must either add suppressor materials to the blood or destroy pressor materials formed in organs other than the kidneys. Loss of these functions in chronic renal disease might contribute to hypertension.

Summary

The kidneys of a normal man at rest are perfused with some 1,200 ml of blood per minute—a volume equivalent to one quarter to one fifth of the cardiac output. The renal nerves are solely vasoconstrictor in function. They become active in states of emergency, reduce renal blood flow and shunt blood to other organs more immediately essential to existence. As much as 1 extra liter of blood per minute can thus be provided to perfuse heart, brain and skeletal muscles at the expense of the kidneys. In less demanding situations, renal blood flow and glomerular capillary pressure are regulated by adjustments of afferent and efferent arteriolar tone to maintain relative constancy of the rate of glomerular filtration, despite modest reduction of blood flow.

The renal vasculature also exhibits an intrinsic capacity to adjust its resistance in response to a change in arterial pressure, to keep blood flow and filtration rate essentially constant. This autoregulation of flow and filtration is independent of renal nerves and extrinsic hormones. It is effective over a range of arterial pressure of 80–180 mm Hg. It may depend on a direct response of smooth muscle to the pressure distending afferent and efferent arterioles or on a neural or hormonal system of control operating wholly within the kidney.

Evidence is accumulating that the polkissen, or polar pad, a specialized segment of the afferent arteriole just ahead of the glomerulus, is a pressure-sensing secretory organ that liberates renin into the blood stream in response to a reduction in blood pressure. Renin is a proteolytic enzyme that attacks an α_2-globulin of plasma to liberate a decapeptide, angiotensin I. Angiotensin II is a highly vasoconstricting octapeptide formed from angiotensin I by a plasma enzyme. This substance causes a sustained increase in blood pressure and serves to compensate the fall in pressure that initiated its production.

The kidneys also contribute to the regulation of blood pressure in another way. They may destroy certain pressor substances that originate in other organs, or they may produce a depressor or moderator substance. Nephrectomy, by removing these influences, results in a sustained increase in blood pressure.

REFERENCES

1. Smith, H. W.: *The Kidney: Structure and Function in Health and Disease* (New York: Oxford University Press, 1951).
2. Van Slyke, D. D., Rhoads, C. P.; Hiller, A., and Alving, A. S.: Relationships between urea excretion, renal blood flow, renal oxygen consumption and diuresis: The mechanism of urea excretion, Am. J. Physiol. 109: 336, 1934.
3. Deetjen, P., and Kramer, K.: Na-Rückresorption und O_2-Verbrauch der Niere, Klin. Wchnschr. 38:680, 1960.
4. Thurau, K.: Renal Na reabsorption and O_2 uptake in dogs during hypoxia and hydrochlorothiazide infusion, Proc. Soc. Exper. Biol. & Med. 106:714, 1961.
5. Gottschalk, C. W., and Mylle, M.: Micropuncture study of pressures in proximal tubules and peritubular capillaries of the rat kidney and their relation to ureteral and renal venous pressures, Am. J. Physiol. 185:430, 1956.
6. Kramer, K., Thurau, K., and Deetjen, P.: Hämodynamik des Nierenmarks, Arch. ges. Physiol. 270:251 and 270, 1960.
7. Thorburn, G. D., Kopald, H. H., Herd, J. A., Hollenberg, M., O'Morchoe, C. C. C., and Barger, A. C.: Intrarenal distribution of nutrient blood flow determined with ^{85}Kr in the unanesthetized dog, Circulation Res. 13:290, 1963.
8. Barger, A. C.: Renal hemodynamic factors in congestive heart failure, Ann. New York Acad. Sc. 139:276, 1966.
9. Reubi, F.: Objections à la théorie de la séparation intrarénal des hématies et du plasma (Pappenheimer), Helvet. med. acta 25:516, 1958.
10. Pilkington, L. A., Binder, R., deHaas, J. C. M., and Pitts, R. F.: Intrarenal distribution of blood flow, Am. J. Physiol. 208:1107, 1965.
11. Smith, H. W.: Physiology of the renal circulation, Harvey Lect. 35:166, 1939–40.
12. Kamm, D. E., and Levinsky, N.: The mechanism of denervation natriuresis, J. Clin. Invest. 44:93, 1965.
13. Selkurt, E. E., Hall, P. W., and Spencer, M. P.: Influence of graded arterial pressure decrement on renal clearance of creatinine, p-amino hippurate and sodium, Am. J. Physiol. 159:369, 1949.
14. Shipley, R. E., and Study, R. S.: Changes in renal blood flow, extraction of inulin, glomerular filtration rate, tissue pressure and urine flow with acute alterations of renal artery blood pressure, Am. J. Physiol. 167:676, 1951.
15. Forster, R. P., and Maes, J. P.: Effect of experimental neurogenic hypertension on renal blood-flow and glomerular filtration rate in intact denervated kidneys of unanesthetized rabbits with adrenal glands demedullated, Am. J. Physiol. 150:534, 1947.
16. Thurau, K.: Renal hemodynamics, Am. J. Med. 36:698, 1964.
17. Langston, J. B., Guyton, A. C., and Gillespie, W. J., Jr.: Acute effects of changes in renal arterial pressure and sympathetic blockade on kidney function, Am. J. Physiol. 197:595, 1959.
18. Pappenheimer, J. R., and Kinter, W. B.: Hematocrit ratio of blood within mammalian

kidney and its significance for renal hemodynamics, Am. J. Physiol. 185:377, 1956.

19. Winton, F. R.: Present concepts of the renal circulation, A.M.A. Arch. Int. Med. 103:495, 1959.

20. Hinshaw, L. B., Day, S. B., and Carlson, C. H.: Tissue pressure as a causal factor in the autoregulation of blood flow in the isolated perfused kidney, Am. J. Physiol. 197:309, 1959.

21. Hinshaw, L. B., Flaig, R. D., Logemann, R. L., and Carlson, C. H.: Intrarenal venous pressure, tissue pressure and autoregulation of renal blood flow in the isolated perfused kidney, Am. J. Physiol. 198:891, 1960.

22. Gottschalk, C. W.: An experimental and comparative study of renal interstitial pressure, Am. J. Physiol. 169:180, 1952.

23. Thurau, K., and Kramer, K.: Weitere Untersuchungen zur myogen Natur der Autoregulation des Nierenkreislaufes, Arch. ges. Physiol. 269:77, 1959.

24. Thurau, K.: Influence of sodium concentration at macula densa cells on tubular sodium load, Ann. New York Acad. Sc. 139:388, 1966.

25. Page, I. H., and Corcoran, A. C.: *Experimental Renal Hypertension* (Springfield, Ill.: Charles C Thomas, Publisher, 1948).

26. Page, I. H., and Bumpus, F. M.: Angiotensin, Physiol. Rev. 41:331, 1961.

27. Skeggs, L. T., Lentz, K. E., Gould, A. B., Hochstrasser, H., and Kahn, J. R.: Biochemistry and kinetics of the renin angiotensin system, Fed. Proc. 26:42, 1967.

28. Goldblatt, H., Lynch, J., Hanzal, R. F., and Summerville, W. W.: Studies on experimental hypertension: I. The production of persistent elevation of systolic blood pressure by means of renal ischemia, J. Exper. Med. 59:347, 1934.

29. Wakerlin, G. E.: Antibodies to renin as proof of the pathogenesis of sustained renal hypertension, Circulation 17:653, 1958.

30. Tobian, L.: Physiology of the juxtaglomerular cells, Ann. Int. Med. 52:395, 1960.

31. Tobian, L.: Interrelationship of electrolytes, juxtaglomerular cells and hypertension, Physiol. Rev. 40:280, 1960.

32. Laragh, J. H., Angers, M., Kelly, W. G., and Lieberman, S.: Hypotensive agents and pressor substances. The effect of epinephrine, norepinephrine, angiotensin II, and others on the secretory rate of aldosterone in man, J. A. M. A. 174:234, 1960.

33. Laragh, J. H.: Renin, angiotensin, aldosterone and hormonal regulation of blood pressure and salt balance, Fed. Proc. 26:39, 1967.

34. Vander, A. J.: Inhibition of distal tubular sodium reabsorption by angiotensin. II. Am. J. Physiol. 205:133, 1963.

35. Vander, A. J.: Control of renin release, Physiol. Rev. 47:359, 1967.

36. Grollman, A., Muirhead, E. E., and Vanatta, J.: Role of the kidney in pathogenesis of hypertension as determined by a study of the effects of bilateral nephrectomy and other experimental procedures on the blood pressure of the dog, Am. J. Physiol. 157:21, 1949.

Buffer Mechanisms of
Tissues and Body Fluids

THE MAJOR IONIC COMPONENTS of the blood plasma and interstitial fluid of all vertebrate species are sodium, chloride and bicarbonate. Equally ubiquitous is carbon dioxide, which is continuously produced by cells and no less continuously removed from the body fluids by lungs or gills. Characteristically, 1 – 1.5 mM of dissolved carbon dioxide and 20 – 30 mEq of bicarbonate ion are contained in each liter of extracellular fluid. Accordingly, the reaction of extracellular fluid throughout the vertebrate subphylum is slightly alkaline.

According to Macallum (1), these similarities in body fluid composition of distantly related vertebrates stem from common protovertebrate ancestors, who lived in Paleozoic seas some 500 million years ago. The oceans were then more dilute, because the leaching of salt had not progressed to its present extent and the polar ice caps had not formed, to reduce the volume of the oceans and thus to concentrate the brine. The air was more heavily charged with carbon dioxide than is the atmosphere today, for the forests that gave rise to the coal deposits of the Carboniferous Period had not yet come into existence. Because the great sedimentary limestone beds were incompletely formed, the seas contained more bicarbonate than is present today. During this period, our aquatic ancestors perfected the physical properties of their cell membranes, determined cell permeability relationships and established

pH optima for the activity of enzymes located intracellularly and at cell surfaces.

With succeeding geologic revolutions, these protovertebrates found it advantageous to enclose a bit of this environment within an integument and to develop mechanisms for rendering its composition stable. It was Claude Bernard's concept that, by so evolving and stabilizing an internal fluid environment, the vertebrates achieved the independence that permitted their development of complex form and function and thus their dominance of the animal kingdom (2).

The importance of the stability of the hydrogen ion concentration of this internal environment is attested by the precision with which it is regulated. Under normal circumstances, the pH of blood plasma of mammals is maintained constant within limits of 7.35 and 7.45 – values corresponding to hydrogen ion concentrations of 4.47 and $3.55 \cdot 10^{-8}$ Eq/L, respectively. Limits compatible with life are generally stated to be pH 7.0 (H^+ = 10^{-7} Eq/L) and pH 7.8 ($H^+ = 1.59 \cdot 10^{-8}$ Eq/L). Although the total range of concentration that can be tolerated above and below the mean average value of $3.98 \cdot 10^{-8}$ (pH = 7.4) is minute, percentagewise the changes are relatively great. Thus, pH 7.0 (H^+ = $10 \cdot 10^{-8}$ Eq/L) represents an increase of 250% in hydrogen ion concentration above the normal, and pH 7.8 ($H^+ = 1.59 \cdot 10^{-8}$ Eq/L) represents a decrease to 40% of nor-

178

mal. It is also obvious that vital cell processes are 100,000 to 1,000,000 times more sensitive to absolute changes in hydrogen ion concentration than to changes in sodium concentration of extracellular fluid.

Precise regulation of reaction is attained through the operation of chemical and physiologic buffering mechanisms. The chemical buffers of tissues and body fluids neutralize acids or bases that are produced in or gain access to the body. Because the body is well buffered, even large quantities of acids or bases cause only minor disturbances in hydrogen ion concentration. The respiratory system eliminates the major acid end product of metabolism, carbon dioxide, as rapidly as it is produced, regulates its partial pressure and thus determines the concentration of carbonic acid in the body fluids. The kidneys eliminate the fixed (nonvolatile) acid and base end products of metabolism and precisely regulate the concentration of bicarbonate in the body fluids.

This chapter will be devoted to a discussion of the chemical buffers of tissues and body fluids (3, 4) and to certain respiratory compensations that occur in metabolic acidosis and alkalosis (5). The succeeding chapter will be devoted to a consideration of the renal mechanisms of regulation of acid-base balance.

The Nature of Buffer Action

IONIZATION

An ion is formed when an atom of one species permanently donates the electrons of its outer valence shell to an atom of another species, which completes its valence shell by accepting those electrons. The donor becomes a positively charged ion, or cation; the recipient becomes a negatively charged ion, or anion. The sodium atom has one electron in its outer shell; the chloride atom has seven. The sodium atom, by giving up its electron, becomes a positively charged sodium ion; the chloride atom fills its outer octet and becomes a negatively charged chloride ion. The hydrogen atom also has one electron it can donate to a chloride atom to become a hydrogen ion; in turn, the chloride atom becomes a chloride ion.

STRONG ELECTROLYTES

The crystal lattice of solid sodium chloride is made up of regularly arranged sodium and chloride ions. When sodium chloride is dissolved in water, these ions become relatively independent in their behavior. Hydrochloric acid also dissociates more or less completely in aqueous solution, to yield hydrogen and chloride ions. Those substances that dissociate into electrically charged ions are termed "electrolytes," because their solutions are capable of carrying an electric current. Strong electrolytes, which include most soluble salts and inorganic acids and bases, dissociate completely. However, because of electrostatic attractive forces, they behave as though they were only 80–90% dissociated in solutions having the ionic strength of the body fluids. The effective ion concentration or activity is thus slightly less than the chemical concentration. The activities of ions, rather than molar concentrations, determine equilibria in mass actions and establish the colligative properties of solutions. However, to simplify matters, we shall use the term "concentration" as though it were synonymous with activity.

WEAK ELECTROLYTES

The weak electrolytes, which include most organic acids and bases, are only partly ionized in solution. Acetic acid is a relatively weak acid; in $0.1-N$ concentration, about 1% of the molecules are dissociated while 99% exist as intact molecules.

$$100\ HCl \xrightarrow{} 100\ H^+ + 100\ Cl^-$$

$$100\ CH_3COOH \underset{\rightarrow}{\xleftarrow{}} \quad 1\ H^+ + 1\ CH_3COO^-$$

DEFINITIONS OF ACIDS AND BASES

According to the Brønsted formulation, an acid is any compound capable of donating a hydrogen ion (proton) to a base. A base is any substance that will accept a hydrogen ion (proton). Thus, HCl, H_2SO_4, H_3PO_4, CH_3COOH and H_2CO_3 are all conventional acids, because each dissociates hydrogen ions. In aqueous solutions, these acids donate hydrogen ions to water, which is, therefore, considered to be a weak base.

$$HCl + H_2O \longrightarrow H_3O^+ + Cl^-$$

Hydrogen ions actually exist in solution in hydrated form as hydronium ions, H_3O^+; but, for the sake of simplicity, we shall consider them free ions (H^+). Somewhat less conventional is the Brønsted view that the ammonium ion (NH_4^+) is an acid, in that it can donate a H^+ ion to a strong base.

$$NH_4^+, Cl^- + Na^+, OH^- \longrightarrow NH_3 + Na^+, Cl^- + H_2O$$

Bases include water, hydroxyl ions, ammonia (NH_3), and the anions of the salts of weak acids, all of which can bind free H^+ ions.

$$NH_3 + H^+, Cl^- \longrightarrow NH_4^+, Cl^-$$
$$Na^+, OH^- + H^+, Cl^- \longrightarrow Na^+, Cl^- + H_2O$$
$$Na^+, HCO_3^- + H^+, Cl^- \longrightarrow Na^+, Cl^- + H_2CO_3$$
$$Na^+, CH_3COO^- + H^+, Cl^- \longrightarrow Na^+, Cl^- + CH_3COOH$$

HYDROGEN ION CONCENTRATION

This may be expressed either in absolute terms of equivalents per liter or in pH units. A 0.1-M solution of a strong acid, such as hydrochloric acid, has a H^+ ion concentration of nearly 0.1 Eq/L, because it is completely dissociated and the activity coefficient of hydrogen ions, in such a solution at least, approaches unity. In contrast, a 0.1-M solution of a relatively weak acid, such as acetic acid, has a H^+ ion concentration of 0.001 Eq/L, for only 1 in 100 molecules dissociate. When one deals with alkaline solutions or acid solutions near neutrality, hydrogen ion concentrations become so small as to be unwieldy if expressed arithmetically. In 1909, Sorensen proposed the expression "pH" and defined it as the negative logarithm, to the base 10, of the hydrogen ion concentration:

$$pH = -\log(H^+)$$

Actually, the instruments, and even the indicators, used to measure pH measure not the true hydrogen ion concentration but the activity of hydrogen ions. The hydrogen ion concentration of blood plasma normally averages 0.0000000398 Eq/L, or $3.98 \cdot 10^{-8}$ Eq/L. To convert to pH units,

$$pH = -\log(H^+)$$
$$pH = -\log(3.98 \cdot 10^{-8})$$
$$pH = -\log 3.98 - \log 10^{-8}$$

The logarithm of 3.98 = 0.60, and that of $10^{-8} = -8$. Hence,

$$pH = -0.60 + 8$$
$$pH = 7.40$$

The positive whole numbers of the pH scale are more readily comprehended than the negative exponents or the minute decimal equivalents of the absolute concentration scale.

In moderately severe acidosis, the pH of blood plasma may decrease to 7.15. To convert to hydrogen ion concentration,

$$pH = -\log(H^+)$$
$$\log(H^+) = -7.15$$

Taking the antilogarithm of both sides,

$$(H^+) = \text{antilog}(-7.15)$$

This latter expression can also be written: antilog $(0.85 - 8)$. The antilogarithm of 0.85 = 7.08; that of $-8 = 10^{-8}$. The product of the two gives $(H^+) = 7.08 \cdot 10^{-8}$ Eq/L.

The hydrogen ion concentration of pure distilled water at 25° C is 10^{-7} Eq/L. The hydroxyl ion concentration is the same; hence, pure distilled water is neutral. In other words, a very small proportion of water molecules, $18 \cdot 10^{-7}$ Gm/kg, dissociates to yield equal numbers of H^+ and OH^- ions. If the concentration of H^+ ions exceeds 10^{-7} Eq/L, the solution is acid; if less than this value, the solution is alkaline. The product of hydrogen and hydroxyl ion concentrations always equals 10^{-14} Eq/L, for if the concentration of one ion increases, that of the other decreases in proportion, to keep the product constant.

$$(H^+) \cdot (OH^-) = K_W = 10^{-14} \text{ Eq/L}$$

Each unit change in pH represents a 10-fold change in hydrogen ion concentration. The pH scale ranges from 0 (H^+ = 1 Eq/L) to 14 (H^+ = 10^{-14} Eq/L) — from the reaction of 1-N strong acid to that of 1-N strong base. Obviously, as the solution becomes more acid, pH decreases; as it becomes more alkaline, pH increases.

LAW OF MASS ACTION

The law of mass action states that the velocity of a reaction is proportional to the product of the molar concentrations of the reactants. In a reversible reaction, such as the following,

$$(A)+(B) \underset{V_2}{\overset{V_1}{\rightleftharpoons}} (C)+(D)$$

the velocity to the right is proportional to the product of (A) and (B) and that to the left is proportional to the product of (C) and (D). At equilibrium, which is the condition attained when the velocities in the two directions are equal and no further net changes in the concentrations of the reactants occur,

$$\frac{(C)\cdot(D)}{(A)\cdot(B)} = K$$

The value of K at equilibrium is always the same, regardless of the proportions or concentrations of the reactants initially present.

IONIZATION CONSTANTS

Applying the mass law to the ionization of a weak acid, $HA \rightleftharpoons H^+ + A^-$ yields the equation

$$\frac{(H^+)\cdot(A^-)}{(HA)} = K_A$$

The constant K_A is the ionization or dissociation constant* of the weak acid. The stronger the acid, the greater is the proportion of ions to undissociated molecules and the larger is the value of K_A. Values of K_A for representa-

TABLE 10–1.— DISSOCIATION CONSTANTS OF ACIDS AND BASES (37° C)

SUBSTANCE	K_A	pK_A
Acetic acid	$2.0 \cdot 10^{-5}$	4.7
Acetoacetic acid	$1.6 \cdot 10^{-4}$	3.8
Carbonic acid, A_1	$7.95 \cdot 10^{-7}$	6.1
β-Hydroxybutyric acid	$1.6 \cdot 10^{-5}$	4.8
Lactic acid	$1.3 \cdot 10^{-4}$	3.9
Phosphoric acid, A_2	$3.0 \cdot 10^{-7}$	6.8
	K'_B	pK'_{AB}
Ammonia	$2.35 \cdot 10^{-5}$	9.37

tive weak acids are given in Table 10 − 1.† Because these values are very small, it is customary to express them as negative logarithms and to use the designation pK_A, analogous to pH.

$$pK_A = -\log K_A$$

The stronger the acid and the larger the K_A value, the smaller is the pK_A.

IONIZATION OF WEAK BASES

The ionization of weak bases, like that of weak acids, is incomplete. The mass law, applied to the ionization of a weak base, such as ammonium hydroxide, yields the following expression:

$$\frac{(NH_4^+)\cdot(OH^-)}{(NH_3)} = K_B$$

K_B is a measure of the extent to which a weak base dissociates hydroxyl ions; it increases in value with increasing strength of the base. Converting the dissociation constant K_B to its negative logarithm yields the constant pK_B; i.e., $pK_B = -\log K_B$. The constants K_B and pK_B of weak bases relate to the hydroxyl ion concentrations and pOH values of their solutions, respectively. Because, in physiology, one customarily expresses the

---

*The dissociation constant of a weak acid or base can be determined from the measured electrical conductivity of a solution of known concentration or from the pH of a solution half neutralized with a strong base or acid.

†The dissociation constants and their negative logarithms given in Table 10–1 are actually K′ and pK′ values. These values refer to 38° C and the ionic strength of body fluids. In contrast, K and pK values should refer to infinite dilution and 25° C. Since all of this discussion is concerned with body fluids at 38° C we have arbitrarily used K and pK instead of the proper K′ and pK′ designation merely as a simplification.

reaction of an alkaline solution in terms of pH rather than of pOH, it is convenient to use the constant pK_{AB}, which relates dissociation of a weak base to pH rather than to pOH. The constant pK_{AB} is simply derived from pK_B by the expression $pK_{AB} = 14 - pK_B$.

COMMON ION EFFECT

The ionization of a weak acid or a weak base is greatly reduced by the addition of a compound that dissociates a common ion. For example, the ionization of acetic acid is depressed by the addition of hydrochloric acid, which dissociates the common hydrogen ion, or by the addition of sodium acetate, which dissociates the common acetate ion. Similarly, the ionization of ammonium hydroxide is depressed by the addition of sodium hydroxide, which dissociates the common hydroxyl ion, or by the addition of ammonium chloride, which contributes the common ammonium ion. It is evident from an inspection of the mass law equation, $\dfrac{(H^+) \cdot (A^-)}{(HA)} = K_A$, that increasing the concentration of acetate ions by the addition of highly dissociated sodium acetate must reduce the concentration of hydrogen ions to maintain constancy of K_A. Similar considerations apply to the effects of the addition of ammonium chloride on the dissociation of ammonium hydroxide.

pH OF A SOLUTION CONTAINING EITHER A WEAK ACID OR A WEAK BASE AND ITS SALT

In either of these cases, the pH is determined by the proportion of salt to acid or base. Owing to the common ion effect, the pH of a salt-acid mixture will be higher, and that of a salt-base mixture will be lower, than the pH of the acid or base alone. The Henderson-Hasselbalch equation, which relates pH to the proportion of salt to acid or base,

may be derived from the mass law equation, as follows:

$$\frac{(H^+) \cdot (A^-)}{(HA)} = K_A \tag{1}$$

Rearranging equation 1 yields

$$(H^+) = K_A \cdot \frac{(HA)}{(A^-)} \tag{2}$$

Taking the negative logarithm of both sides and inverting the last term yields

$$-\log(H^+) = -\log K_A + \log \frac{(A^-)}{(HA)} \tag{3}$$

Substituting pH and pK for the negative logarithms of (H^+) and K_A yields the Henderson-Hasselbalch equation,

$$pH = pK_A + \log \frac{(A^-)}{(HA)}$$

To use this equation, certain simplifying assumptions must be made: that anions are derived solely from the dissociation of salt, that anion activity is equivalent to salt concentration and that all of the weak acid is present in undissociated form. These assumptions introduce no appreciable error except when the ratio of salt (anion) to weak acid is either very high or very low. The usable form of the Henderson-Hasselbalch equation becomes

$$pH = pK + \log \frac{salt}{acid}$$

This equation not only breaks down at very high and very low salt-acid ratios; it also is unusable if the salt is insoluble or poorly dissociated.

It is possible to generalize this equation even further by applying the Brønsted formulation of acids and bases, as follows:

$$pH = pK + \log \frac{base}{acid}$$

The anion of the salt of a weak acid is a base, in that it can bind a hydrogen ion. The cation of the salt of a weak base—e.g., the ammonium ion (NH_4^+)—is an acid, in that it can dissociate a hydrogen ion. Ammonia (NH_3), on the other hand, is a base in that it can bind a hydrogen ion. The Henderson-Hasselbalch equation can therefore be used to calculate the pH of a solution containing a mixture of a weak base and its salt, as well as that of a mixture of a weak acid and its salt. In the former instance the pK_{AB} must be used; in the latter, the pK_A. However, the user of this equation must keep in mind just which component is the acid and which is the base.

BUFFER CURVES

The principles of buffer action are best understood in terms of the following equation and the data presented in Table 10–2 and Figure 10–1.

Weak base + Strong acid ⇌ Neutral salt
+ Weak acid

In essence, this equation states that a weak base binds the hydrogen ions dissociated from the strong acid to form a weak, poorly dissociated acid, thereby buffering (i.e., mitigating) the change in hydrogen ion concentration.

TABLE 10–2. – BASE/ACID RATIOS RESULTING FROM THE TITRATION OF 100 mEQ OF WEAK BASE WITH STRONG ACID

STRONG ACID (mEq)	BASE / ACID	LOG BASE / ACID
1	99	1.996
5	19	1.279
10	9	0.954
20	4	0.602
30	2.333	0.368
40	1.500	0.176
50	1.000	0.000
60	0.667	−0.176
70	0.428	−0.368
80	0.250	−0.602
90	0.111	−0.954
95	0.0526	−1.279
99	0.0101	−1.996

If one measures 100 ml of 1-N weak base (100 mEq) into each of a series of 1-L volumetric flasks and then adds from 1 to 99 ml of 1-N strong acid (1 mEq/ml) to each and dilutes to 1,000 ml, a series of ratios of base/acid may be established, such as that shown in column 2 of Table 10–2. These ratios are calculated as follows: The weak base remaining in the equilibrium mixture equals

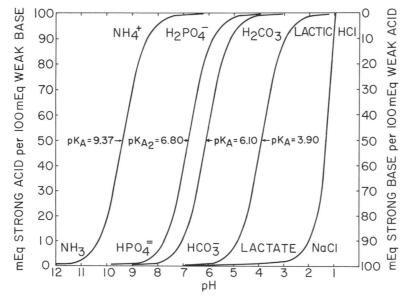

Fig. 10–1. — Titration curves of buffers. *Left to right*, titration of weak bases with strong acid; *right to left*, titration of weak acids with strong base.

100 mEq minus the milliequivalents of strong acid added. The weak acid present in the equilibrium mixture is equal to the milliequivalents of strong acid added. The logarithms of these equilibrium ratios are given in the last column of Table 10–2 and are, of course, the same for all weak acids or bases, because they are determined solely by equivalence. According to the Henderson-Hasselbalch equation, the pH of the equilibrium mixture is equal to the sum of the appropriate pK_A or pK_{AB} and the logarithm of the base/acid ratio. The pH will, of course, vary with the pK value, which is determined by the nature of the weak acid or base.

The relationships between pH and milliequivalents of strong acid added are shown in Figure 10–1 for four weak bases: ammonia, secondary phosphate, bicarbonate and lactate. These curves should be compared with the results obtained on the addition of equal amounts of a strong acid to a neutral salt, such as sodium chloride, which is devoid of buffer properties.

A liter of a solution containing 100 mEq of sodium chloride is neutral and has a pH of 7 (Fig. 10–1, curve beginning at pH 7 and remaining flat and close to the base line to pH 2). The addition of only 0.1 mEq of hydrochloric acid shifts the pH to 4 (10^{-4} Eq of hydrogen ion per liter). The addition of 10 mEq further increases the acidity to pH 2 (10^{-2} Eq of hydrogen ion per liter). Because the pH changes drastically with the addition of a strong acid, the solution is said to be unbuffered.

In contrast, each of the three salts of weak acids – sodium lactate, sodium bicarbonate and secondary sodium phosphate – and the weak base, ammonia, exhibit buffer properties. The addition of successive increments of strong acid causes only minor changes in pH over the range of effective buffer action. The most effective buffering, in each instance, is exerted within limits of ± 1 pH unit to either side of the pK_A or pK_{AB}.

Let us consider the sodium phosphate curve in more detail. The pure secondary salt forms an alkaline solution, owing to the fact that it ionizes completely to form Na^+ and $HPO_4^=$ ions. Pure water contains equal numbers of H^+ and OH^- ions (10^{-7} mEq/L of each at 25° C). The $HPO_4^=$ ions exhibit properties of a weak base and bind some of these hydrogen ions to form $H_2PO_4^-$ ions, shifting the ionization equilibrium of water and resulting in a relative excess of hydroxyl ions. Methods for calculating the pH of pure solutions of such buffer salts are given in standard biochemistry texts and do not concern us in a discussion of physiologic buffering mechanisms. Suffice it to say that the Henderson-Hasselbalch equation cannot be used. The pH changes rapidly with the addition of the first 0.1 mEq of strong acid and much more slowly with successive increments. Again, as the titration progresses to near completion, the pH changes rapidly. The pH change per unit of added acid is least at a pH corresponding to half neutralization; i.e., 6.8. Buffer action is nil at pH values more than 1.5 units removed from the pK. It is apparent that secondary phosphate is a moderately effective chemical buffer at the pH of extracellular fluid. However, the concentration in extracellular fluid is low (1 mM/L), and the role it plays in the buffering of hydrogen ions is, accordingly, small. Bicarbonate is a much less effective chemical buffer, because the pH of extracellular fluid is far removed from the pK_A of the bicarbonate system; i.e., 6.1. However, concentration is high (26–28 mM/L); and because the weak acid, carbonic acid, is potentially volatile and is removed as carbon dioxide by the lungs, bicarbonate is remarkably effective in the physiologic buffering of hydrogen ions.

PHYSIOLOGIC BUFFERING OF STRONG ACID BY BICARBONATE

The titration of bicarbonate with strong acid shown in Figure 10–1 is based on closed-system conditions; i.e., the carbonic acid formed is retained in the buffer mixture. In the body, such relationships do not hold. Instead, the carbonic acid is removed by the lungs as rapidly as it is formed. Because the weak acid does not accumulate, buffering action is greatly enhanced. Furthermore, as the concentration of bicarbonate decreases, breathing is stimulated and the concentration of carbonic acid in body fluids is still further reduced.

Figure 10–2 illustrates the role of the respiratory system in the buffering of strong acid by bicarbonate. Each liter of extracellular fluid contains 24–28 mEq of bicarbonate ion and 1.2–1.4 mEq of carbonic acid. The base/acid ratio is 20; the log of 20 is 1.30, which, added to the pK_A of the bicarbonate system, yields a pH of 7.40. If to each liter of extracellular fluid were added 14 mEq of strong acid, the base/acid ratio would decrease to $14/15.4 = 0.91$. The pH of the mixture would be 6.06. Because the 14 mEq of carbonic acid is removed by the lungs, one might expect the base/acid ratio to increase to $14/1.4 = 10$. The pH of extracellular fluid would then be 7.10. However, compensation begins at once, breathing is stimulated and alveolar ventilation stabilizes at a value between 1.5 and 2 times the normal. The P_{CO_2} of extracellular fluid is reduced from about 40 mm Hg to 23–25 mm Hg, and the carbonic acid concentration to about 0.8 mEq/

L. As a consequence of hyperventilation, the pH of extracellular fluid is returned toward normal; i.e., to 7.34 (compensated metabolic acidosis). Because of pulmonary elimination of carbonic acid as rapidly as it is formed and because of hyperventilation, which stabilizes the carbonic acid concentration at a subnormal value, the poor chemical buffer, bicarbonate, is transformed into a remarkably effective physiologic one.

Not only do the curves of Figure 10–1 describe the buffering of strong acids by weak bases; they equally well describe the buffering of strong bases by weak acids. If one starts with a solution of weak acid (top of the curve) and adds successive increments of strong base (sodium hydroxide), the titration proceeds to the left, along exactly the same curve but in the reverse direction. The reason is obvious: one can arrive at exactly the same base/acid ratio by adding base to acid as by adding acid to base. The base/acid ratio and the pK_A or pK_{AB} determine the pH.

PROTEIN BUFFERS

Plasma proteins and tissue proteins, including hemoglobin, are buffers by virtue of a series of titratable groups within the molecule. These include terminal carboxyl and terminal amino groups of the protein chain, the phenolic group of tyrosine, the sulfhydryl group of cysteine, the free carboxyl group of glutamic acid and aspartic acid, and the free basic groups of lysine, arginine and histidine. The peptide linkages binding the many amino acids into a protein molecule exhibit no buffer characteristics, nor do the amide groups and disulfide groups of the molecule. The pKs of the several titratable groups of plasma proteins cover a fairly wide range; and, because of their overlap, the titration curve is essentially linear within the physiologic range of pH (6). The buffer characteristics of hemoglobin within this range are almost entirely dependent on the imidazole groups of histidine (7). Titration curves for plasma proteins and oxyhemoglobin are shown in Figure 10–3.

Fig. 10–2. — Comparison of bicarbonate as a chemical buffer and as a physiologic buffer of strong acid.

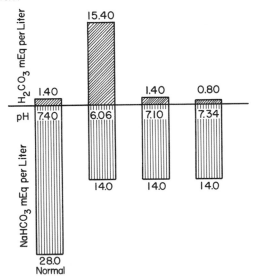

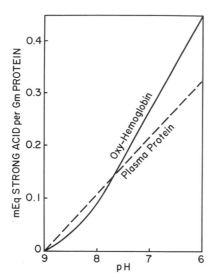

Fig. 10–3. — The buffering of strong acid by plasma proteins and by hemoglobin. (Adapted from Cohn, E. J.: Physiol. Rev. 5:349, 1925, and German, B., and Wyman, J., Jr.: J. Biol. Chem. 117:533, 1937.)

If one first adjusts the reaction of a solution containing 1 Gm of plasma protein to pH 9 by the addition of a strong base and then titrates with strong acid, an essentially linear relationship obtains between milliequivalents of strong acid added and pH of the solution. The same is true for solutions of hemoglobin, except in the alkaline range between pH 9 and pH 8. Figure 10–4 illustrates the mechanism of buffer action of plasma proteins and hemoglobin. At pH 9 the free carboxyl groups of plasma proteins are completely ionized; the basic groups, largely un-ionized. Hydrogen ions liberated in the solution by the addition of strong acid are bound first by the more basic groups and then by the more acidic carboxyl groups. The imidazole groups of histidine account for most of the binding of hydrogen ions by hemoglobin.

One gram of plasma protein binds 0.110 mEq of hydrogen ion when titrated from pH 7.5 to pH 6.5. One gram of oxyhemoglobin binds 0.183 mEq of hydrogen ion. One liter

Fig. 10–4. — Mechanism of buffering of acids and bases by plasma proteins and by the imidazole groups of the histidine contained in hemoglobin. (Adapted from Davenport, H. W.: *The ABC of Acid-Base Chemistry* [4th ed.; Chicago: University of Chicago Press, 1958].)

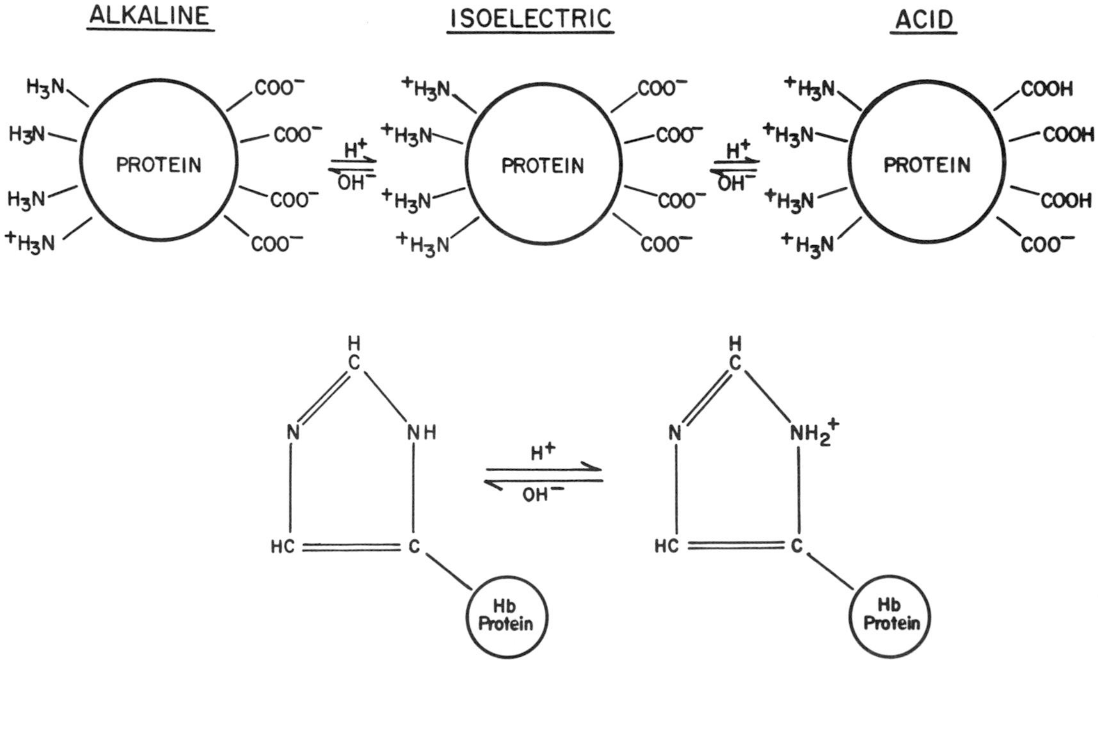

ALKALINE   ISOELECTRIC   ACID

of blood contains 150 Gm of hemoglobin and 38.5 Gm of plasma protein. Accordingly, the oxyhemoglobin of 1 L of blood can buffer $0.183 \cdot 150 = 27.5$ mEq of hydrogen ion between pH 7.5 and 6.5, whereas the plasma protein of 1 L of blood can buffer $0.110 \cdot 35.5 = 4.24$ mEq of hydrogen ion. The hemoglobin of 1 L of blood, therefore, is capable of buffering 6.5 times as much strong acid as the plasma protein. The buffering of the weak acid, carbonic acid, although extremely important in the transport of carbon dioxide from tissues to lungs, is a respiratory problem and will not be considered here. Other body buffers include the proteins and organic phosphate complexes of cells, bone, cartilage, and connective tissues. Their contributions to total body buffering will be considered below.

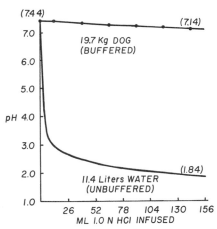

Fig. 10–5.—Comparison of the changes in pH induced by the intravenous infusion of 156 ml of 1N HCl into a 19.7-kg dog with the addition of the same quantity of acid to 11.4 L of water. (From Pitts, R. F.: Harvey Lect. 48:172, 1952–53.)

BUFFERING IN A MULTICOMPONENT SYSTEM

In a solution containing a mixture of buffer acids and bases, the acid/base ratio of each buffer pair is determined by its K_A and by the hydrogen ion concentration of the medium. The blood plasma contains three buffer acids—H_2CO_3, $H_2PO_4^-$ and HPr—and three buffer bases—HCO_3^-, $HPO_4^=$ and Pr^-. Equilibrium is established as follows:

$$(H^+) = K_{A1}\frac{(H_2CO_3)}{(HCO_3^-)} = K_{A2}\frac{(H_2PO_4^-)}{(HPO_4^=)} = K_{A3}\frac{(HPr)}{(Pr^-)}.$$

If the hydrogen ion concentration is altered, the acid/base ratios of all buffers change. If the ratio of the components of any buffer pair is altered, the ratios of all other pairs are altered in proportion.

Chemical Buffering of Strong Acids and Bases in the Body

MECHANISMS FOR BUFFERING STRONG ACIDS

The significance of the several mechanisms for the buffering of strong acid in the body is illustrated in Figure 10–5. Over a period of 90 minutes, 156 mEq of hydrochlo-

ric acid, diluted to 0.3 N, was infused intravenously into a normal dog.* The pH of blood plasma decreased from 7.44 to 7.14, which was indicative of a moderately severe, but by no means fatal, metabolic acidosis. An animal weighing 19.7 kg contains 11.4 L of water. If a similar volume of hydrochloric acid is gradually added to 11.4 L of distilled water, the pH decreases precipitously with the addition of the first few milliliters, reaching a final level of 1.84. The difference in the change of the acidity in these two experiments is related to the fact that the dog is well buffered, whereas distilled water is not.

Because the acid was infused intravenously, one might assume that it was largely neutralized by circulating blood buffers; i.e., by buffers contained in blood plasma and erythrocytes. Actually, nothing could be further from the truth. Van Slyke and Cullen (8), Swan and Pitts (9) and others (10, 11) have

*In this experiment, buffering of the acid load depends almost entirely on the binding of hydrogen ions by the weak bases of blood, interstitial fluid and cell fluid, on the respiratory elimination of carbon dioxide set free in the reaction of acid with bicarbonate and on the respiratory stabilization of the carbonic acid content of the body fluids at the subnormal value. The renal excretion of acid is a relatively slow process, and negligible quantities are eliminated in the urine in the course of 90 minutes.

shown that only 15–20% is neutralized by blood buffers, that a somewhat larger proportion is neutralized by interstitial fluid buffers and that the major fraction is neutralized by buffers of cells and bone.

The means by which strong acid is buffered in the body are described in experiments summarized in Table 10–3 and Figure 10–6. The nature of the experimental approach is illustrated by the data contained in Table 10–3. Animals were nephrectomized at the start of an experiment, to simplify the measurement of extracellular fluid volume and to abolish renal compensations that might otherwise occur during the course of the study. The volume of extracellular fluid—3,990 ml in the control periods and 4,695 ml after the infusion of acid—was measured as the volume of distribution of $^{35}SO_4^{=}$, administered in tracer doses as the sodium salt. The volume of plasma water was calculated from the measured plasma protein concentration and the volume of distribution of Evans blue. Plasma concentrations of sodium, potassium, bicarbonate and chloride were measured and expressed as millimoles per liter of plasma water. Extracellular stores of ions were calculated as the product of the volume of extracellular fluid and the concentration of the several ions in plasma water, appropriately corrected for Donnan distribution across capillary membranes.

It is apparent that extracellular chloride increased by 160 mEq following the infusion of 161 mEq of hydrochloric acid. The chloride obviously remained within the extracellular compartment in this experiment, although in other experiments small amounts entered cells—more specifically, erythrocytes. As a consequence of the infusion of acid, the quantities of sodium and potassium in the extracellular compartment increased by 55 and 31 mEq, respectively, and the quantity of bicarbonate decreased by 67 mEq.

The results obtained in five similar experiments were averaged, and the data are summarized in Figure 10–6. The mean quantity of acid infused was 180 mEq; i.e., 9.5 mEq/kg. The total height of the column represents 100% of the administered acid load. The column is subdivided to indicate the contributions of the several cellular and extracellular mechanisms to the buffering of the acid load.

As a consequence of the decrease in plasma pH from 7.40 to 7.10, about 1% of the acid was buffered by plasma proteins, according to the following equation:

$$Na^+, Pr^- + H^+, Cl^- \longrightarrow Na^+, Cl^- + HPr$$

Extracellular bicarbonate, including both plasma and interstitial fluid moieties, buffered 42% of the acid.

$$Na^+, HCO_3^- + H^+, Cl^- \longrightarrow Na^+, Cl^- + H_2CO_3$$

The concentration of bicarbonate decreased from 26 to 7 mEq/L of water. Carbonic acid was eliminated by the lungs as rapidly as formed. Breathing was stimulated, and the carbonic acid concentration of arterial blood

TABLE 10–3.—Effects of Infusion of Strong Acid on Total Extracellular Stores of Monovalent Ions*

Time (hr)	Plasma Water Volume (ml)	Extra-cellular Volume (ml)	Concentration in Plasma Water (mEq/L)					Total Extracellular Store (mEq)			
			Plasma pH	Na	K	HCO₃	Cl	Na	K	HCO₃	Cl
			CONTROL OBSERVATIONS—16.8-KG DOG								
3.00	660	3,990	7.40	156	4.0	24.6	119	594	15	102	496
4.00	660	3,990	7.42	157	4.1	24.5	119	597	15	102	496
		4.16–6.50 INFUSION OF 550 ML OF 0.291-N HCL (161 MEQ)									
7.75	675	4,695	7.11	145	10.3	6.7	134	652	46	34	658
8.45	675	4,695	7.09	144	10.3	7.3	133	650	46	36	654
							ΔmEq	+55	+31	−67	+160

*From Swan, R. C., and Pitts, R. F.: J. Clin. Invest. 34:205, 1955.

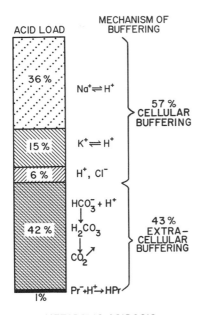

$$H^+, Cl^- \dashv\vdash \to + K^+, Hb \longrightarrow K^+, Cl^- + H \cdot Hb$$

or by the exchange of extracellular chloride for intracellular bicarbonate,

$$Cl^- \rightleftharpoons\vdash HCO_3^-$$

The end result of either operation is the same. Most of the relatively small amount of chloride that left the extracellular fluid entered erythrocytes.

By far the greatest fraction of the infused acid was buffered by the exchange of cellular potassium (15%) and cellular sodium (36%) for extracellular hydrogen ions.

These exchange reactions,

$$H^+ \rightleftharpoons\vdash K^+, A^- \longrightarrow HA \text{ and } H^+ \rightleftharpoons\vdash Na^+, A^- \longrightarrow HA,$$

occurring across the cell membranes of all tissues, make the large stores of intracellular protein and organic phosphate complexes available for the buffering of extracellular hydrogen ions (12).

The hydrogen ions that enter cells are bound by these buffer anions to form poorly dissociated acids. The sodium and potassium ions that leave cells balance the chloride ions, which, for the most part, remain in the extracellular fluid. Had the kidneys been intact, the potassium would have been excreted promptly and no increase in plasma concentration would have occurred. The exchange of cellular potassium for hydrogen and the subsequent excretion of potassium account for the depletion of cellular potassium stores that accompanies clinical metabolic acidosis.

It is probable that some fraction of the sodium ions exchanged for hydrogen ions may actually have come from bone, not from cells. Sodium ions bound on the surfaces of the apatite crystals of bone exchange for hydrogen ions according to the following equation (13):

$$-Ca-O-CO_2-Na + H^+, Cl^- \longrightarrow -Ca-Cl + Na^+, HCO_3^-$$

The buffering of acid by bone appears to be somewhat more significant in chronic

Fig. 10—6.—Mechanisms of buffering of strong acid infused intravenously in the dog. (Adapted from Swan, R. C., and Pitts, R. F.: J. Clin. Invest. 34:205, 1955.)

was maintained at a level roughly half of normal. Had hyperventilation not occurred, plasma pH would have decreased to 6.80 instead of 7.10. The basis for this statement is as follows: The normal ratio of HCO_3^-/H_2CO_3 is 20:1; i.e., 24 mEq/L to 1.2 mEq/L. If the HCO_3^- concentration were reduced to 7 mEq/L without change in the H_2CO_3 concentration, the ratio would decrease to 5:1, corresponding to pH 6.80. Because hyperventilation reduced the H_2CO_3 concentration to 0.7 mEq/L, the ratio HCO_3^-/H_2CO_3 equaled 10, corresponding to pH 7.10. Accordingly, the increase in alveolar ventilation played a prominent role in mitigating the acidosis.

A small fraction of the infused acid (6%) was buffered within cells, either by the penetration of hydrochloric acid,*

---

*The parallel lines in the equation are meant to represent the cell membrane separating interstitial fluid (left) from cell contents (right).

acidosis than in acute acidosis of the nature described here.

Of the total acid infused, only 18% was buffered by plasma bicarbonate and by the hemoglobin of the circulating erythrocytes; i.e., less than one fifth of the acid was neutralized within the vascular compartment. More was neutralized by bicarbonate in the interstitial fluid compartment, and nearly half was neutralized by intracellular buffers other than the hemoglobin of erythrocytes.

Schwartz et al. (14) showed that if acid is infused intermittently for 45 minutes and a period of recovery of 2 hours is permitted before the next acid load is administered, buffering by extracellular bicarbonate is predominant during the infusion, whereas cellular buffering partially restores the plasma bicarbonate level during each interval between acid infusions.

Yoshimura et al. (15) carried out similar studies on dogs with normal renal function and observed changes in the sites of acid buffering with the passage of time following acid administration. On the day of administration, the acid was buffered essentially as described in Figure 10–6. Twenty-four hours later, about one quarter of the acid had been excreted in the urine as titratable acid and combined with ammonia. At this time, the composition of plasma and extracellular fluid had returned nearly to normal. Accordingly, three quarters of the acid administered was now buffered within cells or by bone. Over the succeeding 2–6 days, this acid was gradually returned to the extracellular fluid and excreted in the urine. It is evident that the renal excretion of strong acid, although highly significant, is a relatively slow process. In sharp contrast, the pulmonary excretion of carbonic acid, a weak acid, occurs quite rapidly. The immediate mitigation of change in hydrogen ion concentration when strong acid is liberated in the body thus depends on the buffers of tissues and body fluids and the pulmonary elimination of carbonic acid. Final correction of such a metabolic acidosis depends on the renal excretion of acid.

Relman and his colleagues (16,17) studied buffering of strong acid and alkali in normal man and in patients with renal acidosis. Both groups were maintained on a liquid diet, the nitrogen source of which was a purified soy phosphoprotein virtually free of mineral ions. An equimolar mixture of $Ca(OH)_2$ and $Mg(OH)_2$ was added to the diet in an amount calculated to be equal to the acid that would be generated by the metabolism of organic phosphate. On such a regimen, the net production of fixed acid is measured by the sum of urinary organic acids and inorganic sulfate.

A study on a normal subject is illustrated in Figure 10–7. Serum carbon dioxide content, shown at the top of the figure, was maintained at a normal level of 30–32 mEq/L throughout the study. Net total acid production, shown below, was 65–70 mEq/day. Essentially all of this acid was excreted each day. Accordingly, acid balance varied slightly above and below zero. In

Fig. 10–7.—Acid balance and serum CO_2 content in a normal subject. (From Lemann, J., Jr., Lennon, E. J., Goodman, A. D., Litzow, J. R., and Relman, A. S.: J. Clin. Invest. 44:507, 1965.)

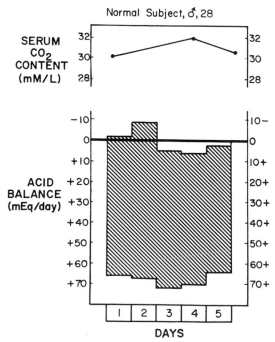

Normal Subject, ♂, 28

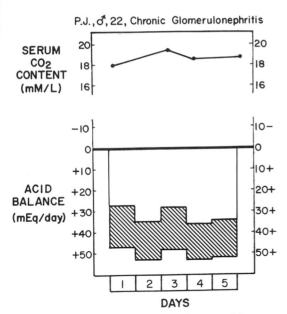

Fig. 10-8.—Acid balance and serum CO_2 content in a patient with chronic glomerulonephritis. (From Goodman, A. D., Lemann, J., Jr., Lennon, E. J., and Relman, A. S.: J. Clin. Invest. 44:495, 1965.)

other words, a normal subject with normal renal function excretes, each day, exactly the same amount of acid as he produces each day. Acid-base balance is maintained.

In contrast, a patient with chronic glomerulonephritis who is in moderate chronic acidosis does not excrete all of the acid he produces each day. This acid is retained and is buffered, most probably, by sodium and calcium largely derived from apatite crystals of cancellous bone. As shown in the upper portion of Figure 10-8, serum carbon dioxide content was maintained throughout this study at levels of 18-19 mEq/l, which are indicative of a modest, stable extracellular acidosis. However, acid production was 48-52 mEq/day, and the acid was only partially excreted. A net positive acid balance of 28-37 mEq/day, indicating a continuous gain of acid within the body, was sustained throughout the study. This deficit of acid excretion, according to Relman, is buffered in the body by cells and by bone. This is emphasized by such bone diseases as nephritic rickets in childhood and osteomalacia in the adult.

A reversal of these processes could account for retention of cation induced by loads of alkali. The prolonged low-grade acidosis characteristic of patients with renal tubular acidosis frequently leads to progressive demineralization of the skeleton.

MECHANISMS FOR BUFFERING BASES

The means by which alkali is buffered in the body are described in Figure 10-9. The experiments upon which this graph is based were performed on nephrectomized dogs in a manner similar to those in which acid was infused (18). Following a control series of observations, 20 mEq/kg of sodium bicarbonate was administered intravenously; and after an interval, to insure equilibration, the observations were repeated. The total height of the column represents 100% of the administered bicarbonate load. The column is subdivided to indicate the contributions of the several cellular and extracellular mechanisms to the buffering of the alkali load.

Fig. 10-9.—Mechanisms of buffering of base infused intravenously in the dog. (Adapted from Swan, R. C., Axelrod, D. R., Seip, M., and Pitts, R. F.: J. Clin. Invest. 34:1795, 1955.)

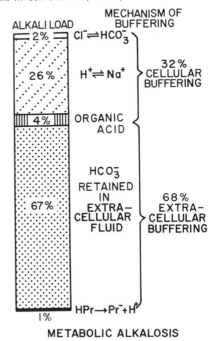

The bicarbonate concentration of plasma increased to 60–70 mEq/L, and plasma pH rose to 7.60–7.65. Owing to the change in pH, plasma proteins buffered about 1% of the alkali; i.e., undissociated protein acid gave up hydrogen ions in an amount sufficient to convert 1% of the bicarbonate to carbonic acid.

$$HPr + Na^+, HCO_3^- \longrightarrow Na^+, Pr^- + H_2CO_3$$

Two thirds of the infused bicarbonate was retained in the extracellular fluid compartment. Respiration was depressed, and the concentration of carbonic acid increased from preinfusion levels of 1.2–1.3 to 2.4–2.6 mEq/L. Had there been no reduction in alveolar ventilation and no increase in the concentration of carbonic acid in extracellular fluid, the pH would have exceeded 7.8. Compensation of metabolic alkalosis by reduction in alveolar ventilation is, of course, limited by increasing hypoxia.

One third of the administered bicarbonate was buffered by one or another of the following cellular mechanisms. About 4% was converted to carbonic acid as a consequence of an outpouring of lactic acid from cells.

$$Na^+, HCO_3^- + H, lactic\ acid \longrightarrow Na^+, lactate^- + H_2CO_3$$

Some 2% of the bicarbonate entered cells in exchange for chloride ions. Most, if not all, of this exchange of bicarbonate for chloride occurred across erythrocyte membranes.

$$HCO_3^- \rightleftharpoons \!\!\!| \!\!\!| \rightleftharpoons Cl^-$$

The remaining 26% was buffered by the exchange of cellular hydrogen ions for extracellular sodium ions. These hydrogen ions were in large part dissociated from intracellular proteins and organic phosphate complexes, although some may have been derived from bone.

$$H_2CO_3 \longleftarrow HCO_3^-, Na^+ \rightleftharpoons \!\!\!| \!\!\!| \rightleftharpoons H^+, A^- \longrightarrow Na^+, A^-$$

Had the kidneys been intact, the rapid urinary excretion of sodium bicarbonate would have restored the composition of the body fluids to normal within a relatively short period of time. The rapidity with which the normal kidney eliminates sodium bicarbonate considerably exceeds that with which it eliminates acid.

Chemical Buffering of Weak Acids In Vivo

RESPIRATORY ACIDOSIS

Inadequate pulmonary clearance of carbon dioxide from the blood produces respiratory acidosis. The P_{CO_2} and carbonic acid concentration rise; the pH falls. Hypoventilation of the whole lung or a major portion of it is the common cause of respiratory acidosis. The condition also develops if ventilation in relation to blood perfusion is very uneven in various portions of the lung. The increase in concentration of carbonic acid in the body fluids is compensated (i.e., buffered) by an increase in the bicarbonate ion concentration. Because the renal mechanisms of ammonia and titratable acid excretion operate slowly to build up bicarbonate reserves, the immediate compensation evident in acute respiratory acidosis must represent the action of chemical buffers, largely those of tissues and bone.

RESPIRATORY ALKALOSIS

Excessive pulmonary clearance of carbon dioxide from the blood results in respiratory alkalosis. The P_{CO_2} and the carbonic acid concentration fall and the pH rises, as a consequence of hyperventilation. The decrease in concentration of carbonic acid in the body fluids is compensated by a decrease in bicarbonate ion concentration. Because increased renal excretion of bicarbonate operates slowly to reduce bicarbonate reserves, the immediate compensation evident in acute respiratory alkalosis must represent the action of chemical buffers, again almost entirely those of tissues and bone.

ROLE OF BODY BUFFERS IN RESPIRATORY ACIDOSIS AND ALKALOSIS

The role of body buffers in mitigating respiratory acidosis and alkalosis is illustrated by the data summarized in Table 10–4 (19). This experiment was performed on a nephrectomized dog and used the volumes of distribution of Evans blue and of $^{35}SO_4^=$ as measures of plasma and extracellular fluid volumes, respectively. During the initial two periods of the experiment, the animal breathed room air spontaneously. Hyperventilation was then instituted with a mechanical pump at a rate sufficient to lower the P_{CO_2} of arterial blood to a value about one fifth of

that observed in the control periods. Two more control periods followed, during which the animal again breathed room air spontaneously. Respiratory acidosis was then induced by the administration of a mixture of 20% carbon dioxide and 80% oxygen as the inspired gas. The P_{CO_2} of arterial blood increased to a level 4–5 times that observed during the spontaneous breathing of room air.

The increase in plasma pH and the decrease in plasma bicarbonate during hyperventilation are characteristic of acute respiratory alkalosis. The decrease in plasma pH and the increase in plasma bicarbonate during hypercapnia are characteristic of acute respiratory acidosis. Because the animal was nephrectomized, alterations in the ionic structure of the plasma were obviously independent of changes in renal function.

In respiratory alkalosis, extracellular stores of sodium, potassium and bicarbonate decreased, whereas those of chloride and lactate increased. In respiratory acidosis, extracellular stores of sodium, potassium and bicarbonate increased, whereas those of chloride and lactate decreased.

TABLE 10-4.—EFFECTS OF ACUTE RESPIRATORY ALKALOSIS AND ACIDOSIS ON TOTAL EXTRACELLULAR STORES OF MONOVALENT IONS*

TIME (Min)	PLASMA WATER VOLUME (ml)	EXTRA-CELLULAR VOLUME (ml)	PLASMA		CONCENTRATION IN PLASMA WATER (mEq/L)					TOTAL EXTRACELLULAR STORE (mEq)				
			P_{CO_2} (mm Hg)	pH	Na	K	HCO_3	Cl	Lact.	Na	K	HCO_3	Cl	Lact.
SPONTANEOUS BREATHING OF ROOM AIR—35.9-KG DOG														
150	1,487	6,545	29.9	7.42	155	3.9	20.8	116	1.0	972	25	142	793	6
210	1,487	6,545	26.7	7.45	154	3.9	19.8	115	1.2	969	26	136	781	8
HYPERVENTILATION														
270	1,284	6,545	6.7	7.57	151	3.9	7.5	124	5.9	960	25	47	850	39
330	1,284	6,545	6.1	7.54	150	3.5	6.9	125	6.7	952	22	43	854	44
									Δ mEq	−15	−2	−94	+65	+35
SPONTANEOUS BREATHING OF ROOM AIR														
390	1,281	6,545	33.2	7.30	154	3.8	17.2	115	3.1	974	24	118	785	20
450	1,281	6,545	33.2	7.34	154	4.2	19.2	116	1.2	980	27	132	793	8
									Δ mEq	+21	+2	+80	−63	−28
BREATHING 20% CO_2 AND 80% O_2														
510	1,233	6,545	146	6.87	160	4.7	28.0	113	1.4	1,006	29	190	777	9
570	1,233	6,545	143	6.92	163	6.5	30.0	113	0.2	1,028	41	205	783	1
									Δ mEq	+40	+9	+72	−9	−9

*From Giebisch, G., Berger, L., and Pitts, R. F.: J. Clin. Invest. 34:231, 1955.

Mechanisms for Buffering Increased Carbonic Acid Content of the Body

The means by which an increase in the carbonic acid content of the body is buffered are described in Figure 10–10. This graph summarizes the results obtained in four experiments in which respiratory acidosis was induced by the inhalation of 20% carbon dioxide. The height of the column is equal to the increase in the extracellular store of bicarbonate. The several mechanisms responsible for this increase are indicated by the subdivisions of the column.

As a consequence of the marked increase in the acidity of the blood, plasma proteins buffer some 2–3% of the carbonic acid; i.e., they account for 2–3% of the increase in the bicarbonate content of extracellular fluid.

$$Na^+, Pr^- + H, HCO_3 \longrightarrow Na^+, HCO_3^- + HPr$$

This reaction represents the sole mechanism of extracellular buffering of carbon dioxide. All other mechanisms involve the participation of cells in one way or another.

Lactate is removed from extracellular fluid and replaced by bicarbonate, a process that accounts for 6% of the increase in extracellular buffer stores.

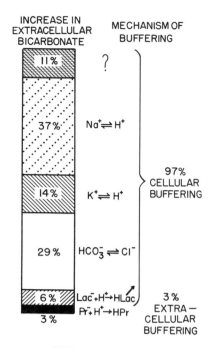

RESPIRATORY ACIDOSIS

Fig. 10–10. — Mechanisms of buffering of CO_2 in respiratory acidosis in the dog. (Adapted from Giebisch, G., Berger, L., and Pitts, R. F.: J. Clin. Invest. 34:231, 1955.)

form carbonic acid; (2) the hydrogen ions dissociated from carbonic acid are bound to hemoglobin anion to form poorly dissociated

$$Na^+, Lactate^- + H, HCO_3 \longrightarrow H, Lactic\ acid + Na^+, HCO_3^-$$

The lactic acid either undergoes complete metabolic degradation within cells or is converted to a nonacidic substance, such as glucose or glycogen.

Twenty-nine per cent of the buffering of carbonic acid is accomplished by the entry of chloride into cells in exchange for bicarbonate.

$$Cl^- \rightleftharpoons HCO_3^-$$

Essentially all of the exchange of chloride occurs across erythrocyte membranes and involves the following steps: (1) carbon dioxide diffuses into red cells and is hydrated to

hemoglobin acid; and (3) equivalent numbers of intracellular bicarbonate ions are exchanged for extracellular chloride ions, increasing the extracellular bicarbonate by 29%.

A reaction of even greater significance is the exchange of intracellular sodium and potassium ions for extracellular hydrogen ions. The exchange of sodium accounts for 37% of the increase in extracellular bicarbonate; the exchange of potassium accounts for 14%. The hydrogen ions that enter cells are bound by protein and organic phosphate anions to form poorly dissociated acids.

$$Na^+, HCO_3^- \longleftarrow HCO_3^-, H^+ \rightleftharpoons Na^+, A^- \longrightarrow HA$$

In part, these ion exchange reactions may involve the apatite crystals of bone. The source of about 11% of increased extracellular bicarbonate has not been defined.

COMPENSATION IN INCREASED BICARBONATE CONCENTRATION

The compensatory nature of the increase in bicarbonate concentration of the extracellular fluid in respiratory acidosis is evident from the following considerations: On breathing 20% carbon dioxide, the plasma concentration of carbonic acid increased to 5 mEq/L. If the concentration of bicarbonate had remained unchanged, the normal ratio of HCO_3^- to H_2CO_3, of 20:1, would have decreased to 4:1. The pH of arterial blood would have been 6.75. Because the plasma bicarbonate increased some 10 mEq/L, the ratio of HCO_3^- to H_2CO_3 decreased only to 6:1. Accordingly, plasma pH was 6.9, not 6.75.

Normal renal function is essential for maximum compensation of respiratory acidosis. In severe chronic respiratory acidosis, the concentration of bicarbonate in extracellular fluid may increase to 50–60 mEq/L as a result of increased excretion of titratable acid and ammonia and of retention of cation as sodium bicarbonate. Because of increased bicarbonate concentration, the ratio of HCO_3^- to H_2CO_3 more nearly approaches the normal, and the acidosis is much less severe than that observed in acute carbon dioxide retention. The renal mechanisms involved will be described in the next chapter.

MECHANISMS FOR BUFFERING REDUCED CARBONIC ACID CONTENT OF THE BODY

The means by which a reduction in the carbonic acid content of the body is buffered are described in Figure 10–11. This graph summarizes the results obtained in five experiments in which respiratory alkalosis was induced by mechanical hyperventilation sufficient to lower the plasma P_{CO_2} to about 6 mm Hg. The height of the column is equal to the decrease in the extracellular store of bicarbonate. The several mechanisms responsible for this decrease are indicated by the subdivisions of the column.

As a consequence of the marked increase in alkalinity of the blood, plasma proteins dissociate hydrogen ions in an amount sufficient to reduce the bicarbonate content of extracellular fluid by about 1%.

$$H^+, Pr^- + Na^+, HCO_3^- \longrightarrow Na^+, Pr^- + H_2CO_3 \nearrow$$

Since this reaction represents the sole extracellular buffer mechanism operative in respiratory alkalosis, it is evident that cellu-

Fig. 10–11.—Mechanisms of buffering of CO_2 in respiratory alkalosis in the dog. (Adapted from Giebisch, G., Berger, L., and Pitts, R. F.: J. Clin. Invest. 34:231, 1955.)

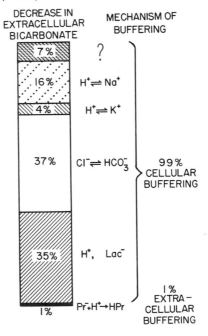

RESPIRATORY ALKALOSIS

lar buffer mechanisms must bear the brunt of change in the reaction of extracellular fluid.

Lactic acid is produced in amounts sufficient to reduce the bicarbonate content of extracellular fluid by 35%. Some 37% of extracellular bicarbonate is replaced by chloride, which is largely derived from red cell stores by ion exchange. Sodium and potassium ions enter a variety of cells in exchange for hydrogen ions, which are buffered by bicarbonate in extracellular fluid. These several mechanisms account for a reduction of 12 – 16 mEq of bicarbonate for each liter of extracellular fluid.

COMPENSATION BY DECREASED BICARBONATE CONCENTRATION

The compensatory nature of the decrease in bicarbonate concentration of extracellular fluid in respiratory alkalosis is evident from the following considerations: Marked hyperventilation reduced the concentration of carbonic acid to about one sixth of its normal value; i.e., to 0.2 mEq/L. If the concentration of bicarbonate had remained unchanged, the ratio of HCO_3^- to H_2CO_3 would have increased from its normal value of 20:1 to more than 120:1. The pH of extracellular fluid, under these circumstances, would have been 8.2. Actually, the bicarbonate concentration was reduced to 8 – 12 mEq/L, corresponding to an HCO_3^-/H_2CO ratio of from 40:1 to 60:1 and a pH of 7.7 – 7.9, not pH 8.2.

Summary

In the normal person, the reaction of the internal fluid environment is kept constant within the narrow limits of pH 7.35 and 7.45. Precise regulation is attained through the operation of both chemical and physiologic buffering mechanisms. The chemical buffers of plasma and interstitial fluid include protein, bicarbonate and inorganic phosphate. Those of tissues include hemoglobin and other intracellular proteins and organic phosphate complexes, such as adenosine triphosphate, adenosine diphosphate and creatine phosphate. The apatite crystals of bone also exhibit buffer properties. The physiologic buffering mechanisms include the respiratory system and the kidneys.

Chemical buffers are mixtures of weak, poorly dissociated organic acids and their highly dissociated salts. Hydrogen ions, dissociated from strong acids formed in the body by the oxidation of sulfur and phosphorus or by the incomplete oxidation of fats, are bound by the anions of buffer salts to form undissociated weak buffer acids. A weak acid is substituted for a strong acid, thus minimizing the increase in hydrogen ion concentration. Hydroxyl ions formed in the body by the oxidation of salts of metabolizable organic acids are buffered by hydrogen ions dissociated from weak buffer acids. The decrease in hydrogen ion concentration that would otherwise occur is minimized. Cells contain large stores of buffer, which they share with extracellular fluid in a variety of ways. A strong acid, such as hydrochloric acid, may penetrate erythrocytes in small quantities and be buffered by hemoglobin in the cell interior. Extracellular chloride ions, which exhibit no buffer characteristics, exchange with cellular bicarbonate ions, restoring the buffer content of extracellular fluid. Extracellular hydrogen ions exchange for cellular sodium and potassium ions and are buffered by cell proteins and organic phosphate complexes. Similar ion shifts occurring in the reverse direction permit the participation of cellular buffers in the neutralization of bases in the extracellular fluid.

The respiratory system participates in the buffering of strong acids liberated within the body by eliminating the carbon dioxide formed in the reaction of hydrogen ions with bicarbonate ions and by subsequently maintaining the carbonic acid concentration of the body fluids at a subnormal value. The respiratory system participates, to a limited extent, in the buffering of base liberated within the body. Hypoventilation, which results in the accumulation of carbonic acid in the body fluids, mitigates the alkalosis. Hypoxia limits the extent of respiratory compensation of metabolic alkalosis.

The chemical buffers of cells, extracellular fluid and bone can be considered as a first line of defense, in that they absorb the immediate shock of liberation of acid or alkali in the body. The respiratory system is a second line of defense, capable of compensating, in part, for both metabolic acidosis and alkalosis. Final correction of disturbances in acid-base balance depends on renal excretion of acid or alkali.

REFERENCES

1. Macallum, A. B.: The paleochemistry of the body fluids and tissues, Physiol. Rev. 6:316, 1926.
2. Bernard, C.: *Leçons sur les phénomenes de la vie communs aux animaux et aux végétaux* (Paris: Baillière, 1885).
3. Westerfeld, W. W.: *Fundamentals of Acid-Base and Electrolyte Biochemistry* (Syracuse: State University of New York College of Medicine at Syracuse, 1953).
4. Clark, W. M.: *The Determination of Hydrogen Ions* (Baltimore: Williams & Wilkins Company, 1928).
5. Gamble, J. L.: *Chemical Anatomy, Physiology and Pathology of Extracellular Fluid* (Cambridge, Mass.: Harvard University Press, 1947).
6. Cohn, E. J.: The physical chemistry of the proteins, Physiol. Rev. 5:349, 1925.
7. German, B., and Wyman, J., Jr.: The titration curves of oxygenated and reduced hemoglobin, J. Biol. Chem. 117:533, 1937.
8. Van Slyke, D. D., and Cullen, G. E.: Studies of acidosis: I. The bicarbonate concentration of the blood plasma; its significance and its determination as a measure of acidosis, J. Biol. Chem. 30:289, 1917.
9. Swan, R. C., and Pitts, R. F.: Neutralization of infused acid by nephrectomized dogs, J. Clin. Invest. 34:205, 1955.
10. Schwartz, W. B., Jenson, R. L., and Relman, A. S.: The disposition of acid administered to sodium-depleted subjects: The renal response and the role of whole body buffers, J. Clin. Invest. 33:587, 1954.
11. Tobin, R. B.: Plasma, extracellular and muscle electrolyte responses to acute metabolic acidosis, Am. J. Physiol. 186:131, 1956.
12. Cooke, R. E., and Segar, W. E.: A proposed mechanism of extracellular regulation of muscle composition, Yale, J. Biol. & Med. 25:83, 1952.
13. Bergstrom, W. H., and Wallace, W. M.: Bone as a sodium and potassium reservoir, J. Clin. Invest. 33:867, 1954.
14. Schwartz, W. B., Orning, K. J., and Porter, R.: The internal distribution of hydrogen ions with varying degrees of metabolic acidosis, J. Clin. Invest. 36:373, 1957.
15. Yoshimura, T., Fujimoto, M., Okumura, O., Sugimoto, J., and Kuwada, T.: Three step regulation of acid-base balance in body fluids after acid load, Japanese J. Physiol. 11:109, 1961.
16. Goodman, A. D., Lemann, J., Jr., Lennon, E. J., and Relman, A. S.: Production, excretion, and net balance of fixed acid in patients with renal acidosis, J. Clin. Invest. 44:495, 1965.
17. Lemann, J., Jr., Lennon, E. J., Goodman, A. D., Litzow, J. R., and Relman, A. S.: The net balance of acid in subjects given large loads of acid or alkali, J. Clin. Invest. 44:507, 1965.
18. Swan, R. C., Axelrod, D. R., Seip, M., and Pitts, R. F.: Distribution of sodium bicarbonate infused into nephrectomized dogs, J. Clin. Invest. 34:1795, 1955.
19. Giebisch, G., Berger, L., and Pitts, R. F.: The extra renal response to acute acid-base disturbances of respiratory origin, J. Clin. Invest. 34:231, 1955.

11

Renal Regulation of Acid-Base Balance

THE BICARBONATE-CARBONIC ACID buffer system plays a key role in the stabilization of reaction of the body fluids. The importance of this system does not derive from the fact that it is an especially effective chemical buffer at the pH of the body fluids, for it is not; its pK is too far removed from the pH for optimum stabilization of reaction. Rather, it derives from the fact that the concentrations of the two components of this buffer system are regulated and stabilized by remarkably effective physiologic mechanisms: the carbonic acid concentration (Pco_2) is regulated by the respiratory system, and the bicarbonate ion concentration is regulated by the kidneys. Because determination of the concentrations of one buffer pair fixes the hydrogen ion concentration, it also fixes the ratio of all other buffer pairs, because they are in equilibrium at the same pH.

The respiratory system and the kidneys primarily regulate the carbonic acid and bicarbonate concentrations of the arterial blood plasma. Because a dynamic equilibrium exists between blood plasma and interstitial fluid across capillary walls, they stabilize fluid reaction throughout the extracellular compartment. Carbon dioxide diffuses rapidly and hydrogen ions and cations exchange more slowly across cell membranes. Accordingly, the respiratory system and the kidneys participate in the regulation of the reaction of intracellular fluid, although they do so indirectly. Intracellular hydrogen ion concentration is neither equal to nor necessarily direct-

ly related to extracellular hydrogen ion concentration. Rather, it is determined by the distribution of ions across cell membranes, which in turn is conditioned by the composition of extracellular fluid.

This chapter is concerned with the renal processes involved in the regulation of the bicarbonate ion concentration of the extracellular fluid; namely, with (1) the conservation of the normal circulating stores of bicarbonate that enter the renal tubules in the glomerular filtrate; (2) the excretion of any excess bicarbonate that gains access to or is produced in the body; and (3) the replenishment of depleted stores of bicarbonate by the renal excretion of titratable acid and ammonia.

The respiratory system is commonly considered to play the dominant role in regulation of acid-base balance. This view is based on the fact that the lungs of man excrete some 13,000 mEq/day of carbonic acid as CO_2, whereas the kidneys excrete only 40–80 mEq/day of nonvolatile acids as titratable acid and as ammonium salts. Two fallacies in this line of reasoning are evident. First, in a quantitative sense, the major contribution of the kidneys to maintenance of acid-base balance is conservation of the circulating extracellular stores of bicarbonate. In man, some 5,100 mEq of bicarbonate ion are reabsorbed each day from the glomerular filtrate by the secretion into the tubular urine of equivalent numbers of hydrogen ions. In this light, the quantitative disparity between the activities

198

of lungs and kidneys is reduced. Second, the hydrogen ion concentration of body fluids is no more dependent on the concentration of carbonic acid than on that of bicarbonate ion. Indeed, it is determined by their ratio and therefore is equally dependent on lungs and kidneys.

The thesis will be developed that the tubular secretion of hydrogen ions in exchange for sodium ions is the key mechanism underlying the reabsorption of bicarbonate, the generation of titratable buffer acid and the excretion of ammonium salts. The extent to which this ion exchange mechanism is engaged in each of these processes is determined by the nature and concentration of buffers delivered into the urine in the glomerular filtrate. If the bicarbonate concentration of the filtrate is normal or above normal, the mechanism will be largely engaged in the reabsorption of this anion; little ammonia and titratable acid will be excreted. If the bicarbonate concentration is below normal, the mechanism will be only partially engaged in the reabsorption of this anion, and more titratable acid and ammonia will be excreted. Finally, if the concentrations of all

buffers in the filtrate are low or if their pK values are unfavorable (β-hydroxybutyrate and acetoacetate), the buffer deficit will be made up largely by the tubular synthesis and secretion of ammonia into the urine at the sites of hydrogen-sodium exchange.

Renal Reabsorption and Excretion of Bicarbonate

GROSS CHARACTERISTICS

The gross characteristics of the processes of renal reabsorption and excretion of bicarbonate in man are illustrated in Figure 11–1 (1). If ammonium chloride is ingested for several days before an experiment, the plasma concentration of bicarbonate is reduced from a normal value of 26–28 mM/L to about 13–15 mM/L. If sodium bicarbonate is infused slowly, the plasma concentration gradually increases. All bicarbonate filtered through the glomeruli is reabsorbed, and none is excreted until the plasma level attains a value of 26–28 mM/L, which is the so-called renal bicarbonate threshold. As still more bicarbonate is infused and the plas-

Fig. 11–1.—Filtration, reabsorption and excretion of bicarbonate as functions of plasma concentration in normal man. (From Pitts, R. F., Ayer, J. L., and Schiess, W. A.: J. Clin. Invest. 28:35, 1949.)

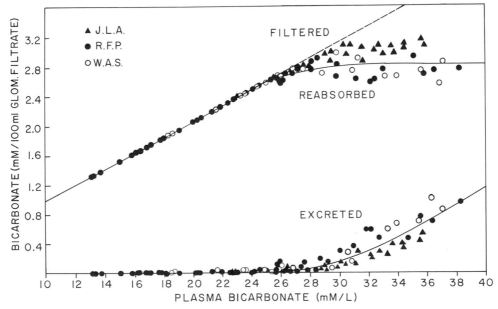

ma concentration increases above 28 mM/L, a limited amount of bicarbonate, equal to 2.8 mM/100 ml, or 28 mM/L, of glomerular filtrate, is reabsorbed. All filtered in excess of this quantity is excreted in the urine. Processes of reabsorption and excretion of bicarbonate in the dog are essentially similar to those in man, except that the threshold is slightly lower, 24–26 mM/L, and the transport rate slightly less, 2.6 mM/100 ml, or 26 mM/L, of glomerular filtrate (2).

Under normal conditions in man, the plasma concentration of bicarbonate is poised at a value slightly below the renal plasma threshold–perhaps 27 mM/L. If the filtration rate is 125 ml/min, 180 L of plasma are filtered per day, delivering into the tubules some 5,100 mM of bicarbonate. Only 1–2 mM is excreted in 1.5 L of urine of pH 6. Accordingly, more than 99.9% of the filtered bicarbonate is reabsorbed.

If the plasma concentration of bicarbonate were to exceed the renal threshold, owing to the ingestion of bicarbonate or to the metabolism of salts of organic acids, the continued reabsorption of 26–28 mM of bicarbonate per liter of filtrate and excretion of the excess would gradually lower the plasma and interstitial fluid concentrations to the normal range. Excretion would then cease. If there always was an excess of inorganic cations in the diet, as there is in herbivorous animals, the processes of reabsorption and excretion alone would serve to stabilize the bicarbonate ion concentration of the body fluids within the usual limits of normal.

The reabsorption in man of 28 mM of bicarbonate per liter of glomerular filtrate, or in the dog of 26 mM/L, should not be construed as indicating that bicarbonate reabsorption is Tm-limited in the same sense that glucose is. The infusion of bicarbonate in both man and dog progressively increases the filtration rate. Constancy of reabsorption, when plasma concentration exceeds the renal threshold, obtains only if reabsorption is factored by filtration rate, not by time. The teleologic significance of this relationship is evident, even though the mechanism is not. If an ani-

mal with a very labile filtration rate, such as a dog, were to be in bicarbonate balance in the fasting state and if bicarbonate reabsorption were truly Tm-limited in terms of millimoles per minute, the ingestion of a large meal of meat and the attendant increase in filtration rate would rapidly deplete the circulating bicarbonate stores. Actually, an increase in filtration rate is accompanied by no increase in bicarbonate excretion; the increased filtered load is reabsorbed. Because both chloride and bicarbonate exhibit this reabsorptive characteristic and since they are the major anions associated with sodium in the filtrate and tubular urine, it is probable that this characteristic is imposed on them by the sodium reabsorptive mechanism (see Chapter 7).

BICARBONATE REABSORPTIVE MECHANISM

The reabsorption of bicarbonate is depressed and excretion is increased by the administration of a variety of N'-unsubstituted sulfonamide compounds, all of which are inhibitors of the enzyme carbonic anhydrase. This fact suggests that the enzyme plays a key role in the reabsorptive mechanism.

CARBONIC ANHYDRASE. — In 1935, Roughton discovered carbonic anhydrase in red blood cells (3). This enzyme greatly increases the rate of attainment of equilibrium in step 1 of the following reaction:

$$CO_2 + H_2O \underset{}{\overset{1}{\rightleftharpoons}} H_2CO_3 \underset{}{\overset{2}{\rightleftharpoons}} H^+, HCO_3^-$$

In the absence of enzyme, step 1 is slow. Step 2, on the other hand, is inherently rapid and is uninfluenced by the presence or absence of enzyme. Catalysis by carbonic anhydrase facilitates the rapid conversion of bicarbonate ion into carbon dioxide in the brief interval that any given unit of blood spends in a pulmonary capillary. It likewise facilitates the rapid conversion of carbon dioxide into bicarbonate ion in the tissue capillaries.

Carbonic anhydrase is a zinc-containing metalloprotein enzyme having a molecular weight of 30,000. Mann and Keilin, in 1940, demonstrated that it is inhibited by N'-unsubstituted sulfonamides. Shortly thereafter, Davenport observed that the enzyme is present in renal tubules in high concentration, and Hoeber maintained that it is involved in some manner in the tubular reabsorption of bicarbonate (4).

Acetazolamide is a highly active inhibitor of carbonic anhydrase. When administered intravenously, the drug depresses the reabsorption and increases the excretion of bicarbonate and sodium ions, alkalizes the urine and enhances the secretion of potassium ions. These effects, illustrated by an experiment on a dog, are summarized in Table 11–1.

PROXIMAL MECHANISM.—A proximal mechanism is specialized to reabsorb the bulk of the filtered bicarbonate from the tubular urine against a relatively low gradient. The basic elements of the mechanism are illustrated in Figure 11–2 (4). Sodium and bicarbonate ions enter the proximal tubule in the glomerular filtrate. Sodium ions diffuse into the tubular cells down a concentration and electrical gradient and are actively extruded into the peritubular fluid by a pump, which maintains intracellular sodium concentration at a low value. Hydrogen ions move from the interior of the cell to the tubular lumen in exchange for sodium ions against an electrical gradient. They associate

PROXIMAL TUBULAR CELL

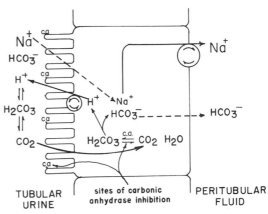

Fig. 11–2. — Schematic representation of bicarbonate reabsorption in a proximal tubular cell. *Dashed lines,* passive diffusion down electrochemical gradients; *solid lines,* active transport.

with bicarbonate ions to form carbonic acid, which decomposes into carbon dioxide and water. The carbon dioxide diffuses into the cell, where it undergoes hydration to form carbonic acid; this reaction is catalyzed by carbonic anhydrase. Subsequent dissociation provides the hydrogen ions, which are exchanged for sodium ions across the luminal membrane, and the bicarbonate ions, which diffuse down a potential gradient into the peritubular fluid. According to this concept, bicarbonate ions are reabsorbed indirectly by conversion within the tubular lumen to carbon dioxide. The key element of the reabsorptive process is the exchange, across the luminal membrane, of intracellular hydrogen ions for sodium ions in the tubular fluid.

As pointed out in Chapter 7, the entry of sodium ions into proximal tubular cells is passive and involves diffusion down a concentration gradient. In contrast, the movement of hydrogen ions in the reverse direction is active and demands a secretory pump—a fact established by Rector *et al.* (5). Whether the passive influx of sodium ions and active efflux of hydrogen ions are carrier-linked is not known. However, they are linked operationally by the necessity to

TABLE 11–1.—EFFECT OF ACETAZOLAMIDE ON EXCRETION OF IONS IN A MILDLY ACIDOTIC DOG (26 KG)*

URINE		RATE OF EXCRETION (mEq/min)			
Flow (ml/min)	pH	Titr. Acid	HCO_3^-	Na^+	K^+
0.81	5.58	0.105	0.0002	0.085	0.068
0.77	5.41	0.154	0.0002	0.085	0.061
0.94	5.38	0.164	0.0003	0.116	0.052
INJECTION OF ACETAZOLAMIDE (10 MG/KG)					
8.06	7.82	0	0.920	1.654	0.264
6.21	7.80	0	0.750	1.315	0.248
4.17	7.73	0	0.456	0.935	0.184

*From Berliner, R. W.: Fed. Proc. 11:695, 1952.

maintain electroneutrality, because the luminal membranes of tubular cells seem to be relatively impermeable to bicarbonate ions as such.

Walser and Mudge (6), in the critique of the mechanism of bicarbonate reabsorption, pointed out the following pertinent facts: The dehydration of H_2CO_3 is inherently slow in the absence of enzymatic catalysis. If no carbonic anhydrase (c.a., in the accompanying equation) is present within the tubular lumen, for dehydration to proceed at a rate equal to the known rate of reabsorption of bicarbonate and thus to account for reabsorption of HCO_3^- as CO_2, the concentration of H_2CO_3 in the tubular fluid would have to be some 8–10 times higher than it would be if it were in equilibrium with CO_2 at its tension in plasma (compare upper and lower lines of the equation). The pH of the fluid

would increase. Rector, Carter and Seldin developed microglass electrodes that could be introduced into the tubular lumen to measure the pH of flowing tubular urine in situ; by this means they could determine whether or not a disequilibrium pH exists.

If no disequilibrium pH were observed, two explanations would be possible. First, HCO_3^- might be reabsorbed by a mechanism other than H^+ secretion and H_2CO_3 generation; namely, by a specific anion transport mechanism. Second, HCO_3^- might be reabsorbed by a H^+ secretory mechanism, but the dehydration of H_2CO_3 could be catalyzed within the tubular lumen by carbonic anhydrase fixed to the luminal membrane. No free carbonic anhydrase is present in plasma or tubular urine. However, if a disequilibrium pH of the proper order of magnitude were observed, reabsorption of HCO_3^-

LUMEN   CELL BLOOD

Uncatalyzed $HCO_3^- + H^+ \rightleftharpoons H_2CO_3$

(filtered) (secreted)   no
                                   c.a.

                        c.a.
Catalyzed $HCO_3^- + {}_{H^+} \rightleftharpoons {}_{H_2CO_3} \rightleftharpoons {}_{H_2O} + {}_{CO_2} \rightleftharpoons {}_{CO_2} \rightleftharpoons {}_{CO_2}$

flowing along the tubule would therefore be 0.85–1 pH unit more acid than it would be after it had come into equilibrium with CO_2 at the tension of plasma. This lower pH of luminal fluid relative to the equilibrium value has been termed a disequilibrium pH.

Prior to the work of Rector *et al.* (5), all measurements of tubular fluid pH were equilibrium values, for fluid was withdrawn in micropipets and protected from CO_2 loss by sealing with oil equilibrated with 5% CO_2 (equal to a plasma tension of approximately 40 mm Hg). During the time of collection and measurement, any excess H_2CO_3 in the sample would dehydrate, and the CO_2 would diffuse into the large volume of oil to equilibrate with CO_2 at plasma tension; thus, pH

by H^+ secretion and H_2CO_3 generation would be established.

Rector *et al.* (5) observed that the pH in situ of distal tubular urine of the rat averaged 0.85 unit more acid than the equilibrium value; this indicated the generation of H_2CO_3 within the tubular fluid by H^+ secretion. Following the intravenous infusion of carbonic anhydrase, a low-molecular-weight protein that enters the glomerular filtrate, the pH of urine in situ rose to equal the equilibrium value; this indicated that the slow, uncatalyzed dehydration of H_2CO_3 accounts for the disequilibrium pH normally observed. In contrast, the pH in situ of proximal tubular urine was identical with the equilibrium pH. However, when a potent inhibitor of carbonic anhydrase was given intravenously, the pH in situ decreased to a value some 0.85 unit less than the equilibrium value. These findings demonstrate that the reabsorption of bicarbonate in the proximal tubule, like that in the distal tubule, is brought about by the secretion of H^+ ions. Furthermore, the magnitude of the disequilibrium pH necessitates the active transport of H^+ ions. No transcellular potential difference exists across the proximal tubule. Even in the distal tubule, it is insufficient to account for passive accumulation of H^+ ions to the extent demanded by the disequilibrium pH. The difference between the proximal and distal tubular mechanisms—that the dehydration of the H_2CO_3 is catalyzed in the proximal tubule, whereas in the distal tubule it is uncatalyzed—is supported by histochemical evidence. Under proper conditions, the precipitation of cobalt carbonate in frozen sections of kidney demonstrates the presence of carbonic anhydrase in the brush border of proximal tubules but not on the luminal surface of distal tubules.

As shown in Figure 11–3, the filtrate is moderately acidified in the kidney of the rat as it flows along the proximal tubule, and the major acidification occurs beyond the distal tubule; i.e., in the collecting duct. If one assumes that the proximal tubule is freely permeable to carbon dioxide and that the P_{CO_2} of tubular fluid is only moderately higher than that of peritubular fluid and arterial blood, one may estimate that the bicarbonate concentration is reduced to about 10 mM/L in proximal tubular urine. If volume is reduced to one fifth of that of the filtrate, some 90% of the filtered bicarbonate must be reabsorbed in the proximal tubule. However, the gradient against which reabsorption occurs is not great: approximately 2:1 or 3:1 (7).

The presence of carbonic anhydrase on the brush border of proximal tubules no doubt facilitates the bulk reabsorption of bicarbonate, for it reduces by a factor of 10 the gradient against which hydrogen ions must be secreted and correspondingly reduces the energy cost of bicarbonate conservation. In a quantitative sense, the distal reabsorption of bicarbonate is a minor fraction of that in the proximal tubule.

DISTAL TUBULE AND COLLECTING DUCT MECHANISMS. — As implied above, the mechanisms for reabsorption of bicarbonate in distal tubules and collecting ducts are qualitatively the same as that in proximal tubules. They differ quantitatively in two respects:

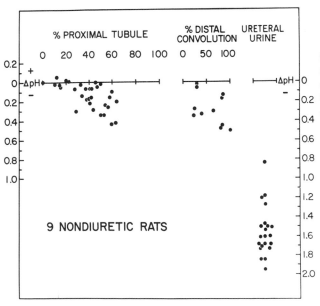

Fig. 11–3.—Change in pH of tubular fluid along the nephron of the rat; measurements made under equilibrium conditions. (From Gottschalk, C. W.; Lassiter, W. E., and Mylle, M.: Am. J. Physiol. 198:581, 1960.)

(1) together they account for only 10% of total bicarbonate reabsorption and (2) they are capable of salvaging essentially all of the bicarbonate remaining in the tubular fluid when plasma concentration is normal or low. To accomplish this latter end, the collecting ducts, specifically, must be able to secrete hydrogen ions against much steeper gradients than either the proximal or the distal tubules. Also, sodium ions may have to be pumped from lumen into cells to accomplish their nearly complete removal in states of sodium depletion. Accordingly, a more tightly coupled hydrogen-sodium exchange pump may be present in collecting ducts.

The limiting gradient against which hydrogen ions can be pumped in forming urine of maximum acidity is about 1000:1, a value which relates blood pH of 7.4 to urine pH of 4.4. Because final acidification of the urine is accomplished in the collecting ducts, maximal gradients are developed in this portion of the nephron. The low rate of bicarbonate transport and the capacity to develop a steep hydrogen ion gradient makes luminal carbonic anhydrase unnecessary. Rector, Carter and Seldin maintained that no luminal enzyme is present in distal tubules and the data of Ochwadt and Pitts (8) suggested that none is present in collecting ducts.

ROLE OF CARBONIC ANHYDRASE. — The role of carbonic anhydrase in the intracellular mechanism for reabsorption of bicarbonate, outlined above — that of providing a steady supply of hydrogen ions to a sodium-hydrogen exchange mechanism — is not accepted by all investigators. Some maintain that hydrogen ions are actively secreted by a redox (oxidation-reduction) ion pump, in which the ferric iron of the cytochrome system oxidizes hydrogen atoms to hydrogen ions:

$$4\ Fe^{+++} + 4H \rightleftharpoons 4Fe^{++} + 4H^{+}$$

The ferrous iron is then reoxidized, as follows, to regenerate ferric iron and to produce equivalent numbers of hydroxyl ions:

$$4\ Fe^{++} + O_2 + 2\ H_2O \rightleftharpoons 4\ Fe^{+++} + 4OH^{-}$$

The role of carbonic anhydrase (c.a.) in such a system would be that of facilitating the neutralization of hydroxyl ions:

$$4\ OH^{-} + 4\ CO_2 \xrightleftharpoons{c.\ a.} 4\ HCO_3^{-}$$

This system is similar to one that has been proposed as the mechanism of secretion of gastric acid. It is capable of elevating the electrochemical potential of hydrogen ions to a value several orders of magnitude greater than that required in either the proximal tubule or the collecting duct of the amphibian and mammalian kidney. Although the mechanism of transport of hydrogen ions has not been experimentally defined, the author prefers the view of the role of carbonic anhydrase initially presented. According to this view, inhibitors of carbonic anhydrase reduce the rate of formation of hydrogen ions within tubular cells and therefore reduce their availability to the luminal exchange mechanism.

In the proximal tubule, these inhibitors also reduce the rate of dehydration of carbonic acid within the tubular lumen, increase the gradient against which hydrogen ions must be secreted and, accordingly, depress reabsorption. It must be clearly understood that carbonic anhydrase is not an integral part of the hydrogen ion pump. The enzyme merely serves to supply H^{+} to the pump and to speed their removal from proximal tubular urine.

FACTORS AFFECTING BICARBONATE TRANSPORT

The renal bicarbonate threshold of 24–26 mM/L in the dog and of 28 mM/L in man is by no means an unvarying constant. At least four factors influence it: (1) changes in the carbon dioxide tension of the arterial blood, (2) variations in the body store of potassium; (3) variations in the plasma level of chloride and (4) variations in the secretion of adrenocortical hormones.

BICARBONATE TRANSPORT AND CHANGES IN P_{CO_2} OF ARTERIAL BLOOD. — The effects

TABLE 11–2.—EFFECT OF BREATHING 6% CO_2 ON REABSORPTION
AND EXCRETION OF BICARBONATE IN THE DOG*

			PLASMA			BICARBONATE			
GAS BREATHED	URINE FLOW (ml/min)	GFR (ml/min)	HCO_3^- (mEq/L)	pH	P_{CO_2} (mm Hg)	Filtered (mEq/min)	Excreted (mEq/min)	Reabsorbed (mEq/min)	Reabsorbed (mEq/100 ml)
Air	5.80	65.2	37.4	7.55	44.2	2.44	0.81	1.63	2.50
Air	6.40	62.5	37.4	7.56	43.2	2.34	0.81	1.53	2.45
CO_2	4.70	64.0	43.4	7.32	86.7	2.78	0.61	2.17	3.40
CO_2	4.60	65.2	44.5	7.31	91.1	2.90	0.62	2.28	3.50
Air	5.65	59.0	42.9	7.51	55.5	2.53	0.88	1.65	2.81
Air	5.85	61.5	44.3	7.44	67.2	2.72	0.98	1.74	2.83

*From Pitts, R. F.: Harvey Lect. 48:172, 1952–53.

of changes in P_{CO_2} of arterial blood on bicarbonate transport are dramatic and of obvious clinical import for an understanding of the renal compensations in respiratory acidosis and alkalosis. Table 11–2 summarizes an experiment on a dog in which bicarbonate reabsorption was studied under normal conditions and in acute respiratory acidosis induced by the breathing of 6% carbon dioxide in air. The plasma concentration of bicarbonate was elevated by the infusion of sodium bicarbonate to a level sufficient to saturate the reabsorptive mechanism under all conditions. In the two control periods during the breathing of room air, 2.50 and 2.45 mM of bicarbonate were reabsorbed per 100 ml of filtrate. During inhalation of carbon dioxide, reabsorption increased promptly to 3.40 and 3.50 mM/100 ml of filtrate; on the restoration of air breathing it declined to 2.81 and 2.83 mM/100 ml. Two significant changes occurred during carbon dioxide inhalation which might have stimulated the renal tubules to reabsorb more bicarbonate: (1) the pH of the arterial blood fell and (2) the P_{CO_2} of the arterial blood rose (9).

The experiment summarized in Table 11–3 indicates that the significant factor increasing the reabsorption of bicarbonate is the increased P_{CO_2} of arterial blood, not the decreased pH. During the first three clearance periods, sodium bicarbonate was infused at a low rate, and the plasma bicarbonate and pH increased moderately, to 34 mM/L and pH

7.49. Bicarbonate reabsorption amounted to 2.8 mM/100 ml of glomerular filtrate. Sodium bicarbonate was then infused at a high rate, and the plasma concentration increased to 90 mM/L. The administration of 12% carbon dioxide, which increased the P_{CO_2} of arterial blood to 120–130 mm Hg, compensated almost exactly the enhanced metabolic alkalosis. Arterial blood pH did not change significantly. Because bicarbonate reabsorption rose from 2.8 to 3.6 mM/100 ml of filtrate, it is evident that increased P_{CO_2}, not decreased pH of the arterial blood, is the significant stimulus.

Presumably, an increase in P_{CO_2} of arterial blood is accompanied by an equivalent increase in P_{CO_2} within tubular cells, resulting in enhanced formation of carbonic acid and

TABLE 11–3.—EFFECT OF INCREASED P_{CO_2} AT
CONSTANT pH ON REABSORPTION AND EXCRETION
OF BICARBONATE IN THE DOG*

	PLASMA			BICARBONATE	
				Reabsorbed	
GFR (ml/min)	HCO_3^- (mEq/L)	pH	P_{CO_2} (mm Hg)	(mEq/min)	(mEq/100 ml)
SLOW INFUSION OF $NaHCO_3$; ROOM AIR INHALED					
50.9	34.8	7.49	47.3	1.44	2.82
51.0	34.9	7.50	46.3	1.44	2.82
46.9	34.2	7.49	46.3	1.31	2.80
RAPID INFUSION OF $NaHCO_3$; 12% CO_2 INHALED					
54.4	89.1	7.49	121	1.86	3.42
55.4	92.3	7.48	128	2.01	3.64
53.0	94.5	7.48	131	1.93	3.64

*From Pitts, R. F.: Harvey Lect. 48:172, 1952–53.

elevated intracellular hydrogen ion concentration. With more hydrogen ions available to the exchange mechanism, bicarbonate is reabsorbed at a higher rate. Thus, ultimately the stimulus for increased reabsorption of bicarbonate is increased hydrogen ion concentration of the contents of tubular cells.

Figure 11–4 describes the effects of acute variations in arterial P_{CO_2} on bicarbonate reabsorption in the dog. When animals are hyperventilated, reducing the P_{CO_2} to values less than the normal 40 mm Hg, the reabsorption of bicarbonate is reduced. When animals breathe carbon dioxide–air mixtures, so that the P_{CO_2} is increased to values above the normal 40 mm Hg, the reabsorption of bicarbonate is increased. At very high levels of P_{CO_2}, bicarbonate reabsorption more than doubles (10). Chronic exposure of animals to high partial pressures of carbon dioxide still further enhances the tubular reabsorption of

bicarbonate, the major response occurring within the first 48 hours (11). The mechanism of this delayed increase in reabsorptive capacity has not been defined.

RENAL COMPENSATIONS IN RESPIRATORY ACIDOSIS AND ALKALOSIS. — In chronic pulmonary insufficiency with retention of carbon dioxide, the plasma concentration of bicarbonate increases. Although plasma pH is reduced, the extent of the reduction is much less than it would be if there were no increase in the plasma level of bicarbonate. From the Henderson-Hasselbalch equation,

$$pH = pK + \log \frac{(HCO_3^-)}{(H_2CO_3)}$$

it is evident that, if the plasma concentration of carbonic acid were to increase twofold, to 2.8 mM/L, as a consequence of failure of pulmonary elimination of carbon dioxide, doubling of the plasma concentration of

Fig. 11–4. — The relationship between P_{CO_2} of arterial blood and reabsorption of bicarbonate in the dog. (From Rector, F. C., Jr., Seldin, D. W., Roberts, A. D., Jr., and Smith, J. S.: J. Clin. Invest. 39:1706, 1960.)

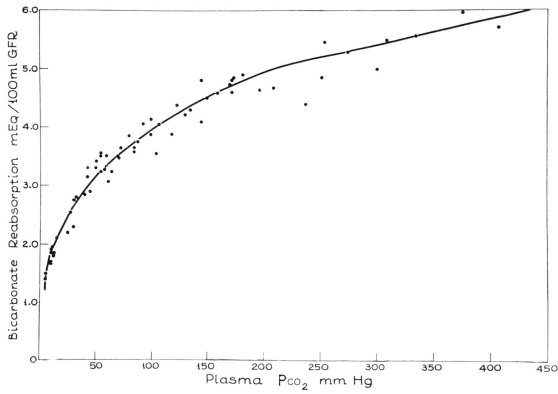

bicarbonate to 56 mM/L would maintain a constant ratio of 20:1, and no pH change would occur. Because the reabsorption of bicarbonate is enhanced by an increase in arterial Pco_2, plasma concentration tends to stabilize at a supernormal level. Of course, increased renal production of bicarbonate by enhanced excretion of titratable acid and ammonia is necessary initially to elevate plasma bicarbonate to supernormal levels. However, compensation is never perfect; i.e., plasma bicarbonate does not increase sufficiently to prevent a decrease in plasma pH.

In chronic respiratory alkalosis resulting from prolonged hyperventilation, the plasma concentration of bicarbonate decreases. It is evident from the Henderson-Hasselbalch equation that, if the plasma concentration of carbonic acid were to be reduced by one half as a consequence of doubling alveolar ventilation, halving of the plasma concentra-

tion of bicarbonate would maintain a constant ratio of 20:1, and no pH change would occur. Because the reabsorption of bicarbonate is reduced and excretion is increased by a reduction in arterial Pco_2, plasma concentration stabilizes at a subnormal value. However, compensation is never perfect, and plasma pH increases in respiratory alkalosis.

BICARBONATE REABSORPTION AND VARIATIONS IN BODY STORES OF POTASSIUM.—It has long been known that the oral administration of potassium chloride increases the excretion and reduces the plasma concentration of bicarbonate. Figure 11–5 illustrates the effects, in the dog, of the intravenous infusion of potassium salts on the rate of tubular reabsorption of bicarbonate (12). When the plasma concentration of potassium falls below the normal value of 4 mEq/L, bicarbonate reabsorption is elevated above the normal value of 2.4–2.6 mEq/100 ml of filtrate. When, in consequence of the infusion

Fig. 11–5.—The relationship between plasma potassium concentration and bicarbonate reabsorp-

tion in the dog. (From Fuller, G. R., MacLeod, M. B., and Pitts, R. F.: Am. J. Physiol. 182:111, 1955.)

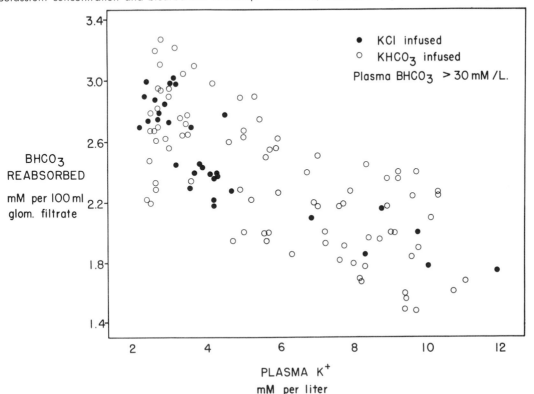

of potassium salts, the plasma potassium concentration exceeds 4 mEq/L, bicarbonate reabsorption is reduced below the normal value.

It is probable that the significant factor controlling bicarbonate reabsorption is not the plasma but the intracellular concentration of potassium. Cooke, Darrow and others have shown that infused potassium rapidly enters all cells in exchange for hydrogen ions, raising the intracellular potassium concentration and reducing the intracellular hydrogen ion concentration. The hydrogen ions leaving tissue cells are buffered by extracellular bicarbonate, and plasma bicarbonate concentration decreases. Presumably, the renal tubular cells respond in a similar manner—accumulating potassium ions from, and extruding hydrogen ions into, the peritubular fluid. As a consequence of reduced intracellular hydrogen ion concentration, fewer hydrogen ions are secreted and less bicarbonate is reabsorbed. The urine becomes alkaline and contains large amounts of potassium bicarbonate. Loading with potassium salts therefore results in hyperkalemic metabolic acidosis. The acidosis is extracellular; the cell contents are relatively alkaline. However, despite reduction in extracellular bicarbonate, the urine is alkaline.

More significant, clinically, is hypokalemic metabolic alkalosis. If body potassium stores are depleted in consequence of reduced intake or increased gastrointestinal or urinary losses due to vomiting, diarrhea, hyperadrenocorticism (13) or prolonged alkali therapy, the capacity of the renal tubules to reabsorb bicarbonate increases, and plasma concentration is stabilized at a higher-than-normal value. Presumably, tubular cells lose potassium and gain hydrogen ions in hypokalemia. As a consequence of increased intracellular hydrogen ion concentration, more hydrogen ions are secreted and more titratable acid and ammonia are excreted. Accordingly, the kidneys build up the bicarbonate stores of the body and maintain them at supernormal values by virtue of increased reabsorptive capacity. The urine is acidic despite the elevated plasma bicarbonate concentration. Little potassium is excreted.

The reciprocal relationship between hydrogen ion and potassium ion secretion has been interpreted as evidence for competition of these two ion species for a common secretory mechanism. This concept, developed by Berliner *et al.* (14), has been widely accepted in the past. Present views, based on observations of Rector *et al.* (15) and Giebisch *et al.* (16), are that the two mechanisms are independent and therefore noncompetitive. Hydrogen ion secretion and, thus, bicarbonate reabsorption are increased by hypokalemia and decreased by hyperkalemia along the entire length of the nephron, due to the changes in cellular hydrogen ion concentration described above. Because filtered potassium is almost entirely reabsorbed in the proximal tubule, no competition between potassium ions and hydrogen ions for secretory transport could occur at this site. The potassium that is excreted is secreted in the distal part of the nephron. The secretory mechanism is passive, and the distribution of potassium ions is determined in large part by the transtubular potential gradient. However, some reabsorption continues in the terminal nephron, even in the presence of net secretory transport. Thus, electrochemical equilibrium is never attained. In potassium deficiency, the transtubular potential at the secretory site is low, and little potassium is excreted. In hyperkalemia, the potential is high, and much potassium is excreted. Furthermore, the concomitant depression of reabsorption and increase in excretion of bicarbonate in hyperkalemia results in the delivery of unreabsorbed anions to the secretory site—a condition that, in itself, increases the transtubular potential gradient and potassium secretion.

BICARBONATE REABSORPTION AND PLASMA CHLORIDE CONCENTRATION.—When the body is depleted of chloride and hypochloremia develops, plasma bicarbonate increases. Bicarbonate reabsorption increases, sustaining a higher plasma concentration. Conversely, when body chloride stores are expanded and hyperchloremia develops, plasma bicarbonate decreases. Bicarbonate reabsorption is reduced, and plasma concentration is maintained at a subnormal level. When the chloride deficit is replaced or when the chloride excess is excreted, the plasma level of bicarbonate rapidly returns to normal.

These reciprocal relationships between plasma concentrations of chloride and bicarbonate were once thought to be due to an ill-defined competition in tubular reabsorption. They are now known to be due to the operation of a mechanism that relates reabsorption to extracellular volume (17). Sodium chloride and sodium bicarbonate are the only two salts that, when infused, cause appreciable expansion of extracellular fluid. When isotonic sodium bicarbonate is infused intravenously, extracellular volume expands at the same rate as the increase in plasma concentration of bicarbonate; reabsorption of bicarbonate decreases below the normal threshold level of 25 mM/L of glomerular filtrate. If plasma bicarbonate is increased with minimal expansion of extracellular volume by infusion of hypertonic sodium bicarbonate, little change in reabsorption per liter of glomerular filtrate occurs. On the other hand, if extracellular volume is contracted by hemodialysis against a low-chloride, high-bicarbonate bath, reabsorption increases with plasma bicarbonate concentration. When expansion of volume is exaggerated by simultaneous infusion of isotonic sodium chloride, reabsorption of bicarbonate is further depressed. When volume is depleted even more by simultaneous controlled hemorrhage, still further increase in reabsorption of bicarbonate per liter of filtrate occurs. The rat is less sensitive to changes in extracellular volume than is the dog, although it exhibits qualitatively similar alterations. Man probably exhibits the same phenomena, although they have been less well defined.

Changes in reabsorption per liter of filtrate with expansion and contraction of extracellular volume are not peculiar to the bicarbonate system alone; they are observed for reabsorption of chloride and sodium as well. Perhaps most significant is the fact that the secretion of hydrogen ions (reabsorption of bicarbonate) is an inverse function of extracellular volume.

BICARBONATE REABSORPTION AND SECRETION OF ADRENOCORTICAL HORMONES. — Variations in secretion of adrenal cortical hormones must affect bicarbonate reabsorption, although the mechanism of action is not entirely clear. In Cushing's syndrome and in hyperaldosteronism, the plasma concentration of bicarbonate is moderately elevated; i.e., hypersecretion of gluco- and mineralocorticoids induces metabolic alkalosis associated with increased bicarbonate reabsorption. In contrast, in Addison's disease, the plasma concentration of bicarbonate is moderately reduced; i.e., a deficiency of adrenocortical hormones induces metabolic acidosis associated with reduced bicarbonate reabsorption.

In the dog, the administration of ACTH, cortisone or deoxycorticosterone has no demonstrable acute effect on bicarbonate reabsorption. When deoxycorticosterone is administered in high dosage over prolonged periods of time, bicarbonate reabsorption is enhanced. The effect is increased by a high-sodium, potassium-poor diet; it is abolished by the addition of potassium to the diet. Increased reabsorption of bicarbonate due to excessive amounts of a mineralocorticoid such as deoxycorticosterone therefore appears to be secondary to potassium depletion; i.e., it is a consequence of hypokalemic alkalosis (13). Reduced reabsorption of bicarbonate in adrenalectomized animals is presumably an expression of hyperkalemic metabolic acidosis.

RENAL TUBULAR ACIDOSIS

Renal tubular acidosis (RTA) is a clinical syndrome of hyperchloremic acidosis associated with a normal or only slightly reduced glomerular filtration rate. Indeed, acidosis of renal disease, whatever its cause, is always renal tubular in origin. However, RTA is distinguished as a specific deficiency of the renal tubules in the secretion of hydrogen ions or the maintenance of a normal hydrogen ion gradient between blood and urine. It occurs in the absence of azotemia or uremia. As a consequence of reduced secretion of hydrogen ions, plasma concentration of bicarbonate is lower than the normal 26–28 mM/L, and the plasma concentration of chloride is higher than the normal 103–106 mM/L.

The classification of RTA into proximal and distal nephron types is probably an oversimplification, but there is physiologic justification for such a distinction. In proximal RTA, the proximal tubules, which normally account for the reabsorption of 85–90% of the filtered load of bicarbonate, now secrete fewer hydrogen ions and reabsorb less bicarbonate. Maximal proximal reabsorption of bicarbonate is reduced. As a consequence, the distal nephron segments, which normally reabsorb only 10–15% of the filtered load, are flooded with bicarbonate. Bicarbonate is excreted, and plasma concentration falls to acidotic levels. Eventually, plasma concentration stabilizes at some subnormal value such that the filtered load can be entirely reabsorbed by the proximal system (reduced hydrogen ion secretion) and the distal system (normal hydrogen ion secretion). Under these circumstances, the urine becomes acidic, and titratable acid and ammonia are secreted in normal amounts. If the patient is subjected to the stress of oral administration of ammonium chloride, which reduces the plasma concentration of bicarbonate still further, urine pH falls below 5.4 and titratable acid and ammonia excretion become appropriate to the degree of acidosis. The extent of acidosis is thus self-limited.

Distal RTA is characterized by an inability to reduce urine pH below 6.6–7. It must be remembered that this is essentially the pH at which the tubular fluid leaves the proximal segment. In other words, few additional hydrogen ions are added to the final urine. In fact, passive back diffusion of hydrogen ions from urine to blood may occur and might be causal. Normally, the last traces of bicarbonate are abstracted from the urine by establishing a hydrogen ion gradient reaching 1,000:1 between urine and blood (pH 4.4:pH 7.4). Because the loss of some fraction of filtered bicarbonate continues and because the urine pH remains in the neutral or alkaline range despite developing acidosis, the excretion of titratable acid and ammonia remains low (see succeeding sections of this chapter). Accordingly, the excretion of acid is less than the net production of acid, and acidosis develops. If large amounts of bicarbonate are administered orally or intravenously, essentially normal rates of reabsorption of bicarbonate may be attained (26–28 mM/L of glomerular filtrate). Thus, in either proximal or distal RTA the basic deficiency is in net secretion of hydrogen ions and therefore in net reabsorption of bicarbonate. However, the clinical manifestations of proximal and distal RTA differ, as do the orders of magnitude of base required for their treatment.

In primary or idiopathic proximal RTA, symptoms and signs may be minimal and limited to retarded growth. In the secondary form of the disease associated with the Fanconi syndrome, cystinosis, glycogenosis, myeloma, galactosemia, Wilson's disease, cadmium toxicity, etc., symptoms and signs are largely those of the causal disease. Treatment is effective but may require large doses of alkali—as much as 10 mEq/kg of sodium bicarbonate or sodium citrate per day, if normal plasma bicarbonate levels are to be maintained. As plasma concentration decreases, proximal reabsorption becomes more nearly complete, distal flooding ceases, and the final urine is acidified. Secretion of ammonia and titratable acid become equal to metabolic acid production.

In contrast, symptoms and signs of either primary or secondary distal tubular acidosis are protean. The secondary form of the disease is seen in association with malnutrition, hyperparathyroidism, vitamin D deficiency or intoxication, phenacetin and amphotericin B nephropathies, and a variety of hyperglobulinemic states. Symptoms and signs include anorexia, constipation, polyuria, retarded growth, nephrocalcinosis, nephrolithiasis, rickets, osteomalacia, spontaneous fractures, hyperkaluria, and hypokalemia. Most of these manifestations of distal tubular RTA are consequences of severe and prolonged metabolic acidosis and dehydration. If instituted adequately before irreversible renal damage occurs, therapy is effective. Again, the disease is treated by administration of alkali: sodium and potassium bicarbonate or sodium and potassium citrate in doses of 1–

neutral salts are transported to the kidneys by the blood stream. If the neutral salts were excreted as such, the bicarbonate reserves would suffer progressive depletion.

The kidneys perform two types of operations on salts of metabolic acids (20–22). Buffer salts that enter the renal tubules in the glomerular filtrate are transformed into acid salts or into free acids. In the example below, disodium phosphate is shown as reacting with carbonic acid to form monosodium phosphate and sodium bicarbonate:

$$Na_2HPO_4 + H_2CO_3 \longrightarrow NaH_2PO_4 \text{ (excreted)} + NaHCO_3 \text{ (reabsorbed)}$$

3 mEq/kg per day. The bony changes and the associated secondary calcifications, as well as hyperkaluria and hypokalemia, are obviously due to the prolonged acidosis and the persistent positive acid balance with bone buffering of the excess acid (see p. 191). This sketchy survey of RTA can be supplemented by a number of excellent reviews; as sources, two are cited (18, 19).

RENAL RESTORATION OF DEPLETED BICARBONATE RESERVES

Not only are the renal tubules charged with the reabsorption of the bicarbonate normally present in the glomerular filtrate and with the excretion of any excess; they must also replenish bicarbonate stores depleted by the neutralization of strong acids, such as sulfuric acid and phosphoric acid. These acids, formed in the metabolism of proteins and phospholipids, are buffered in the following manner:

$$H_2SO_4 + 2\,NaHCO_3 \longrightarrow Na_2SO_4 + 2H_2O + 2CO_2\nearrow$$

$$H_3PO_4 + 2\,NaHCO_3 \longrightarrow Na_2HPO_4 + 2H_2O + 2CO_2\nearrow$$

Strong acids are replaced by neutral salts and

The reaction is driven to the right by the reabsorption of sodium bicarbonate. The original filtrate, which has a slightly alkaline reaction, is thereby converted into acidic urine. If urine is collected for 24 hours and titrated from its initial· acid reaction to the reaction of the blood, the amount of alkali that must be added is exactly equal to the amount of bicarbonate restored to the body by the formation of titratable acid. The capacity of the kidney to form titratable acid is limited. The tubules can salvage, at most, one of the two sodium ions of disodium phosphate. To salvage the second would necessitate the formation of urine of pH 2.5. Because the kidney cannot elaborate urine more acidic than pH 4.4, negligible quantities of strong acids, such as sulfuric acid and hydrochloric acid, can be eliminated in free titratable form.

These strong acids must be excreted fully neutralized. The kidney accomplishes this without sacrifice of sodium ions, by combining them with ammonium ions. In the example below, sodium sulfate present in the filtrate is shown as reacting with carbonic acid and ammonia to form ammonium sulfate and sodium bicarbonate:

$$Na_2SO_4 + 2H_2CO_3 + 2NH_3 \longrightarrow (NH_4)_2SO_4 \text{ (excreted)} + 2NaHCO_3 \text{ (reabsorbed)}$$

carbonic acid; the latter is eliminated through the lungs as carbon dioxide. The

The reaction is driven to the right by the reabsorption of bicarbonate. The ammonia content of the 24-hour urine sample, expressed in milliequivalents, is equal to the quantity of bicarbonate restored to the body by ammonia excretion. The sum of the urinary titratable acid and ammonia is a measure of total renal replenishment of buffer reserves.

REGULATION OF ACID-BASE BALANCE BY TITRATABLE ACID AND AMMONIA EXCRETION.—The contribution of these two processes to the homeostasis of the buffer content and reaction of the body fluids is summarized in Table 11–4. A normal person on an average mixed diet excretes 30–50 mEq of acid per day in combination with ammonia and 10–30 mEq as titratable acid. In this manner, he eliminates, each day, the excess of fixed (nonvolatile) acid formed metabolically. His body buffer stores and the reaction of his body fluids are maintained at optimum levels.

The uncontrolled diabetic patient in severe ketosis produces much more metabolic acid than does the normal person. Not only does he metabolize his own body proteins and lipids at a high rate, producing increased quantities of phosphoric acid and sulfuric acid; he also produces large quantities of β-hydroxybutyric acid and acetoacetic acid. The excessive drain on buffer reserves to neutralize this load of metabolic acid is reflected in a 5–10-fold increase in the rate of excretion of titratable acid and ammonia. Because renal compensation is never complete, moderate to severe metabolic acidosis develops. Buffer stores are depleted, and body fluids become more acid.

In chronic renal disease, the production of metabolic acid is within normal limits, or even reduced, if the patient is maintained on a low-protein diet. However, the capacity of the kidneys to eliminate acid and to replenish buffer reserves is reduced. In terminal Bright's disease, the total acid excretion may fall to 2.5 mEq/day – 0.5 mEq in combination with ammonia and 2 mEq as titratable acid. The normal kidney excretes 1–2.5 times as much acid combined with ammonia as is excreted in free titratable form. The diseased kidney excretes a lesser proportion combined with ammonia. Reduction in titratable acid and ammonia excretion ultimately accounts for the acidosis of renal failure.

EXCRETION OF TITRATABLE ACID

Tubular fluid could be acidified and titratable acid formed in either of two ways. The alkaline components of buffer mixtures filtered through the glomeruli might be reabsorbed, leaving the acid components to be excreted in the urine. Alternatively, the alkaline components of buffer mixtures filtered through the glomeruli could be converted into acid components by hydrogen ions secreted into the renal tubules. The operation of these hypothetical mechanisms is illustrated in Figure 11–6. Only the dibasic-monobasic phosphate and the bicarbonate-carbonic acid buffer systems need be considered under normal conditions, for they alone enter the filtrate in significant quantities.

If, as is shown in the upper diagram of Figure 11–6, dibasic phosphate were preferentially reabsorbed, the excreted monobasic phosphate could be titrated as acid in the urine. Additionally, bicarbonate must be completely reabsorbed from the tubular fluid, to prevent it from titrating the monobasic phosphate as rapidly as it is formed. If, as shown in the second diagram, bicarbonate were completely reabsorbed and if the tubules were impermeable to carbonic acid, as

TABLE 11–4.—EXCRETION OF ACID BY MAN*

	MEQ OF ACID EXCRETED PER DAY	RATIO NH₃/TITRATABLE ACID
Normal man:		
Acid combined with ammonia	30–50	
		1–2.5
Titratable acid	10–30	
Diabetic ketosis:		
Acid combined with ammonia	300–500	
		1–2.5
Titratable acid	75–250	
Chronic Bright's disease:		
Acid combined with ammonia	0.5–15	
		0.2–1.5
Titratable acid	2.0–20	

*From Pitts, R. F.: Science 102:49 and 81, 1945.

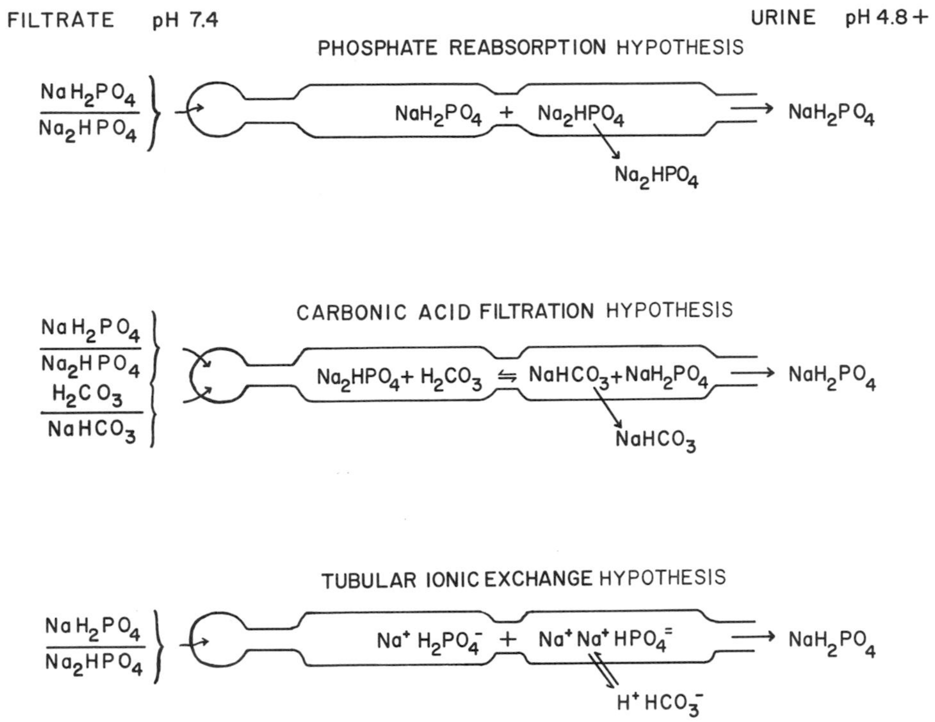

FILTRATE   pH 7.4   URINE   pH 4.8 +

PHOSPHATE REABSORPTION HYPOTHESIS

$$\left.\frac{NaH_2PO_4}{Na_2HPO_4}\right\}$$

$$NaH_2PO_4 + Na_2HPO_4 \longrightarrow NaH_2PO_4$$

$$Na_2HPO_4$$

CARBONIC ACID FILTRATION HYPOTHESIS

$$\left.\begin{array}{c}\dfrac{NaH_2PO_4}{Na_2HPO_4}\\[2pt]\dfrac{H_2CO_3}{NaHCO_3}\end{array}\right\}$$

$$Na_2HPO_4 + H_2CO_3 \rightleftharpoons NaHCO_3 + NaH_2PO_4 \longrightarrow NaH_2PO_4$$

$$NaHCO_3$$

TUBULAR IONIC EXCHANGE HYPOTHESIS

$$\left.\frac{NaH_2PO_4}{Na_2HPO_4}\right\}$$

$$Na^+ H_2PO_4^- + Na^+ Na^+ HPO_4^= \longrightarrow NaH_2PO_4$$

$$H^+ HCO_3^-$$

Fig. 11–6. — Hypotheses to account for acidification of the urine. (From Pitts, R. F., and Alexander, R. S.: Am. J. Physiol. 144:239, 1945.)

originally claimed by Sendroy, Seelig and Van Slyke, this acid would react with alkaline buffer salts to convert them into titratable buffer acids.

Conversely, two mechanisms of tubular secretion of hydrogen ions have been proposed. Molecular acid, secreted by tubular cells, might ultimately account for the titratable acid appearing in the urine. On the other hand, as first proposed by Homer Smith (23),

the exchange of hydrogen ions for cations across the tubular epithelium could accomplish the same end. Much evidence in favor of this latter mechanism has been advanced, and it is now generally accepted.

EVIDENCE FOR TUBULAR SECRETION OF HYDROGEN IONS. — An experiment on normal man that illustrates one type of evidence supporting this view is summarized in Table 11–5. The significant features of the experi-

TABLE 11–5. — EXPERIMENT DESIGNED TO TEST POSSIBLE MECHANISMS OF ACID EXCRETION IN MAN*

PLASMA CONCENTRATION					URINE	PHOSPHATE		URINARY TITRATABLE ACID				
								Measured	Calculated from —			
									PO$_4$ Reabsorbed		H$_2$CO$_3$ Filtered	
GFR	HCO$_3^-$	H$_2$CO$_3$	PO$_4$	pH	pH	Excreted	Reabsorbed		mEq/min	% Obs.	mEq/min	% Obs.
(ml/min)	(mEq/L)					(mM/min)	(mM/min)	(mEq/min)				
102	14.8	0.86	5.45	7.34	4.64	0.419	0.137	0.328	0.031	9.5	0.087	26.5
101	14.8	0.86	6.04	7.34	4.63	0.455	0.155	0.348	0.035	10.0	0.087	25.0
98.7	14.6	0.82	6.49	7.35	4.60	0.486	0.154	0.371	0.034	9.2	0.081	21.8
100	14.8	0.83	6.73	7.35	4.56	0.516	0.157	0.395	0.035	8.9	0.083	21.0
							Av.	0.361	0.034	9.4	0.085	23.6

*From Pitts, R. F., Lotspeich, W. D., Schiess, W. A., and Ayer, J. L.: J. Clin. Invest. 27:48, 1948.

ment are the following: A moderately severe metabolic acidosis (plasma bicarbonate 14.8 mEq/L, pH 7.34) was induced by the ingestion of ammonium chloride for 3 days prior to the experiment. Neutral sodium phosphate was infused at such a rate as to increase plasma concentration 5–6-fold and to cause the excretion of 0.4–0.5 mM of phosphate per minute. The urine was highly acidic, and the rate of excretion of titratable acid* was comparable to that observed in severe diabetic acidosis. The glomerular filtration rate, the rate of filtration, reabsorption and excretion of phosphate, and the rate of filtration of carbonic acid were all measured.

The rate of excretion of titratable acid may be calculated in two ways, in order to test the adequacy of the phosphate reabsorption hypothesis and the carbonic acid filtration hypothesis as explanations of the measured rate of excretion of titratable acid. The measured rate of reabsorption of phosphate was found to vary from 0.137 to 0.157 mM/min. On the assumption that only disodium phosphate is reabsorbed, the contribution of the corresponding excess of filtered monosodium salt to titratable acid excretion has been calculated.† The phosphate reabsorption hypothesis can account for 10% or less of the observed excretion of titratable acid. If it is assumed that all the filtered carbonic

acid appears in the urine as titratable buffer acid, the product of the rate of glomerular filtration and the plasma concentration of carbonic acid should yield the rate of excretion of titratable acid. The carbonic acid filtration hypothesis can account for only 21–26.5% of the observed rate of titratable acid excretion. Obviously, the tubules must secrete hydrogen ions, either as molecular acid or in exchange for sodium ions.

In all fairness, it must be pointed out that either the phosphate or the bicarbonate reabsorption hypothesis is adequate to explain the excretion of titratable acid by the normal person. Only when titratable acid excretion is greatly enhanced by acidosis and the infusion of phosphate can the inadequacies of the two hypotheses be demonstrated.

MECHANISM OF FORMATION OF TITRATABLE ACID.—The mechanism illustrated in Figure 11–7 was proposed to explain the formation of titratable acid by ion exchange in the dog (24) and in man (25). At first, it was thought to be restricted to the distal convoluted tubule, for in the frog and in *Necturus* acidification of the urine is confined to the distal segment. Subsequently it was recognized as a general mechanism, concerned not only with the formation of titratable acid but also with the reabsorption of bicarbonate. If the tubular urine contains a mixture of buffer salt and nonvolatile buffer acid, the exchange of hydrogen ions for sodium ions results in the formation of titratable acid. If the buffer is a mixture of bicarbonate and carbonic acid, the exchange of hydrogen ions for sodium ions results indirectly in the reabsorption of bicarbonate. The mechanism is now thought to be distributed throughout the length of the nephron. Present views hold that the bulk of the filtered bicarbonate is reabsorbed in the proximal tubule. Because the urine is only moderately acidified in the proximal segment, the major fraction of the titratable acid represented by buffers of low pK, such as β-hydroxybutyrate, must be formed in the collecting ducts; i.e., at the site of major acidification. However, the titratable acid represented by phosphate (high pK)

---

*High urinary level of titratable acid is the result of acidosis and the high rate of excretion of a buffer of favorable pK. If no phosphate had been administered, the rate of excretion of titratable acid would have been relatively low.

†The calculation is straightforward, although moderately complicated. Recalculation of the data is a good exercise for the student in the use of the Henderson-Hasselbalch equation. The method is as follows: The quantities of Na_2HPO_4 and NaH_2PO_4 filtered each minute are calculated from the total quantity of PO_4 filtered and the plasma pH. Subtracting the PO_4 reabsorbed from the Na_2HPO_4 filtered (i.e., assuming that all of the phosphate reabsorbed is the disodium salt) yields the Na_2HPO_4 apparently excreted. The remainder of the PO_4 excreted must be NaH_2PO_4. Using this calculated ratio of Na_2HPO_4/NaH_2PO_4 presumably remaining in the urine, one then computes the amount of alkali that must be added to adjust the ratio to that existing at the pH of the blood. This amount of alkali is equivalent to the titratable acid that could be formed by the preferential reabsorption of disodium phosphate.

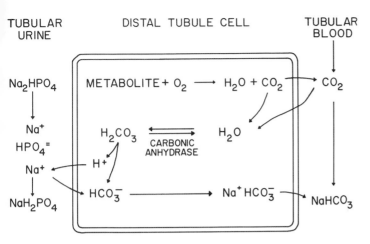

TUBULAR URINE   DISTAL TUBULE CELL   TUBULAR BLOOD

Fig. 11—7.—Mechanism of formation of titratable acid in tubular cells. (From Pitts, R. F., and Alexander, R. S.: Am. J. Physiol. 144:239, 1945.)

is, probably, formed chiefly in the proximal tubule. Although the proximal mechanism and the collecting-duct mechanism are basically the same, the former is specialized to exchange a large quantity of hydrogen ions against a low gradient, and the latter is specialized to exchange a small quantity of hydrogen ions against a high gradient.

RATE OF TITRATABLE ACID FORMATION. — Three major factors affect the rate of forma-tion of titratable acid: (1) the rate of excretion of buffer, (2) the pK' of the buffer and (3) the degree of acidosis. The significance of the first two factors is illustrated in Figure 11–8. In each of the three experiments, acidosis was induced by the ingestion of ammonium chloride. In one experiment, neutral sodium phosphate, in a second, creatinine, and in a third, sodium p-aminohippurate, were infused at such rates as to cause

Fig. 11—8.—Relationship of rate of excretion of titratable acid to rate of excretion of buffer and to pK' of the buffer in acidotic men. (From Schiess, W. A., Ayer, J. L., Lotspeich, W. D., and Pitts, R. F.: J. Clin. Invest. 27:57, 1948.)

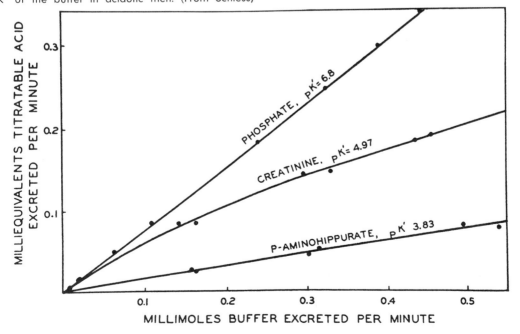

equimolar increases in rates of excretion. It is evident that the rate of excretion of titratable acid progressively increases with the presentation of increasing quantities of buffer to the ion exchange mechanism. It is also evident that phosphate, having the highest pK, is the most effective buffer. The range of effective buffering by any compound extends 1 pH unit to either side of the pK value. More hydrogen ions can therefore be buffered by a mole of phosphate with the development of a lower transtubular hydrogen ion gradient than by a mole of creatinine or p-aminohippurate. Accordingly, phosphate is a more effective urinary buffer than the other two compounds. The pK value of β-hydroxybutyrate is somewhat less than that of creatinine but greater than that of p-aminohippurate. The kidney can use β-hydroxybutyrate much less effectively in the buffering of hydrogen ions than it can use phosphate. However, because the molar rate of excretion of β-hydroxybutyrate is far greater than that of phosphate in diabetic acidosis, it is the major urinary buffer in this condition.

Figure 11–9 illustrates the increase in the rate of excretion of titratable acid in acidosis in comparison with normal acid-base balance. What is surprising is that the kidneys of a person in normal acid-base balance eliminate so much titratable acid when creatinine is infused. It seems that the normal person is, in reality, in a state of moderate acidosis, as

far as his renal response to buffer infusion is concerned.

INTERRELATIONS IN ACID EXCRETION AND BICARBONATE REABSORPTION. — Figure 11–10 illustrates an experiment in which a person in metabolic acidosis was restored to normal acid-base balance and then made alkalotic by the infusion of sodium bicarbonate. Creatinine was infused throughout, to maintain a high and constant rate of urinary excretion of buffer.

For the first 60 minutes of this experiment, during which plasma bicarbonate rose from 15.5 to 20 mM/L, the rates of excretion of titratable acid and ammonia were sustained at constant high levels. As plasma bicarbonate further increased, from 20 to 25 mM/L, the rates of excretion of titratable acid and ammonia progressively declined. No significant bicarbonate excretion occurred until the 10th period, at a plasma bicarbonate concentration of 26.7 mM/L. Further increases in plasma concentration profoundly increased bicarbonate excretion and reduced titratable acid and ammonia excretion to negligibly low values.

It is evident that, over a range of 20–25 mM of bicarbonate per liter of plasma, rates of excretion of titratable acid and ammonia decrease with increasing filtered load of bicarbonate, without any corresponding increase in bicarbonate excretion. One may infer that at plasma levels below 20 mM/L,

Fig. 11–9.—Excretion of titratable acid by the same subject in acidosis and in normal acid-base balance at a series of comparable rates of excretion of buffer. (From Schiess, W. A., Ayer, J. L., Lotspeich, W. D., and Pitts, R. F.: J. Clin. Invest. 27:57, 1948.)

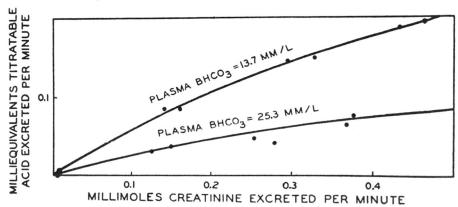

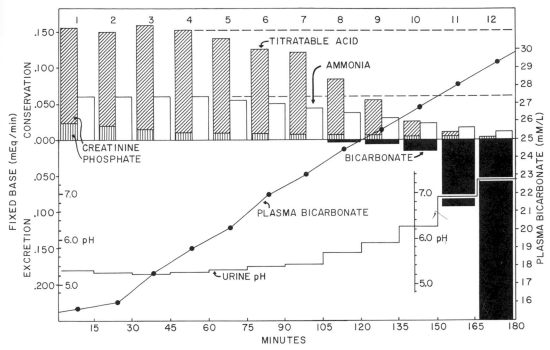

Fig. 11-10. — Relationship between acid and ammonia excretion, bicarbonate excretion and plasma concentration of bicarbonate in man. (From Pitts, R. F., Ayer, J. L., and Schiess, W. S.: J. Clin. Invest. 28:35, 1949.)

so large a proportion of the filtered load of bicarbonate is reabsorbed early in the proximal tubules that the late proximal, distal and collecting-duct mechanisms are occupied almost entirely with titratable acid and ammonia secretion. At plasma levels of 20–25 mM/L, increasing amounts of bicarbonate escape early proximal reabsorption and are delivered into more distal parts of the nephron. Here the competition between bicarbonate reabsorption and titratable acid and ammonia secretion leads to progressive reduction in the latter. At plasma levels above 27 mM/L, the exchange mechanism throughout the length of the nephron is concerned solely with bicarbonate reabsorption.

EXCRETION OF AMMONIA

As pointed out above, the titratable acid of normal urine is largely monobasic phosphate, and its rate of excretion is basically limited by the phosphate content of the diet. However, under conditions of acid stress, phosphate may be withdrawn in moderate amounts from stores in bone and cells, but only at the expense of altered structure and function. Ammonia, in contrast, is a buffer that is potentially available in much larger amount, theoretically equivalent to that of the nitrogen derived from the metabolism of protein. Under normal conditions, most of this nitrogen is excreted as urea. In acidosis, ammonia excretion increases and urea excretion decreases. This does not mean that urinary ammonia is derived from urea; rather, it means that the nitrogen of amino acids, deaminated in the liver, is converted in increased amount to ammonia precursors, rather than to urea. In the kidney these precursors give rise to urinary ammonia. Their nature will be considered later.

AMMONIA AS A BUFFER

According to the Bronstedt formulation,

$$NH_3 + H^+ \rightleftharpoons NH_4^+$$

NH_3 is a base, which in acid solution binds or buffers a hydrogen ion to form an ammonium ion. Conversely, NH_4^+ is an acid, which in alkaline solution dissociates a hydrogen ion to form the base, ammonia. Jacobs, many years ago, pointed out that the free base, NH_3, is uncharged, is lipid-soluble, and penetrates cell membranes readily, whereas the ammonium ion is charged, is water-soluble and penetrates cell membranes with difficulty, if at all. These properties are causally related to the mechanism of ammonia secretion, which is now generally believed to be one of passive, nonionic diffusion.

NATURE OF THE SECRETORY MECHANISM: NONIONIC DIFFUSION. — A bare outline of the nature of the secretory mechanism for ammonia is illustrated in Figure 11 – 11. Glutamine and other amino acids are extracted from blood by the renal tubules. They undergo deamidation and deamination within tubular cells, to liberate ammonia. The highly permeant free base, NH_3, diffuses in both directions; i.e., into urine and into peritubular capillary blood. In acidic urine, the base buffers hydrogen ions to form impermeant ammonium ions. One can therefore describe the mechanism as one of nonionic diffusion, for it is the un-ionized species that diffuses from cell to urine. One may also describe it

Fig. 11–11. — Simplified schema of the renal secretion of ammonia. The free base, NH_3, formed within tubular cells from glutamine and other amino acids, diffuses passively down a gradient of concentration into urine and into blood. Only the free base diffuses rapidly; the ammonium ion is relatively nondiffusible. (From Pitts, R. F.: Physiologist 9:97, 1966.)

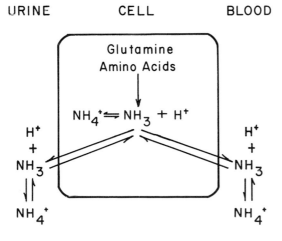

URINE   CELL   BLOOD

as a diffusion-trapping mechanism, for the free base diffuses into acidic urine, where it is trapped as nondiffusible ammonium ion. The free base diffuses into peritubular blood to a lesser extent and is carried out of the kidney in the venous blood stream — a fact demonstrated by Nash and Benedict more than 50 years ago (26).

A key feature of this secretory mechanism is that no energy is directly expended in moving ammonia from cell to urine or blood. Transport is downhill, the free base diffusing passively down a gradient of concentration from cell into acidic urine and into blood. However, energy is expended in transporting hydrogen ions and in maintaining a pH gradient between cells and urine.

The pK of the ammonia buffer system is 9.2 – 9.3. Therefore, at the pH of blood (7.4) or of the cytoplasm of tubular cells (estimated to be approximately 7), some 99 of each 100 molecules of total ammonia exist as ammonium ions. Only one exists as the diffusible free base, NH_3. However, if that one diffuses to a site of lower concentration, it is immediately replaced by the dissociation of a H^+ ion from an NH_4^+ ion. Because the free base is lipid-soluble, it can dissolve in and diffuse rapidly through the lipid cell membrane. The entire cell surface is thus available for base diffusion; ammonia is not restricted to aqueous channels. It behaves in this respect as do oxygen and carbon dioxide. The ammonium ion is water-soluble, not lipid-soluble, and is restricted to aqueous channels. Furthermore, its charge additionally restricts diffusion. Accordingly, cells are effectively impermeable to ammonium ions.

Within recent years, several lines of evidence have provided support for the thesis of nonionic diffusion as the mechanism of ammonia secretion. The first, the simplest, and perhaps the most conclusive of these arguments is illustrated by the two experiments shown in Figure 11 – 12 (27). A dog was made chronically acidotic by the administration of 10 Gm of ammonium chloride each day for 3 days. The ureters were separately catheterized, and a fine needle was

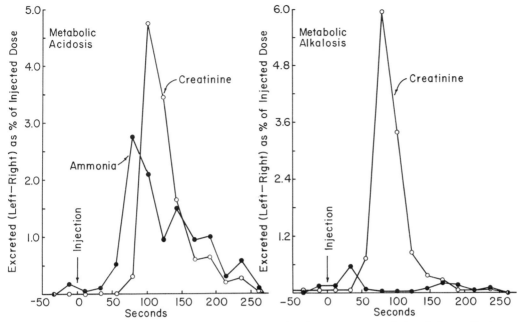

Fig. 11—12. — Time course of the urinary excretion of ammonia and creatinine, following their rapid injection into one renal artery of a dog. **Left,** dog in chronic metabolic acidosis; all urine samples acidic. **Right,** dog in acute metabolic alkalosis; all urine samples alkaline. (Adapted from Balagura, S., and Pitts, R. F.: Am. J. Physiol. 203:11, 1962.)

inserted in the left renal artery through a small flank incision. Urine was collected at 20-second intervals from each of the two kidneys. At zero time, marked by the arrow, 1 ml of saline solution containing creatinine and ammonium lactate was rapidly injected into the left renal artery.

In the experiment at the left in Figure 11–12, the urine samples were highly acidic: around pH 5. It is apparent that the injected ammonia appeared in the urine at least 20 seconds before the creatinine; namely, at 50 seconds on the time axis. Creatinine first appeared at 70 seconds. This 70-second appearance time for creatinine represents the time of formation of filtrate and its progress along the renal tubule, ureter and catheter to the collecting vial. Earlier appearance of ammonia can only mean passage from peritubular blood into the tubular urine downstream from the glomerulus.

The dog was then given sodium bicarbonate in an amount sufficient to correct the acidosis and to cause the excretion of alkaline urine. The experiment was repeated some 30 minutes later. The major difference in the experiment at the right in Figure 11–12 was that the urine samples were highly alkaline: around pH 8. The time course of excretion of creatinine was essentially the same in alkalosis as in acidosis. However, none of the ammonia appeared in the urine. Even that which must have been filtered, along with creatinine, was reabsorbed from the tubular urine.

These experiments demonstrate two facts: (1) that ammonia diffuses readily and rapidly in both directions across the renal tubules—from blood to tubular urine and from tubular urine to blood; and (2) that the direction of diffusion is along a hydrogen ion gradient, from the more alkaline phase to the more acidic phase. Because these are the two postulates of nonionic diffusion, its participation in ammonia secretion is evident. Somewhat more involved experiments of Denis et al. (28) and Sullivan et al. (31) confirm this point of view.

Stone *et al.* (29) demonstrated that diffusion equilibrium for free-base ammonia in the acidotic dog is attained throughout all parts of the kidney with a transit time no longer than that of the flow of blood through the kidney. The concepts upon which this statement is based are shown in Figure 11–13. The ammonia pool of the kidney is no doubt small but turns over rapidly. The major fraction of this ammonia is produced in the kidney from amino acid precursors, largely glutamine. The minor fraction enters the kidney as preformed ammonia. The turnover of the pool in micromoles per minute is the sum of the ammonia excreted in the urine and that added to renal venous blood.

If ^{15}N-ammonium chloride is infused into one renal artery at a low and constant rate, the isotopic ammonia mixes with the pool, and in part is excreted in the urine and in part removed in renal venous blood. One may calculate the expected dilution of the isotope by factoring its rate of infusion by the turnover rate of the pool. Its dilution may be measured directly by analysis of urinary

ammonia nitrogen with an isotope-ratio mass spectrometer. The urine is farthest from the site of delivery of the isotope, and diffusion must occur from peritubular capillaries across interstitial fluid and cells to reach the urine. If the measured dilution of isotope in urine equals the dilution calculated from rate of infusion factored by turnover rate of the pool, it is obvious that diffusion equilibrium has been achieved.

Table 11–6 presents data obtained in one of a series of similar experiments on dogs in acidosis. The sum of renal venous outflow of ammonia and urinary excretion of ammonia is equal to the turnover of the pool. At a rate of infusion of ^{15}N-ammonium chloride equal to a 1.85-μM excess per minute into the left renal artery, the calculated specific activity of the pool was 3.15 atoms % excess. Isotopic ammonia was measured in the urine formed by the left (infused) kidney and by the right (control) kidney. Subtracting the specific activity of the urine formed by the right kidney from that formed by the left kidney corrects for recirculation of isotope. The

Fig. 11–13. — Schematic representation of the concepts involved in demonstrating diffusion equilibrium in the kidney of the acidotic dog. (From Stone, W. J., Balagura, S., and Pitts, R. F.: J. Clin. Invest. 46:1603, 1967.)

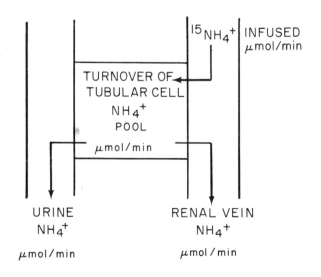

TABLE 11–6.–DATA INDICATING DIFFUSION EQUILIBRIUM FOR AMMONIA THROUGHOUT ALL PHASES OF THE KIDNEY OF THE ACIDOTIC DOG*

	AMMONIA		SPECIFIC ACTIVITY		
Venous Out	Urine Out	Pool Turnover	Pool	Urine (L–R)	Urine ─── Pool
	(μmol/min)		Atoms % excess ^{15}N		
Infuse $^{15}NH_4Cl$ – 1.85 μmol/min					
21.2	37.6	58.8	3.16	3.30	1.04
17.4	37.7	55.1	3.36	3.35	1.00
15.1	37.2	52.3	3.45	3.44	1.00
Infuse $^{15}NH_4Cl$ – 9.27 μmol/min					
20.4	40.0	60.4	15.35	15.39	1.00
19.1	39.0	58.1	15.95	15.85	0.99
17.0	41.3	58.3	15.90	15.91	1.00

*From Stone, W. J., Balagura, S., and Pitts, R. F.: J. Clin. Invest. 46: 1603, 1967.

corrected specific activity measured in the urine from the left kidney was 3.30 atoms % excess. The ratio of measured specific activity to calculated specific activity was 1.04. In two additional periods, agreement was essentially perfect. In the final three periods, the rate of infusion of isotopic ammonia was increased 5 times without change in agreement of measured and calculated specific activities. Thus, a fivefold increase in rate of infusion of isotope did not alter completeness of mixing with the pool. This observation strongly implies that ammonia is distributed by a passive process of diffusion rather than by active transport. Indeed, it would be difficult to conceive of an active system of transport that could account for equilibrium distribution of synthesized and preformed ammonia throughout a heterogenous system of widely differing hydrogen ion concentrations such as the kidney.

Experiments of Oelert *et al.* (30) on the kidney of the rat have demonstrated directly that these inferences are correct. Proximal and distal tubules were micropunctured, fluid was collected and analyzed for ammonia, and hydrogen ion concentration was measured. Carbonic anhydrase was infused intravenously, to prevent the development of disequilibrium pH. As shown in Table 11–7, the ammonia content increased and the pH decreased as the tubular fluid progressed along proximal and distal tubules; yet the pNH$_3$ of tubular urine remained essentially constant along the nephron and did not differ significantly from the pNH$_3$ of renal venous blood.

When proximal and distal tubules were perfused with ammonia-free buffers of pH 6.4, so compounded that gain or loss of fluid was minimal, the pNH$_3$ of the perfusate rose within 0.1–0.2 second to equal that of peritubular blood. Because the transit time of tubular urine through the proximal segment is approximately 10 seconds and the binding of H$^+$ ions by NH$_3$ to form NH$_4^+$ ions is essentially instantaneous, it is obvious that permeability of proximal and distal tubules to free-base NH$_3$ is not a factor that limits transfer and accumulation of ammonia plus ammonium ion in urine. These microperfusion data permit the calculation of a permeability to free base of not less than 1×10^{-2} cm/sec.

SITE OF AMMONIA SECRETION.– In the amphibian kidney, fluid withdrawn by micropuncture of glomeruli or proximal tubules is essentially free of ammonia; i.e., concentration is less than the sensitivity of the method. Ammonia first appears in samples collected from the first part of the distal tubule and increases in concentration as the fluid flows along the terminal parts of the nephron (32). The increase in concentration of ammonia exactly parallels the increase in acidity of the urine (33). Lacking evidence to the contrary, the assumption was made that the secretion of ammonia by the mammalian nephron fol-

TABLE 11–7.–DATA INDICATING DIFFUSION EQUILIBRIUM THROUGHOUT PROXIMAL AND DISTAL TUBULES AND RENAL VENOUS BLOOD*

LOCATION	TUBULAR FLUID		
	Ammonia (mM)	pH	pNH$_3$ (mm Hg $\times 10^{-6}$)
Proximal tubule	0.20	7.22	105 ± 32
First third	0.31	7.08	123 ± 25
Second third	0.45	6.95	125 ± 22
Last third	0.50	6.88	121 ± 29
Distal tubule			109 ± 20
Renal venous blood			

*From Oelert, H., Uhlich, E., and Hills, A. G.: Pflüg. Arch. 300:35, 1968.

lowed a similar pattern. When it was subsequently found, in studies on the rat, that the glomerular filtrate is modestly acidified as it flows along the proximal tubule (see Fig. 11–3), it became apparent that conditions were appropriate for diffusion and trapping of ammonia in proximal tubular urine, if indeed ammonia was formed in proximal tubular cells. The presence of enzymes potentially involved in ammonia formation in high concentration in the renal cortex and, by inference in proximal tubular cells, suggested that this might be true.

Glabman *et al.* (34) showed, in the rat, that ammonia is added to tubular urine in increasing amounts as it flows along the proximal segment (Fig. 11–14). The concentration considerably exceeds that which would result from filtration of ammonia from arterial plasma with subsequent concentration by

reabsorption of water. Additional ammonia is secreted into distal tubules and collecting ducts, although here reabsorption of water contributes significantly to increasing concentration. Three pertinent conclusions were drawn from this study: (1) the entire nephron participates in ammonia secretion; (2) fully half of the ammonia excreted in the urine could be added by proximal tubules; and (3) proximal secretion of ammonia is enhanced in chronic acidosis, in which condition proximal fluid is more intensely acidified. Similar observations have been made on the dog (35).

Evidence of Denis *et al.* (28) suggests that the free base, NH_3, within cortical tubular cells of both proximal and distal tubules is so readily diffusible that it is essentially in equilibrium with the free base in peritubular interstitial fluid and blood and with the free

Fig. 11–14.—Sites of tubular secretion of ammonia in rats. Samples of tubular fluid, collected from proximal and distal segments by micropuncture, and urine collected from the ureter of the same kidney were analyzed for ammonia. (From Glabman, S., Klose, R. M., and Giebisch, G.: Am. J. Physiol. 205:127, 1963.)

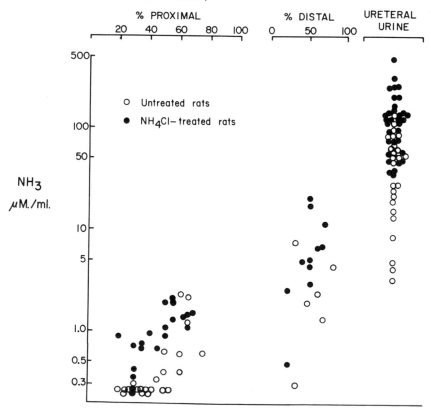

base in tubular urine. The concentration of total ammonia (NH_3 plus NH_4^+) in tubular urine should therefore increase linearly with increasing H^+ ion concentration along the length of the nephron. The rate of removal of ammonia from the kidney in the renal venous blood stream should be largely flow-limited. Both excretion of ammonia from blood and addition of ammonia to blood should be primarily determined by rate of production by tubular cells, not by any limitation of diffusion. Within limits, all three postulates seem to be true. The possible consequences of counter-current accumulation of ammonia in the medulla and papilla, if it occurs, have not been defined, although it is probable that a part of the ammonia formed by proximal cells and carried to the loop of Henle in the tubular urine diffuses directly into collecting ducts, thus by-passing the distal tubule entirely (36).

PRECURSORS OF URINARY AMMONIA.— Nash and Benedict, in 1921 (26), first demonstrated that ammonia is formed in the kidneys of the dog from precursors delivered in the arterial blood. Their evidence included the following points: The concentration of ammonia in arterial blood perfusing the kidney is very low, and, even if all of it were extracted in one circulation through the kidney, the amount would be insufficient to account for that which is excreted in the urine. The concentration of ammonia in arterial blood is unchanged in acidosis, in alkalosis, or following nephrectomy—conditions that drastically alter ammonia excretion. The renal venous concentration of ammonia exceeds the arterial concentration. Thus, the kidney does not extract ammonia from the blood, at least in net amounts; rather, it adds ammonia to the blood. The nitrogen of urea, amino acids and amide groups of proteins were subsequently claimed to be precursors of ammonia.

Some 20 years later, Van Slyke et al. (37) suggested that the amide nitrogen of circulating plasma glutamine is the major precursor of ammonia produced by the kidney of the acidotic dog. They observed that sufficient glutamine was extracted from the blood perfusing the kidney to account for all of the ammonia added to renal venous blood and for two thirds or more of that excreted in the urine. Presumably, the remainder of the ammonia produced by the kidney was derived from the α-amino nitrogen of unspecified amino acids. The induction of acute metabolic alkalosis by the infusion of sodium bicarbonate drastically reduced both the renal extraction of glutamine and the renal production of ammonia.

Twenty more years elapsed before the application of new methods advanced our understanding of renal ammonia metabolism. The development of column chromatography permitted an assessment of the renal metabolism of a variety of amino acids, including glutamine. Van Slyke had used a specific enzymatic method to measure glutamine and a nonspecific α-amino nitrogen method to measure all other amino acids. The introduction of the technic of catheterization of a renal vein under fluoroscopic guidance permitted studies on man as well as on experimental animals. Van Slyke had used dogs in which one kidney had been explanted subcutaneously in the flank and a skin-tube constructed around the renal vein. Blood was withdrawn by puncture of the renal vein.

A study by Shalhoub et al. (38) is summarized in Figure 11–15. Samples of arterial and renal venous plasma were collected simultaneously from 20 acidotic dogs, and the concentrations of some 23 free amino acids were measured following chromatographic separation. Average concentrations are given in this bar graph.

At the left of Figure 11–15, arterial concentrations, expressed in micromoles per milliliter of plasma are shown by the upper black bar of each pair. The renal venous concentrations are shown by the lower white bar. At the right are shown arteriovenous concentration differences: black, if the amino acid is removed from plasma perfusing the kidney; white, if the kidney manufactures the amino acid and adds it to renal venous plasma. Essentially similar findings in man have been reported by Owen and Robinson (39).

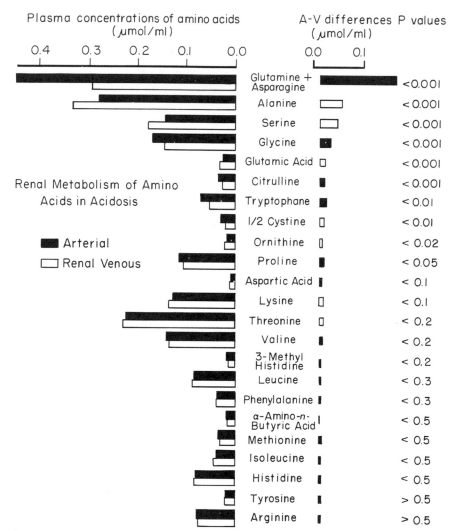

Fig. 11–15.—Renal extraction of amino acids. **Left,** mean concentrations of free amino acids in simultaneously collected samples of arterial and renal venous plasma of 20 acidotic dogs. **Center,** arterio-venous differences in concentration. **Right,** P values: probabilities that arteriovenous differences could have been fortuitous. (From Shalhoub, R., Webber, W., Glabman, S., Canessa-Fischer, M., Klein, J., DeHaas, J., and Pitts, R. F.: Am. J. Physiol. 204:181, 1963.)

The five amino acids at the top of this graph are the most interesting. It is evident that glutamine is extracted in far greater amount than is any other amino acid—a fact that confirms the finding of Van Slyke and his associates. Glycine is also extracted in a much smaller but still significant amount. In contrast, alanine and serine are produced by the kidney and added to renal venous plasma, and the amounts produced suggest that some of the nitrogen of the extracted gluta-mine must have been diverted from ammonia production to the production of alanine and serine. Glutamic acid is also consistently added to renal venous plasma, but it is the smallness of the quantity added that is of special interest. If only the amide nitrogen of glutamine were used for the production of ammonia, then for each micromole of gluta-mine extracted from arterial plasma, 1 μmol of glutamic acid should have been added to renal venous plasma, for essentially no glutamic acid was excreted in the urine. Actually, only 0.07 μmol was added to renal venous plasma. Therefore, 93% of the glutamic acid equivalent of the extracted glutamine disappeared. The amino nitrogen of glutamine does, in fact, appear in part in the ammonia produced in the kidney and in part in the nitrogen of the alanine and serine that are added to renal venous plasma (see below).

If glutamine and other amino acids are the sole sources of ammonia produced by the kidney, then, in the steady state, the net renal extraction of amide and amino nitrogen should equal total ammonia production. Such a renal balance, achieved by measuring simultaneously renal plasma flow, arterial and renal venous concentrations of each of the plasma amino acids, arterial and renal venous concentrations of ammonia, and rate of excretion of ammonia, is illustrated in Table 11–8.

The total amide and amino nitrogen extracted by the kidney averaged 86 μmol/min. This was largely glutamine and glycine. The total amino nitrogen added to renal venous plasma amounted to 31.1 μmol/min. This was largely alanine and serine. The net nitrogen extraction therefore was 54.9 μmol/min. The sum of the ammonia added to renal venous blood and excreted in the urine averaged 57.5 μmol/min. It was therefore pos-

sible to account for 95% of the ammonia produced by the kidney in terms of the net extraction of amino and amide nitrogen. This is essentially equal to 100%, for errors are easily compounded in work of this type. However, from such data it is not possible to assign an absolute percentage contribution of any one precursor, such as the amide nitrogen of glutamine, to ammonia formation. For instance, what is the source of the nitrogen used for the production of alanine and serine? Is it amide or amino nitrogen? The 30 μmol of nitrogen used for these synthetic purposes is more than one third of the total nitrogen extracted by the kidney. Recent studies using amino acids labeled with isotopic nitrogen have clarified sources of ammonia produced in the kidneys and, to some extent, the metabolic pathways involved.

The method used to study directly the origin of ammonia produced in the intact functioning kidney of the dog is illustrated in Figure 11–16. The diagram specifically relates to studies with glutamine, in which 95 of every 100 molecules infused contained ^{15}N in the amide position (95 atoms % ^{15}N amide glutamine). ^{15}N is a heavy nonradioactive isotope of nitrogen, which must be quantified by mass spectrometry. Isotopic glutamine is infused at a constant rate into one renal artery of an acidotic dog, in tracer amounts. In this diagram, G represents isotopic glutamine, and g represents normally occurring ^{14}N glutamine. The ammonia excreted by the infused kidney contains ^{15}N demonstrating its origin within the kidney from the amide nitrogen of glutamine. However, some of the infused ^{15}N glutamine is not extracted from the blood in its first circuit through the kidney and enters the general circulation. This isotopic glutamine is returned equally to both kidneys. Accordingly, the ammonia excreted by the noninfused kidney contains a far smaller but still significant amount of ^{15}N. By appropriate measurements and calculations, which need not concern us here, one may correct for recirculation of isotopic glutamine, and arrive at a precise estimation of the proportion and absolute amount of am-

TABLE 11–8.—RENAL BALANCE OF AMINO, AMIDE AND AMMONIA NITROGEN IN THE DOG IN CHRONIC ACIDOSIS; MEAN OF NINE EXPERIMENTAL STUDIES ON EIGHT DOGS*

Total amide and amino nitrogen extracted from plasma	86.0 μmol/min
Amino nitrogen added to plasma	31.1 " "
Net amide and amino nitrogen extracted from plasma	54.9 " "
Ammonia nitrogen added to renal venous blood	14.4 μmol/min
Ammonia nitrogen excreted in urine	43.1 " "
Total ammonia nitrogen produced in kidney	57.5 " "

NOTE:

$$\frac{\text{Net nitrogen extracted}}{\text{Ammonia produced}} = \frac{54.9}{57.5} \times 100 = 95\%$$

*From Pitts, R. F., DeHaas, J. C. M., and Klein, J.: Am. J. Physiol. 204:187, 1963.

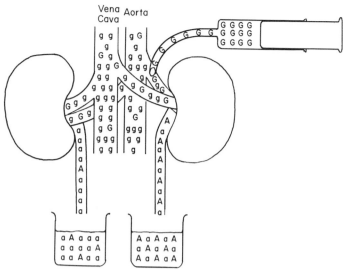

Fig. 11–16.—Use of ^{15}N-amide-labeled gluta-mine in the study of the origin of urinary ammonia in the acidotic dog G, ^{15}N-amide glutamine; g, ^{14}N-glutamine; A, ^{15}N-ammonia; a, ^{14}N-ammonia. (From Pitts, R. F.: Physiologist 9:917, 1966.)

monia derived within the kidney from the amide nitrogen of circulating plasma gluta-mine (40).

Table 11–9 summarizes results of 36 ex-periments with six different labeled com-pounds. In nine experiments, a mean of 43.3% of the ammonia produced by the kid-ney was derived from the amide nitrogen of plasma glutamine, confirming the view of Van Slyke *et al.* (37) that the amide nitro-gen of glutamine is the major precursor of renal ammonia. In six experiments, 18% of the ammonia was derived from the amino nitrogen of plasma glutamine. Thus, on an average, nearly two thirds of the renal am-monia is derived from the two nitrogens of plasma glutamine. Alanine, glycine and glu-tamic acid account for much smaller but still significant proportions of the ammonia. In all, 73% of the ammonia is derived from these 4 amino acids; 35% is derived from preformed arterial ammonia. Because, as stated earlier, ammonia is in diffusion equi-librium throughout all parts of the kidney, the preformed ammonia that enters the kidney in arterial blood, plus that formed from precurs-ors within the kidney, equals the total am-monia that leaves the kidney in venous blood, plus that excreted in the urine. Accordingly, the renal pool of ammonia is well mixed. The sum of all sources of ammonia pro-duced or brought to the kidney (108%) is

TABLE 11–9.—CONTRIBUTIONS OF FIVE PLASMA AMINO ACID PRECURSOR NITROGENS TO URINARY AMMONIA*

NUMBER OF EXPERIMENTS	AMMONIA EXCRETED AND ADDED TO RENAL VENOUS BLOOD		
	Source	Mean (%)	Range (%)
9	Amide nitrogen of glutamine	43.3	35.3 –51.4
6	Amino nitrogen of glutamine	18.3	10.1 –25.5
8	Amino nitrogen of alanine	5.71	3.03 – 8.41
5	Amino nitrogen of glycine	3.76	2.92 – 5.55
2	Amino nitrogen of glutamate	1.88	1.43 – 2.34
6	Arterial ammonia	35.0	23.0 –48.0
TOTAL		108.0	

*Data compiled from Pitts, R. F., Pilkington, L. A., and DeHaas, J. C. M.: J. Clin. Invest. 44:731, 1965; Pitts, R. F., and Pilkington, L. A.; ibid. 45:86, 1966; Pitts, R. F., and Stone, W. J.: ibid. 46:530, 1967; and Stone, W. J., Balagura, S., and Pitts, R. F.: ibid. 46:1603, 1967.

within the limits of error of the measurement.

PATHWAYS OF AMMONIA PRODUCTION. — Renal tubular cells contain a number of enzymes that, potentially, could play some role in the metabolism of amino acids and in ammonia production. The precise contribution of these enzymes and their functional organization can be assessed only by studies on the intact functioning kidney, for slices of renal cortex, isolated tubules and, even more obviously, a homogenate do not represent a kidney. They lack a constantly renewed filtrate, tubular urine and blood supply. The medium in which they are suspended is highly artificial. Cellular products pile up in the medium or in an even more restricted volume of tubular fluid contents. Hormonal controls are lost as are those controls dependent on subtle changes in body fluid composition. Concentrations of substrates added are usually far from the range of normal. Nevertheless, knowledge of renal enzymes and their properties, even under the highly artifi-

tively little is known of the kidney of man.

Glutaminase I is a hydrolytic enzyme that catalyzes the deamidation of glutamine to form glutamic acid and ammonia.

$$
\begin{array}{ccc}
\text{COOH} & & \text{COOH} \\
| & & | \\
\text{CHNH}_2 & & \text{CHNH}_2 \\
| & & | \\
\text{CH}_2 & \xrightarrow[\text{Glu}\cdot\text{NH}_2\text{-ase}]{\text{HOH}} & \text{CH}_2 \\
| & & | \\
\text{CH}_2 & & \text{CH}_2 \\
| & & | \\
\text{CONH}_2 & & \text{COOH} + \text{NH}_3 \\
\text{(Glutamine)} & & \text{(Glutamic acid)}
\end{array}
$$

Its optimal pH is around 7, and it is activated by inorganic phosphate and, to a lesser extent, by sulfate and arsenate. The enzyme is associated with mitochondria. The hydrolysis of glutamine results in a relatively large decrease in free energy (3,420 Cal/mol). The net synthesis of glutamine therefore occurs by a separate biosynthetic pathway powered by ATP and catalyzed by glutamine synthetase.

$$
\begin{array}{ccc}
\text{COOH} & & \text{COOH} \\
| & & | \\
\text{CHNH}_2 & & \text{CHNH}_2 \\
| & & | \\
\text{CH}_2 & \xrightarrow[\text{Synthetase}]{\text{Glu}\cdot\text{NH}_2} & \text{CH}_2 \\
| & & | \\
\text{CH}_2 & & \text{CH}_2 \\
| & & | \\
\text{COOH} + \text{ATP} + \text{NH}_3 & & \text{CONH}_2 + \text{ADP} + \text{P}_i \\
\text{(Glutamic acid)} & & \text{(Glutamine)}
\end{array}
$$

cial conditions of a homogenate or a slice, must constitute the starting point of any attempt to describe the pathways of ammonia production in vivo. The kidney of the rat and the dog differ in certain known respects, and an extrapolation of the findings on one to explain the behavior of the other is, at best, a hazardous procedure. Rela-

Although this enzyme system is present in rat and guinea pig kidneys, it is absent from dog and cat kidneys, which appear to synthesize no glutamine (41).

Glutamate dehydrogenase, also associated with mitochondria, catalyzes the oxidative deamination of glutamate to form α-ketoglutarate and ammonia.

$$
\begin{array}{ccc}
\text{COOH} & & \text{COOH} \\
| & & | \\
\text{CHNH}_2 & & \text{CO} \\
| & \xrightarrow[\text{Glu}\cdot\text{Dehydrogenase}]{\text{HOH}} & | \\
\text{CH}_2 + \text{DPN}^+ & & \text{CH}_2 + \text{NH}_3 + \text{DPNH} + \text{H}^+ \\
| & & | \\
\text{CH}_2 & & \text{CH}_2 \\
| & & | \\
\text{COOH} & & \text{COOH} \\
\text{(Glutamic acid)} & & \text{(α-Ketoglutaric acid)}
\end{array}
$$

Diphosphopyridine nucleotide is the coenzyme involved in kidney tissue. The reaction is reversible, and the equilibrium in vitro favors the synthesis of glutamate. However, in the presence of an adequate supply of oxidized DPN^+; the glutamate formed from glutamine by the action of glutaminase I could be further degraded to α-ketoglutarate, liberating the amino nitrogen as well as the amide nitrogen of the original glutamine as ammonia. The reaction to the right is also favored by the diffusion of ammonia into acid urine and into blood and its removal from the kidney. Glutamate dehydrogenase is present in large amounts in kidney tissue.

A large number of amino acids, when infused into acidotic dogs intravenously, cause the excretion of increased amounts of ammonia in the urine (42, 43). Because L-amino acid oxidases are virtually absent from kidney tissue of the dog, any direct contribution of these amino acids to renal ammonia production is improbable. However, a variety of transaminases, capable of transferring the α-amino nitrogen of these L-amino acids to α-ketoglutarate to form glutamate, are present in kidney tissue.

$$
\begin{array}{c}
\text{COOH} \\
| \\
\text{CHNH}_2 \\
| \\
\text{CH}_2 \\
| \\
\text{CH}_2 \\
| \\
\text{COOH} \\
\text{(Glutamic acid)}
\end{array}
+
\begin{array}{c}
\text{COOH} \\
| \\
\text{CO} \\
| \\
\text{CH}_3 \\
\text{(Pyruvic acid)}
\end{array}
\xrightleftharpoons[\text{-ase}]{\text{Transamin-}}
\begin{array}{c}
\text{COOH} \\
| \\
\text{CO} \\
| \\
\text{CH}_2 \\
| \\
\text{CH}_2 \\
| \\
\text{COOH} \\
(\alpha\text{-Ketoglutaric acid})
\end{array}
+
\begin{array}{c}
\text{COOH} \\
| \\
\text{CHNH}_2 \\
| \\
\text{CH}_3 \\
\text{(Alanine)}
\end{array}
$$

The subsequent deamination of glutamate by glutamic dehydrogenase would contribute amino acid nitrogen to the ammonia pool indirectly.

A specific glutamine transaminase capable of transferring the α-amino nitrogen of glutamine to a variety of α-keto acids is present in the kidney.

$$
\begin{array}{c}
\text{COOH} \\
| \\
\text{CHNH}_2 \\
| \\
\text{CH}_2 \\
| \\
\text{CH}_2 \\
| \\
\text{CONH}_2 \\
\text{(Glutamine)}
\end{array}
+
\begin{array}{c}
\text{COOH} \\
| \\
\text{CO} \\
| \\
\text{CH}_3 \\
\text{(Pyruvic acid)}
\end{array}
\xrightarrow[\text{Transamin-}\atop\text{ase}]{\text{Glu}\cdot\text{NH}_2}
\begin{array}{c}
\text{COOH} \\
| \\
\text{CO} \\
| \\
\text{CH}_2 \\
| \\
\text{CH}_2 \\
| \\
\text{CONH}_2 \\
(\alpha\text{-Ketoglutaramic acid})
\end{array}
+
\begin{array}{c}
\text{COOH} \\
| \\
\text{CHNH}_2 \\
| \\
\text{CH}_3 \\
\text{(Alanine)}
\end{array}
$$

$$
\begin{array}{c}
\text{COOH} \\
| \\
\text{CO} \\
| \\
\text{CH}_2 \\
| \\
\text{CH}_2 \\
| \\
\text{CONH}_2 \\
(\alpha\text{-Ketoglutaramic} \\ \text{acid})
\end{array}
\xrightarrow[\text{Amidase}]{\text{HOH}}
\begin{array}{c}
\text{COOH} \\
| \\
\text{CO} \\
| \\
\text{CH}_2 \\
| \\
\text{CH}_2 \\
| \\
\text{COOH} + \text{NH}_3 \\
(\alpha\text{-Ketoglutaric} \\ \text{acid})
\end{array}
$$

The products of this reaction are α-ketoglutaramate and the amino acid analogues of the keto acids. The α-ketoglutaramate is immediately deamidated to ammonia and α-ketoglutaric acid by tissue amidases. The enzyme complex of glutamine transaminase and tissue amidase is also known as glutaminase II. It was once thought to be a single enzyme, activated by keto acids and having an optimal pH of 8. The end products of the coupled glutaminase II reactions are similar to those of the glutaminase I-glutamate dehydrogenase couplet. It is therefore difficult to distinguish between these two enzyme systems.

Evidence for the participation of each of these enzyme systems in ammonia production by the dog kidney has been obtained, using ^{15}N-labeled amino acids (44, 45). The pathways involved are summarized in Figure 11–17, which represents diagrammatically a tubular cell. In the interest of clarity, ammonia is shown as diffusing only into the urine, although it obviously diffuses in lesser amounts into peritubular blood. Similarly, amino acids are shown as entering the cell only from peritubular blood, whereas it is probable that their major uptake is from the tubular lumen in the course of their reabsorption from glomerular filtrate.

The glutaminase I pathway is shown at the right in Figure 11–16. Although a major pathway of glutamine metabolism, it is not the exclusive one it was once inferred to be. The amide nitrogen of glutamine is split off hydrolytically to yield ammonia and glutamate. This reaction is essentially irreversible for the reason stated earlier: it is associated with a large decrease in free energy. The glutamate is then oxidatively deaminated to yield ammonia and α-ketoglutarate. This latter reaction is reversible; in fact, the equilibrium in vitro favors the synthesis of glutamate. However, in the dog kidney in vivo, little glutamate is formed; the reaction proceeds almost entirely toward production of

Fig. 11–17.—Pathways of ammonia production in renal tubular cells. (From Pitts, R. F.: Am. J. Med. 36:720, 1964.)

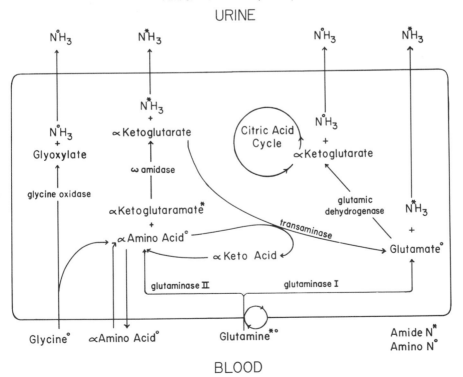

α-ketoglutarate and ammonia. The α-keto-glutarate has several possible fates: (1) it can enter the Krebs cycle and serve as a source of energy to power various transport mechanisms; (2) it can participate in the glutaminase II sequence; (3) it can serve as the substrate in conventional transamination reactions, by which a variety of amino acids contribute their amino nitrogens to the ammonia pool; (4) or, following partial dissimilation, a part of the carbon skeleton can appear in several renal products, notably glucose.

Glutamine may be metabolized to a significant extent by the glutaminase II pathway (49). Oxalacetate, pyruvate, hydroxypyruvate and, probably, α-ketoglutarate could be transaminated directly by glutamine to yield aspartate, alanine, serine and glutamate and the common end product, α-ketoglutaramate. The last-named compound is unstable and is deamidated to yield ammonia and α-ketoglutarate. Alanine and serine are formed in the kidney of both dog and man and are added in net amounts to renal venous blood. Experimental evidence suggests that a significant fraction of renal alanine and, presumably, of renal serine is formed by the glutaminase II reaction, their nitrogens coming from amino groups of glutamine. Aspartate is the second most abundant free amino acid in kidney tissue; the most abundant is glutamate. Renal aspartate may also be formed in significant amounts by the glutaminase II reaction. Insofar as the transaminase step of the glutaminase II reaction contributes to the renal synthesis of amino acids, the succeeding deamidation step must contribute to the ammonia pool of the kidney. Because, in the dog, α-ketoglutarate is not reductively aminated to form glutamate and glutamate is not amidated to form glutamine, the entire ammonia pool of the kidney is dissipated by diffusion either into acid urine, where it buffers H^+ ions to form NH_4^+ ions, or in lesser amounts into peritubular capillary blood.

Although under normal circumstances most of the ammonia formed in the kidney is derived from the amide and, to a lesser extent, from the amino groups of glutamine, other amino acids contribute nominally to the pool (see Table 11–9). This fact is clearly evident in the increased excretion of ammonia observed following the intravenous administration of such amino acids as asparagine, alanine, histidine, aspartate, glycine, leucine, methionine and cysteine. These amino acids probably contribute their nitrogens by transaminating α-ketoglutarate to form glutamate. Oxidative deamination of the latter compound regenerates the α-ketoglutarate and yields the original amino nitrogen as ammonia.

Glycine, which normally provides only a small amount of urinary ammonia, can provide a much greater percentage when plasma concentration is increased. In fact, this is true of all amino acids studied. Thus, although the kidney preferentially uses glutamine as a source of ammonia, it will use many different amino acids if they are presented in excessive amounts. Utilization is probably entirely by transamination to glutamate, except for glycine, which may be oxidatively deaminated by D-amino acid oxidase, and except for asparagine, which has its amide nitrogen removed by asparaginase.

CONTROL OF AMMONIA EXCRETION. – On average, the rate of excretion of ammonia in the urine is nicely attuned to the numbers of excess protons in the body. Normally, some 30–50 mEq of ammonia are excreted in the urine each day – a value that may increase 10-fold in severe acidosis (see Table 11–4). If no proton excess exists (alkalosis), ammonia excretion may cease entirely. The question of how this control of excretion is effected can be answered only in part. We need to know (1) what determines the distribution of ammonia between urine and blood and (2) what determines the rate of production of ammonia within the kidney.

The prime determinants of distribution of ammonia between urine and blood are the pHs of the two phases and their relative rates of flow. The more acid the tubular urine, the greater is the sink into which the free-base NH_3 diffuses to be trapped as ammonium ion (see Fig. 11–11). Because, under the circumstances of normal acid-base balance and acidosis, the acidity of tubular urine is much greater than that of peritubular blood, most of the ammonia enters and is trapped in tubular urine ($\pm 75\%$). Approximately 25% enters the peritubular capillaries and is carried away in the venous stream. If the urine is suddenly alkalized by the intravenous injection of a carbonic anhydrase inhibitor, the ammonia that previously diffused into acid urine now diffuses into the blood. No immediate change occurs in rate of production (46). If the pH of the urine approaches that of the blood, the distribution becomes largely determined by their relative flows. Because the flow of peritubular capillary blood far exceeds that of tubular urine, most of the ammonia enters the blood. However, it must be emphasized that the pH of tubular urine will normally equal that of peritubular blood only if no excess of protons exists. Under such conditions the production of ammonia by the kidney is drastically curtailed.

The interaction of urine acidity and rate of production and excretion of ammonia are shown in Figure 11–18, which relates ammonia excretion to urine pH in the same dog under two different conditions: in normal acid-base balance and in chronic acidosis induced by the daily feeding of ammonium chloride. In both series of experiments, the pH of the urine was progressively elevated by the infusion of sodium bicarbonate. In both, ammonia excretion was inversely related to urine pH. However, at any given urine pH, the rate of ammonia excretion was higher in the acidotic than in the normal animal. From this, it can be inferred that the rate of cellular production of ammonia is increased in chronic acidosis.

CONTROL OF AMMONIA PRODUCTION.— No definitive explanation of increased production of ammonia in acidosis, which is generally applicable, can be advanced. Most studies have been performed on rats and dogs. Dissimilarities of these two species are sufficiently numerous to make an extrapolation to man of dubious value. What does seem certain in man, rat and dog is that avail-

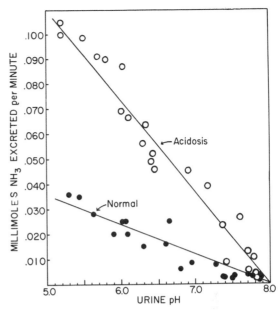

Fig. 11–18. — Relationship between urine pH and ammonia excretion in a single animal under conditions of normal acid-base balance and chronic acidosis. Urine pH was varied by the intravenous infusion of sodium bicarbonate. (From Pitts, R. F.: Fed. Proc. 7:418, 1948.)

ability of the major substrate, glutamine, is not the determining factor. The quantity of glutamine delivered to the kidneys in the arterial blood does not differ significantly in alkalosis and acidosis; i.e., the product of arterial glutamine concentration and renal blood flow. However, the rate of use of glutamine does differ markedly.

The concept that the intracellular concentration of renal ammonia-producing enzymes might be a rate-limiting factor was based on the observation of Davies and Yudkin (47) that a highly significant increase in the activity of glutaminase I in the rat kidney is induced by the daily feeding of ammonium chloride. Rector *et al.* (48) noted an impressive correlation, in rat kidney, of glutaminase I activity and rate of ammonia excretion. However, Rector and Orloff (49) found that no adaptive increase in enzyme activity occurred in the kidney of the dog in response to repeated administration of ammonium chloride, although rate of excretion of ammonia increased progressively, as it did in the rat. Subsequently, Goldstein (50) observed that the administration of an inhibitor of protein synthesis blocked the adaptive increase in glutaminase I activity of the rat kidney, which resulted from the daily feeding of ammonium chloride, yet did not alter the progressive increase in rate of ammonia excretion. Obviously, whatever one measures in vitro as enzyme adaptation is not the factor that determines ammonia excretion in either the rat or the dog. The amounts of enzyme normally present in the kidney are apparently adequate to produce the increased quantities of ammonia excreted under the stress of acidosis.

Because substrate availability is unchanged, yet enzymatic production of ammonia increases in acidosis, the funtional activity of enzymes in vivo must be increased as a consequence of some alteration of the intracellular milieu. The following alterations have been suggested as significantly increasing enzyme activity in acidosis: (1) an increase in cellular acidity; (2) a reduction in cellular concentration of potassium; and (3) a reduction in cellular concentration of glutamate, which would reduce the inhibition of glutaminase by one of its reaction products.

In support of the third hypothesis, Goldstein (51, 52) demonstrated in the rat that the free glutamate of renal tubular cells is an effective inhibitor of phosphate-dependent glutaminase at the concentrations present in the normal kidney: $7-8 \times 10^{-3}$ mol/kg. Indeed, the K_i glutamate (concentration for 50% inhibition of enzyme) is only 1×10^{-3} mol/kg. Chronic acidosis causes approximately a 35% decrease in renal cellular glutamate; i.e., to $4-5 \times 10^{-3}$ mol/kg. This decrease in glutamate concentration would be expected to produce a 20% increase in glutaminase activity, resulting in an increase of ammonia production of comparable magnitude. Instead, one observes an increase of 200–300% in ammonia excretion in the acidotic rat.

A decrease in the concentration of α-ketoglutarate in renal tissue has also been observed in chronic acidosis. Reduction in concentration of this product of the glutamate dehydrogenase reaction, as well as removal of ammonia in acid urine, would favor deamination of glutamate and thus increase ammonia production. Whether or not these several factors increasing the activity of glutaminase and glutamic dehydrogenase are adequate explanations of increased production of ammonia in acidosis remains to be demonstrated.

The theory of control that has received the most attention and support in recent years is that based on an increase in renal gluconeogenesis and an adaptive increase in renal content of phosphoenolpyruvate carboxykinase (PEPCK) in acidosis (53, 54). This enzyme converts oxaloacetate to phosphoenolpyruvate (PEP), thus by-passing the irreversible step, pyruvate to PEP, in reverse glycolysis (Fig. 11–19). As a consequence of the adaptive increase in PEPCK, concentrations of all renal intermediates of the Krebs cycle, back to and including α-ketoglutarate (α-KG), are decreased. Reducing α-KG deinhibits glutamic dehydrogenase and thus increases conversion of glutamate to α-KG and NH_3. Reducing the concentration of glutamate deinhibits glutaminase I and thus increases conversion of glutamine to glutamate and NH_3. Thus, all ammonia produced from glutamine must, according to theory, ultimately be ascribed to an adaptive increase in PEPCK. Although widely accepted, this thesis had not been critically tested until recently. The only test having true validity is one performed on the intact animal with normally functioning kidneys, not on slices of renal cortex. Furthermore, the test should be performed at normal endogenous blood concentrations of glutamine, not at the elevated (10–20 times normal) levels customarily used in studies on slices. These considerations made the use of ^{14}C-uniformly-labeled glutamine mandatory and the dog the experimental animal of choice (55, 56).

In outline, the experiment was as follows: ^{14}C-uniformly-labeled glutamine of high spe-

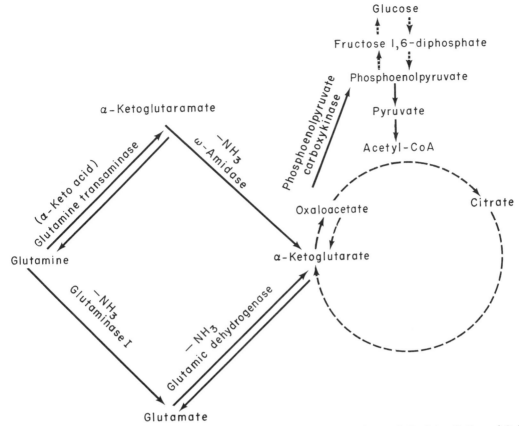

Fig. 11–19.—Relation between renal gluconeogenesis from glutamine and renal production of ammonia. (From Goodman, A. D., Fuisz, R. E., and Cahill, G. F., Jr.: J. Clin. Invest. 45:612, 1966.)

cific activity was infused at a constant rate into a peripheral vein. After some 40 minutes, counts per minute in glutamine per milliliter of arterial blood became relatively constant and adequate for accurate measurement; no measurable increase in blood concentration of glutamine occurred as a consequence of infusion of isotope. Renal venous blood was collected through a catheter introduced into a renal vein under fluoroscopic guidance; arterial blood was collected from the femoral artery. The extraction of glutamine by the kidney could now be measured as the product of the difference in arterial and renal venous blood concentrations and renal blood flow. The conversion of glutamine to glucose and its oxidation to CO_2 were measured simultaneously, using ^{14}C as the tracer. Total production of CO_2 was used

as a measure of the metabolic rate of the kidney.

A mean of 27.7 μmol of glutamine was extracted by the kidney per minute in acidosis; 8.04 μmol/min was extracted in alkalosis. These data are presented in the first pair of columns in Figure 11–20. If both nitrogens of glutamine were converted to ammonia, a total of 55.4 μmol/min of ammonia would be produced in acidosis and 16.08 μmol/min in alkalosis. The excretion of ammonia averaged 41.4 μmol/min in acidosis and 3.43 μmol/min in alkalosis. These data are presented in the last pair of columns in Figure 11–20. On average, about 25% of the ammonia produced in the kidney of the acidotic dog is added to renal venous blood. Subtracting 25% from 55.4 μmol/min left 41.6 μmol/min—essentially the quantity

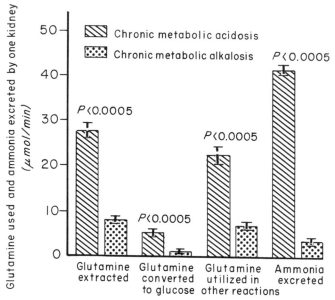

Fig. 11–20.—Comparisons of mean rates of extraction of glutamine, conversion to glucose, use in other reactions and excretion of ammonia in dogs in chronic metabolic acidosis and alkalosis. (From Pitts, R. F., Pilkington, L A., Leal-Pinto, E., and MacLeod, M. B.: J. Clin. Invest. 51:557, 1972.)

excreted in the urine. Assuming that roughly the same absolute amount of ammonia was added to renal venous blood in chronic alkalosis, there remained 3.0 μmol to be excreted. These estimates are presented to show that, within reasonable limits, essentially all of the glutamine extracted by the kidney was converted to α-KG and NH$_3$ in both acidosis and alkalosis.

Figure 11–20 demonstrates that the production of glucose from glutamine is not rate-limiting for the production of ammonia in either acidosis or alkalosis (note second pair of columns). Thus, a relatively small proportion of the glutamine extracted in acidosis was converted to glucose: 5.34 μmol/min, or about 20% of the total glutamine extracted. In alkalosis, 0.78 μmol/min of glutamine was converted to glucose: again, about 20% of the total extracted. Accordingly, it is evident that about 80% of the glutamine extracted is metabolized by reactions other than conversion to glucose (see third pair of columns).

Other data derived from these experiments demonstrate that the major fraction of this glutamine is oxidized completely to CO_2. Of course, for each 2 mol of glutamine converted to 1 mol of glucose, 4 mol of CO_2 and

4 mol of ammonia are formed. When 1 mol of glutamine is oxidized completely, 5 mol of CO_2 and 2 mol of ammonia are produced. Less than 20% of the CO_2 and of the ammonia derived from glutamine is the product of its conversion to glucose. Therefore, gluconeogenesis cannot be rate-limiting for the production of ammonia. A much more likely thesis would be that some factor or factors controlling oxidation of glutamine in the Krebs cycle regulates ammonia production by the kidney.

Although we have not tested the following hypothesis in any direct way, it is possible that the control of ammonia production depends on the control of entry of glutamine to the site of the enzymes responsible for ammonia production. Both glutaminase I and glutamic dehydrogenase are intramitochondrial enzymes. Because filtration rates and plasma glutamine concentrations are the same in acidosis and alkalosis, the amounts of glutamine entering tubular cells in the course of reabsorption from the filtrate are the same. In alkalosis, a major fraction of reabsorbed glutamine traverses tubular cells unchanged. In acidosis, glutamine penetrates mitochondria, where it is exposed to the action of glutaminase I, glutamic dehydrogenase and the enzymes of the Krebs cycle. Penetration may be a consequence of increased active transport into mitochondria in acidosis or increased passive entry dependent on swelling and increased permeability. This concept accounts for most of the presently known facts concerning control of ammonia production.

SITES OF PRODUCTION OF GLUTAMINE. — It is obvious that increased use of glutamine by the kidneys in acidosis must be accompanied by increased production of glutamine in other organs. Production must be closely related to use, for plasma concentration is essentially the same in acidosis and alkalosis. According to Addae and Lotspeich (57), the major site of production in the dog is the liver. They equate the signal for increased hepatic synthesis of glutamine with an increase in ammonia content of the portal blood entering the liver from the gastrointestinal tract. The GI tract is also a major site of breakdown of glutamine to form ammonia — an activity that, presumably, is increased in acidosis — as well as the site of absorption of ammonia in experimental ammonium chloride acidosis. Hills *et al.* (58) have disputed the importance of the liver as a source of replacement of blood glutamine removed by the kidneys; instead, they found skeletal muscle and brain to be the major sources of supply in the dog and the spider monkey. This is an important question, which should be clarified by further work.

RENAL DEFENSES OF ACID-BASE BALANCE IN HEALTH AND DISEASE

The means by which the normal person withstands the initial insult of a suddenly imposed acid load and the way in which his

Fig. 11—21. — Rates of excretion of ions prior to, during and after a period of acidosis induced by the ingestion of ammonium chloride. Subject, a normal young adult. (Adapted from Sartorius, O. W., Roemmelt, J. C., and Pitts, R. F.: J. Clin. Invest. 28:423, 1949.)

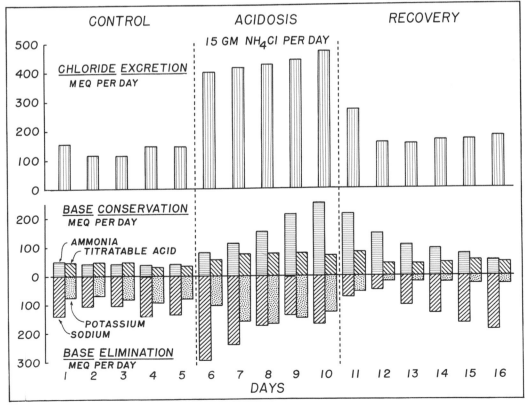

kidneys repair the damage to the acid-base structure of his body fluids are illustrated in Figure 11–21 (59).

For 16 days, the experimental subject was maintained on a diet that was constant with respect to protein, calories and electrolytes. Successive 24-hour urine samples were collected and analyzed for selected ionic constituents. The rates of excretion of these several constituents, expressed in milliequivalents per day, are plotted in block form. During the first 5 days, which constituted the control phase of the experiment, the subject excreted, on average, 130 mEq of chloride per day. Because the diet, like all normal mixed diets, had an acid ash residue, about 40 mEq of ammonia and 40 mEq of titratable acid were eliminated each day, to balance the acid-base budget. These quantities are plotted upward from the base line across the lower half of the figure, to indicate that they represent conservation and restoration of

cation to the body as bicarbonate. Sodium and potassium are plotted downward from the same base line, to indicate cation loss. During the control phase, the excretion of sodium averaged 125 mEq/day; of potassium, 78 mEq/day. Because the subject was in electrolyte balance, these quantities represent the quantities ingested in the diet.

During the second 5-day period, the acid load was increased sharply by the ingestion of 15 Gm of ammonium chloride per day. This constitutes an acid load equal to 290 mEq of strong acid per day. Chloride excretion increased sharply on the first day of this period. Although the excretion of titratable acid and ammonia increased moderately, the excess chloride in the urine was balanced on the first day almost entirely by sodium drawn from buffer reserves of tissues and body fluids. During the succeeding 4 days of acid ingestion, progressively less and less sodium was sacrificed to balance chloride. Instead,

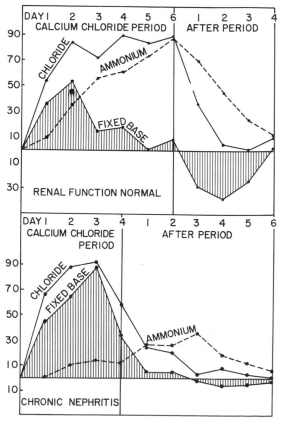

Fig. 11–22.—Comparison of the renal excretion of ions by a subject with normal renal function and by a patient with chronic nephritis during and following the imposition of an acid load in the form of calcium chloride, orally administered. Rates of excretion are plotted as increments over fore-period levels. (Adapted from Gamble, J. L.: *Chemical Anatomy, Physiology, and Pathology of Extracellular Fluid* [5th ed.; Cambridge, Mass.: Harvard University Press, 1947].)

on the second and third days, use was made of potassium, derived from cell buffer reserves. However, during the last few days, the major fraction of the acid was eliminated in combination with ammonia. In fact, this mechanism permitted the achievement of acid-base equilibrium and halted the wastage of sodium and potassium toward the end of the period of acid ingestion.

The repair of the depleted reserves of sodium and potassium is illustrated in the last 6 days of the experiment. The excretion of sodium and potassium decreased to very low levels during the first 2 days of recovery, although the dietary intake remained the same. Acid was eliminated, largely in combination with ammonia, whereas dietary sodium and potassium were retained to replenish depleted reserves. Even after 6 days, the deficit of potassium had not been restored.

Figure 11–22, taken from the work of Gamble et al. (60), illustrates the response of a normal person to a standard acid load, compared with the response of a patient with chronic nephritis. Calcium chloride was administered as the acidifying agent. In each graph, the urinary rates of excretion of chloride, cation (fixed base) and ammonia are plotted as increments over the control period levels. In both the normal and the nephritic subject, it is evident that, early in the period of acid loading, the excess urinary chloride was largely neutralized by fixed cation. However, in the normal subject, ammonia excretion increased promptly and by the sixth day was sufficient to cover the chloride load completely. Loss of cation ceased; in the succeeding recovery period, depleted cation reserves were restored promptly. In contrast, in the nephritic subject, ammonia excretion increased only moderately. Loss of cation continued at a high rate, and it was necessary to terminate the experiment on the fourth day because of severe acidosis. Recovery was slow and inadequate.

Summary

The kidney participates in the regulation of acid-base balance by stabilizing the plasma concentration of bicarbonate at a level of 26–28 mEq/L. The respiratory system participates by stabilizing the plasma concentration of carbonic acid at a level of 1.3–1.4 mEq/L. Together, the concentrations of these two components determine the pH of

Fig. 11–23.—Role of the exchange of cellular H^+ ions for Na^+ ions of tubular fluid in the reabsorption of bicarbonate and in the urinary excretion of titratable acid and ammonia (From Pitts, R. F.: Am. J. Med. 36:720, 1964.)

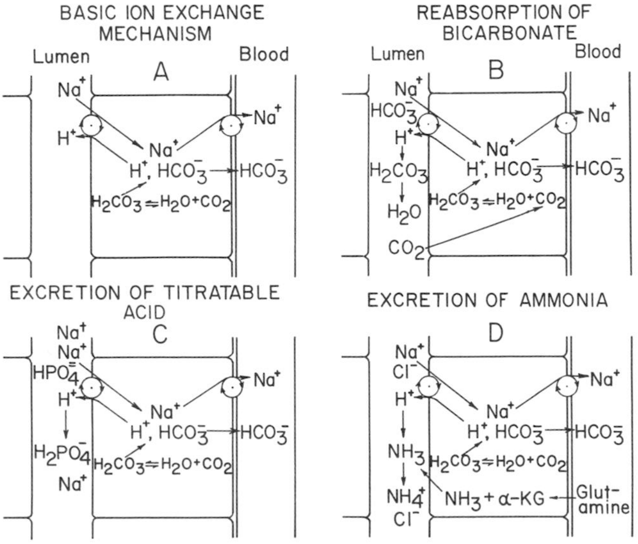

the plasma and interstitial fluid and, indirectly, that of cell contents as well.

Renal stabilization of bicarbonate involves essentially complete reabsorption of the quantities normally filtered, excretion of any excess that may gain access to the body and restoration of depleted reserves by excretion of titratable acid and ammonia (61). Evidence exists that each of these operations is carried out along the length of the nephron by processes involving ion exchange. The basic ion exchange mechanism is illustrated in Figure 11–23, A. Na^+ ions of tubular urine are exchanged for H^+ ions of tubular cells. The H^+ ions, derived within the cell from carbonic acid, are actively secreted into the urine. Na^+ ions enter tubular cells passively and are actively extruded into peritubular capillaries. Just what this mechanism accomplishes is determined by the nature of the buffer in the tubular urine at the site of exchange.

If the buffer is largely bicarbonate (Fig. 11–23, B), the exchange of H^+ ions for Na^+ ions forms carbonic acid in tubular fluid. This carbonic acid dehydrates to CO_2 and water, and the CO_2 diffuses into tubular cells. There it is hydrated to re-form carbonic acid. This cellular carbonic acid is the source of the hydrogen ions secreted into tubular urine and of the bicarbonate ions returned to peritubular blood in association with sodium ions.

Carbonic anhydrase within cells speeds the formation of carbonic acid and insures a steady supply of H^+ ions to the secretory mechanism. In the proximal tubules, where up to 90% of the filtered bicarbonate is reabsorbed, carbonic anhydrase is present within the tubular lumen attached to the brush border. Here it keeps the carbonic acid concentration low and in equilibrium with the CO_2 of tubular cells and blood. Because the carbonic acid concentration is low, the gradient against which H^+ ions must be secreted is also low, and the energy that must be expended in their secretory transport is reduced. Accordingly, the proximal tubules are specialized for the bulk reabsorption of bi-

carbonate, not for the salvage of the last remaining traces of this ion. No carbonic anhydrase is present on luminal surfaces of distal tubules and collecting ducts. Because moderately high hydrogen ion gradients must be established to reabsorb the last traces of bicarbonate and because only a minor fraction of the total filtered load enters these segments, enzyme would not be especially useful.

If the major buffer in the urine is phosphate, the exchange of H^+ ions for Na^+ ions converts the filtered dibasic phosphate to the acid monobasic form (Fig. 11–23, C). The H^+ ions are excreted as the titratable monobasic acid salt. The carbonic acid, which is the source of the cellular hydrogen ions exchanged for sodium ions, is derived in part from CO_2 produced in cellular metabolism and in part from CO_2 brought to the cell in peritubular blood. A relatively large proportion of the titratable acid formed from a buffer of high pK, such as phosphate, has its origin in the proximal segment. Only a small proportion of the titratable acid formed from a buffer of low pK, such as creatinine, β-hydroxybutyrate or acetoacetate, is formed proximally; most is formed distally, where higher hydrogen ion gradients are developed.

If little buffer is present in tubular urine, the exchange of H^+ ions for Na^+ ions ceases, for the accumulation of free unbuffered H^+ ions blocks the pump. Under such circumstances (i.e., low bicarbonate and low phosphate in tubular urine), the free-base NH_3 is formed in increased amounts, diffuses into acid urine, buffers H^+ ions, and prevents their accumulation in high concentration. Removal as NH_4^+ ions permits continued secretion of H^+ ions (Fig. 11–23, D).

When acid is liberated within the body, it is buffered by bicarbonate, CO_2 is expelled by the lungs and the concentration of bicarbonate in body fluids decreases. At first, the acid anions are excreted in the urine in association with nearly equivalent numbers of sodium ions. Later, potassium ions, derived from intracellular buffer stores, assume a greater role. Titratable acid excretion increases as more hydrogen ions are secreted to convert neutral buffer salts to their acid forms. However, the major renal response is a relatively slow adaptive increase in rate of renal production and excretion of ammonia. As ammonia excretion increases, loss of sodium and potassium decreases. Repair of the altered ionic structure of the body fluids is brought about by (1) continued excretion of titratable acid and ammonia and (2) retention of dietary cations as bicarbonate to replenish depleted stores. In chronic renal disease, the capacity to excrete titratable acid and, especially, ammonia is reduced; body stores of cation are depleted; reserves of bicarbonate and other buffers are exhausted; and acidosis and dehydration develop.

REFERENCES

1. Pitts, R. F., Ayer, J. L., and Schiess, W. A.: The renal regulation of acid base balance in man: III. The reabsorption and excretion of bicarbonate, J. Clin. Invest. 28:35, 1949.
2. Pitts, R. F., and Lotspeich, W. D.: Bicarbonate and the renal regulation of acid-base balance, Am. J. Physiol. 147:136, 1946.
3. Berliner, R. W.: Carbonic anhydrase inhibitors, Pharmacol. Rev. 8:137, 1946.
4. Pitts, R. F.: A comparison of the mode of action of certain diuretic agents, Prog. Cardiovas. Dis. 3:537, 1961.
5. Rector, F. C., Jr., Carter, N. W., and Seldin, D. W.: The mechanism of bicarbonate reabsorption in the proximal and distal tubules of the kidney, J. Clin. Invest. 44:278, 1965.
6. Walser, M., and Mudge, G. H.: Renal Excretory Mechanisms, in *Mineral Metabolism* (New York: Academic Press, Inc., 1960) Vol. 1, Pt. A, p. 287.
7. Gottschalk, C. W., Lassiter, W. E., and Mylle, M.: Localization of urine acidification in the mammalian kidney, Am. J. Physiol. 198:581, 1960.
8. Ochwadt, B. K., and Pitts, R. F.: Effects of intravenous infusion of carbonic anhydrase on carbon dioxide tension of alkaline urine, Am. J. Physiol. 185:426, 1956.
9. Pitts, R. F.: Mechanisms for stabilizing the alkaline reserves of the body, Harvey Lect. 48:172, 1952–53.
10. Rector, F. C., Jr., Seldin, D. W., Roberts, A. D., Jr., and Smith, J. S.: The role of plasma CO_2 tension and carbonic anhydrase activity in the renal reabsorption of bicarbonate, J. Clin. Invest. 39:1706, 1960.

11. Sullivan, W. J., and Dorman, P. J.: The renal response to chronic respiratory acidosis, J. Clin. Invest. 34:268, 1955.
12. Fuller, G. R., MacLeod, M. B., and Pitts, R. F.: Influence of administration of potassium salts on the renal tubular reabsorption of bicarbonate, Am. J. Physiol. 182:111, 1955.
13. Giebisch, G., MacLeod, M. B., and Pitts, R. F.: Effect of adrenal steroids on renal tubular reabsorption of bicarbonate, Am. J. Physiol. 183:377, 1955.
14. Berliner, R. W., Kennedy, T. J., Jr., and Orloff, J.: Factors affecting transport of potassium and hydrogen ions by renal tubules, Arch. internat. pharmacodyn. 97:299, 1954.
15. Rector, F. C., Jr., Bloomer, H. A., and Seldin, D. W.: Effects of potassium deficiency on the reabsorption of bicarbonate in the proximal tubule of the rat, J. Clin. Invest. 43:1976, 1964.
16. Giebisch, G., Klose, R. M., and Malnic, G.: Renal Tubular Potassium Transport, in Schreiner, G. (ed.): *Proceedings of the 3rd International Congress on Nephrology, Washington, D. C., 1966* (Basel: Karger, 1967).
17. Seldin, D. W., and Rector, F. C., Jr.: The generation and maintenance of metabolic acidosis, Kidney Internat. 1:306, 1972.
18. Rodriguez-Soriano, J., and Edelmann, C. M.: Renal tubular acidosis, Ann. Rev. Med. 20:363, 1969.
19. Morris, R. C., Sebastian, A., and McSherry, E.: Renal acidosis, Kidney Internat. 1:322, 1972.
20. Pitts, R. F.: The renal regulation of acid base balance with special reference to the mechanism for acidifying the urine, Science 102:49 and 81, 1945.
21. Pitts, R. F.: The renal excretion of acid, Fed. Proc. 7:418, 1948.
22. Pitts, R. F.: Acid base regulation by the kidneys, Am. J. Med. 9:356, 1950.
23. Smith, H. W.: *The Physiology of the Kidney* (New York: Oxford University Press, 1937).
24. Pitts, R. F., and Alexander, R. S.: The nature of the renal tubular mechanism for acidifying the urine, Am. J. Physiol. 144:239, 1945.
25. Pitts, R. F., Lotspeich, W. D., Schiess, W. A., and Ayer, J. L.: The renal regulation of acid base balance in man: I. The nature of the mechanism for acidifying the urine, J. Clin. Invest. 27:48, 1948.
26. Nash, T. P., Jr., and Benedict, S. R.: The ammonia content of the blood and its bearing on the mechanism of acid neutralization in the animal organism, J. Biol. Chem. 48:463, 1921.

27. Balagura S., and Pitts, R. F.: Excretion of ammonia injected into renal artery, Am. J. Physiol. 203:11, 1962.

28. Denis, G., Preuss, H., and Pitts, R. F.: The pNH_3 of renal tubular cells, J. Clin. Invest. 43:571, 1964.

29. Stone, W. J., Balagura, S., and Pitts, R. F.: Diffusion equilibrium for ammonia in the kidney of the acidotic dog, J. Clin. Invest. 46: 1603, 1967.

30. Oelert, H., Uhlich, E., and Hills, A. G.: Messungen des Ammoniakdruckes in den corticalen Tubuli der Rattenniere, Plüger's Arch. ges. Physiol. 300:35, 1968.

31. Sullivan, L. P., and McVaugh, M.: Effect of rapid and transitory changes in blood and urine pH on ammonia excretion, Am. J. Physiol. 204:1077, 1963.

32. Walker, A. M.: Ammonia formation in the amphibian kidney, Am. J. Physiol. 131:187, 1940.

33. Montgomery, H., and Pierce, J. A.: The site of acidification of the urine within the renal tubule in amphibia, Am. J. Physiol. 118:114, 1937.

34. Glabman, S., Klose, R., and Giebisch, G.: Micropuncture study of ammonia excretion in the rat, Am. J. Physiol. 205:127, 1963.

35. Clapp, J. R., Owen, E. E., and Robinson, R. R.: Contribution of the proximal tubule to urinary ammonia excretion by the dog, Am. J. Physiol. 209:269, 1965.

36. Pitts, R. F.: Renal production and excretion of ammonia, Am. J. Med. 36:720, 1964.

37. Van Slyke, D. D., Phillips, R. A., Hamilton P. B., Archibald, R. M., Futcher, P. H., and Hiller, A.: Glutamine as a source material of urinary ammonia, J. Biol. Chem. 150:481, 1943.

38. Shalhoub, R., Webber, W., Glabman, S., Canessa-Fischer, M., Klein, J., DeHaas, J., and Pitts, R. F.: Extraction of amino acids from and their addition to blood plasma, Am. J. Physiol. 204:181, 1963.

39. Owen, E. E., and Robinson, R. R.: Amino acid extraction and ammonia metabolism by the human kidney during the prolonged administration of ammonium chloride, J. Clin. Invest. 42:263, 1963.

40. Pitts, R. F., Pilkington, L. A., and DeHaas, J. C. M.: N^{15} tracer studies on the origin of urinary ammonia in the acidotic dog, with notes on the enzymatic synthesis of labeled glutamic acid and glutamines, J. Clin. Invest. 44: 731, 1965.

41. Lyon, M. L., and Pitts, R. F.: The glutamine synthetase system in the kidney of the rat and dog (unpublished observations).

42. Lotspeich, W. D., and Pitts, R. F.: The role of amino acids in the renal tubular secretion of ammonia, J. Biol. Chem. 168:611, 1947.

43. Kamin, H., and Handler, P.: The metabolism of parenterally administered amino acids: III. Ammonia formation, J. Biol. Chem. 193:873, 1951.

44. Pitts, R. F., and Stone, W. J.: Renal metabolism of alanine, J. Clin. Invest. 46:530, 1967.

45. Stone, W. J., and Pitts, R. F.: Pathways of ammonia metabolism in the intact functioning kidney of the dog, J. Clin. Invest. 46:1141, 1967.

46. Owen, E. E., Tyor, M. P., Flanagan, J. F., and Berry, J. N.: The kidney as a source of blood ammonia in patients with liver disease: The effects of acetazolamide, J. Clin. Invest. 39:288, 1960.

47. Davies, B. M. A., and Yudkin, J.: Studies in biochemical adaptation. The origin of urinary ammonia as indicated by the effects of chronic acidosis and alkalosis on some renal enzymes in the rat, Biochem. J. 52:407, 1952.

48. Rector, F. C., Jr., Seldin, D. W., and Copenhaver, J. H.: The mechanism of ammonia secretion during ammonium chloride acidosis, J. Clin. Invest. 34:20, 1955.

49. Rector, F. C., and Orloff, J.: Ammonia production in acidotic and alkalotic dogs, Fed. Proc. 17:129, 1958.

50. Goldstein, L.: Actinomycin D inhibition of the adaptation of renal glutamine-deaminating enzymes in the rat, Nature, London 205: 1330, 1965.

51. Goldstein, L.: Relation of glutamate to ammonia production in the rat kidney, Am. J. Physiol. 210:661, 1966.

52. Goldstein, L.: Pathways of glutamine deamination and their control in the rat kidney, Am. J. Physiol. 213:983, 1967.

53. Goodman, A. D., Fuisz, R. E., and Cahill, G. E.: Renal gluconeogenesis in acidosis, alkalosis and potassium deficiency: Its possible role in the regulation of renal ammonia production, J. Clin. Invest. 45:612, 1966.

54. Alleyne, G. A. O., and Scullard, G.: Renal metabolic response to acid base changes. I. Enzymatic control of ammonia-genesis in the rat, J. Clin. Invest. 48:364, 1969.

55. Pitts, R. F., Pilkington, L. A., Leal-Pinto, E., and MacLeod, M. B.: Metabolism of glutamine by the intact functioning kidney of the dog, J. Clin. Invest. 51:557, 1972.

56. Pitts, R. F.: Control of renal production of ammonia, Kidney Internat. 1:297, 1972.

57. Addae, S. K., and Lotspeich, W. D.: Relation between glutamine utilization and production in metabolic acidosis, Am. J. Physiol. 215: 269, 1968.

58. Hills, A. G., Reid, E. L., and Kerr, W. D.:

Circulatory transport of L-glutamine in fasted mammals: Cellular sources of urine ammonia, Am. J. Physiol. 223:1470, 1972.

59. Sartorius, O. W., Roemmelt, J. C., and Pitts, R. F.: The renal regulation of acid base balance in man: IV. The nature of the renal compensations in ammonium chloride acido-

sis, J. Clin. Invest. 28:423, 1949.

60. Gamble, J. L., Blackfan, K. D., and Hamilton, B.: The diuretic action of acid producing salts, J. Clin. Invest. 1:403, 1925.

61. Pitts, R. F.: The role of ammonia production and excretion in regulation of acid-base balance, New Engl. J. Med. 284:32, 1971.

12

Regulation of Volume and Osmolar Concentration of Extracellular Fluid

THE BODY WEIGHT of a normal adult in caloric balance is remarkably stable from day to day and relatively independent of intake of salt and water. Stability of weight implies constancy of volume of body fluid—more specifically, of extracellular fluid. The osmolar concentration of extracellular fluid is even more stable, although this fact is less generally appreciated than is constancy of body weight.

The volume of the extracellular compartment is primarily dependent on its sodium content. Gain of sodium induces thirst, and an osmotically equivalent volume of water is retained. Sodium and water are gradually excreted, and volume is restored to normal. Loss of sodium induces the excretion of solute-free water, restoring osmolarity. However, if extracellular volume is seriously compromised by the excretion of water, restoration of normal osmolar concentration is incomplete.

The osmolarity of extracellular fluid depends primarily on water content. Gain of water induces prompt water diuresis; loss of water induces thirst and antidiuresis.

The volume of extracellular fluid is regulated by control of the excretion of both sodium and water. Osmolarity of extracellular fluid, on the other hand, is regulated almost entirely by control of the excretion of water (1, 2, 3). Appetite for salt* and thirst are integral parts of both regulatory mechanisms, because deficits of sodium and water cannot be corrected merely by renal conservation.

Regulation of Extracellular Volume

A function so crucial to existence as the maintenance of volume of extracellular fluid no doubt depends on several interrelated mechanisms of control. However, their nature and even their numbers have not been adequately defined, and no general agreement exists as to the relative significance of the several mechanisms that have been described (3). Volume regulation involves receptors that sense errors in volume, neural and humoral mechanisms that apprise the kidney of those errors and renal mechanisms by which the kidneys compensate for them.

VOLUME RECEPTORS

Volume receptors presumably are sensitive to extracellular volume; to some fraction of that volume, such as plasma or interstitial fluid; to some derivative of volume, such as intravascular or interstitial pressure or distention; or to blood flow. According to Viar et al. (4) and Strauss (5), the receptor mechanism is located in the cephalad portion of

---

*Salt intake in man is conditioned to a greater degree by dietary habit than by appetite for salt. Except under conditions of rigid restriction, the intake of salt is more than adequate to supply normal requirements.

the body and is directly sensitive either to extracellular volume or to venous pressure or distention. Epstein (6), on the other hand, suggested that the receptor mechanism is in the arterial reservoir and that the degree of distention of this reservoir generally, or of some highly sensitive portion of it, initiates the afferent messages that ultimately modulate salt and water excretion. Bartter and Gann (7) adopted the view that the junction of the thyroid and carotid arteries is a baroreceptor organ specifically concerned with the control of salt excretion. Gauer *et al.* (8) suggested that the degree of distention of the left atrium governs water excretion through the antidiuretic mechanism of the posterior pituitary, whereas the degree of distention of the right atrium governs the excretion of sodium through its control of adrenocortical secretion of aldosterone. Borst (9), in contrast, maintained that the receptor mechanism (site unspecified) is sensitive to cardiac output or perhaps to cardiac output relative to the metabolic demands of the body. Davis (10) and others suggested that the juxtaglomerular apparatus of afferent renal arterioles is either flow- or pressure-sensitive and, through secretion of renin with subsequent formation of circulating angiotensin, directly controls the output of aldosterone and, therefore, sodium reabsorption. One may summarize these views in the following terms: Changes in extracellular volume are sensed as changes in pressure or distention of the interstitial, venous or arterial reservoirs or as changes in blood flow. Although some investigators believe that a single type of receptor responsive to a single stimulus activates mechanisms of volume control, the author subscribes to the concept that several types of receptors responsive to as many stimuli probably activate a number of effector mechanisms and provide defense in depth.

STIMULI AFFECTING VOLUME RECEPTORS. — Water diuresis unrelated to change in osmolarity of the body fluids is induced by the assumption of supine posture, by negative-pressure breathing, by mechanical distension of the left atrium and by the infusion of large volumes of isotonic saline solution or iso-oncotic albumin. The presumed stimuli are, respectively, venous distention in cephalad parts of the body, distention of thoracic blood reservoirs (more specifically the left atrium) and either increase in pressure in baroreceptor areas of the arterial tree or increase in cardiac output. Each of these stimuli might have its origin in an increase in extracellular volume, although, of the conditions outlined, only the infusion of saline solution and albumin produce an actual increase in volume. The excretion of water is compensatory, in that it reduces extracellular volume. However, unless accompanied by the excretion of sodium, loss of water is limited by increasing osmolarity of the body fluids.

Antidiuresis unrelated to change in osmolarity of the body fluids is induced by the assumption of erect posture, by positive-pressure breathing, by hemorrhage and by the trapping of blood in the extremities by venous tourniquets. The presumed stimuli are the reverse of those detailed in the preceding paragraph. Each might arise in consequence of a reduction in extracellular volume, although, of the conditions outlined, only hemorrhage results in an actual decrease.

Conservation of sodium to the extent of virtually complete reabsorption of this ion from the urine results from hemorrhage, the trapping of blood in the extremities by venous tourniquets, interference with venous return by the inflation of a balloon catheter in the vena cava and the assumption of erect posture. Reduced venous or atrial distention (more specifically, that of the right atrium), reduced baroreceptor activity and reduced blood flow or cardiac output have all been claimed as stimuli initiating sodium conservation. Each might arise in consequence of a reduction in extracellular volume.

Enhanced sodium excretion (natriuresis), on the other hand, is readily induced only by the expansion of extracellular stores of sodium. Because the infusion of hypo-, iso-, or hypertonic saline solution results in sodium diuresis, the concentration of sodium in extracellular fluid is not the prime factor. Moderate natriuresis results from the assumption of supine posture, but this seems to be nothing more than inhibition of the antinatriuresis of the antecedent erect posture.

The procedures of standing erect and of blocking the return of blood by venous tourniquets or a balloon catheter suggest that an abnormal distribution of extracellular fluid, no less than an actual reduction in volume, may be a significant stimulus to fluid and sodium conservation. However, all the conditions mentioned affect cardiac output; thus, one cannot claim to have distinguished among the several possible factors.

Renal Effector Mechanisms

Renal mechanisms that compensate for errors in volume include those concerned with the excretion and conservation of water and those concerned with the excretion and conservation of sodium. The former will be dealt with in the next section, in relation to the control of osmolarity; the latter concern us here.

Three mechanisms for the precise regulation of sodium excretion have been proposed: (1) hemodynamic alterations in the sodium load presented to the renal tubules, (2) changes in the distribution of filtrate among nephrons of varying reabsorptive capacities and (3) control of completeness of tubular reabsorption of sodium by variations in the rate of secretion of aldosterone by the adrenal cortex.

HEMODYNAMIC MECHANISMS. — Well over a decade ago, Warren, Stead, Merrill, Mokotoff and others observed that renal blood flow and glomerular filtration rate are frequently reduced in patients in severe congestive heart failure who are retaining sodium and becoming edematous. Most of their patients with filtration rates of less than 70 ml/min were frankly edematous; those with filtration rates approaching normal were not. The above-named investigators concluded that reduction in filtration rate without equivalent reduction in tubular reabsorptive capacity leads to retention of salt and water and to an abnormal expansion of extracellular fluid volume. Although it is now generally recognized that a reduction in filtered load is by no means a complete explanation of sodium retention in edematous patients, variations in filtration rate play some role in the control of extracellular volume.

Figure 12 – 1 illustrates the very dramatic changes in sodium excretion caused by acute changes in filtration rate (11). A balloon catheter was introduced into the femoral artery of a dog and positioned in the aorta above the origins of the renal arteries. By varying the degree of distention of the balloon, the renal arterial pressure could be reduced to and stabilized at any desired value. Prior to and during the experiment, isotonic saline solution was administered intravenously at a rate of 10 ml/min, in order to expand the extracellular volume and induce sodium excretion. The reduction of renal arterial pressure from 150 to 90 mm Hg reduced the filtration rate to a minor degree: from 77 to 70 ml/min. However, this 10% reduction in filtration rate was associated with a 50% reduction in urine flow and sodium excretion. Inflation of the balloon a second time, reducing the renal arterial pressure to 70 mm Hg, caused a further decline in the filtration rate and the sodium excretion. Inflation a third time reduced the filtration rate by half (i.e., to 40 ml/min), and the excretion of sodium virtually ceased. Similar results were obtained in adrenalectomized dogs, in dogs with diabetes insipidus induced by section of the pituitary stalk and in animals with denervated kidneys; therefore, it is evident that the reabsorption of an excessive fraction of the filtered sodium is independent of neural and hormonal factors and must be related to a reduction in filtered load.

No precise definition of the relationship between filtered load and tubular reabsorption is possible at present. As was pointed out in Chapter 7, some two thirds to seven eighths of filtered sodium is reabsorbed in the proximal segment of the renal tubule. If

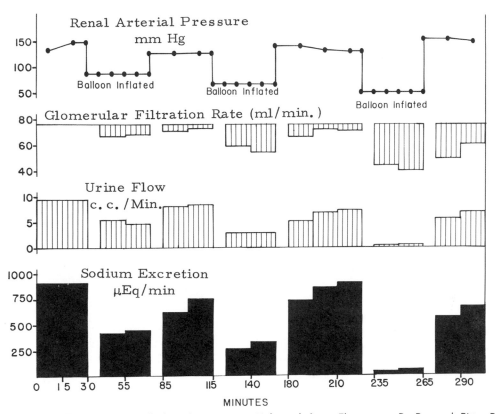

Fig. 12—1. — Effects of controlled reduction of renal arterial pressure in the dog on glomerular filtration rate, urine flow and sodium excretion.

(Adapted from Thompson, D. D., and Pitts, R. F.: Am. J. Physiol. 168:490, 1952.)

the filtration rate increases, the absolute amount of sodium reabsorbed in the proximal segment increases; if the filtration rate decreases, the absolute amount of sodium reabsorbed decreases. However, of more immediate significance is the fact that an increase in the filtration rate results in the delivery of more sodium into distal parts of the nephron, and a decrease in the filtration rate results in the delivery of less sodium. If, as seems probable, the reabsorptive capacity of the distal nephron is limited, the rate of excretion of sodium will vary as some nonlinear function of the filtration rate. When the filtration rate increases, the one third to one eighth of the filtered load that escapes reabsorption in the proximal segment will exceed the reabsorptive capacity of the distal nephron, and sodium will be excreted. When the filtration rate is reduced, the one third to one eighth of the filtered load presented to the distal nephron will be less than its reabsorptive capacity, and sodium will be more or less completely reabsorbed.

MECHANISM OF REDISTRIBUTION OF FILTRATE. — Goodyer and Jaeger (12) proposed that certain rapid alterations in sodium excretion in the absence of significant changes* in glomerular filtration rate could be effected by a shift in activity between long, salt-conserving nephrons and short, salt-wasting nephrons. The over-all rate of glomerular

---

*One of the major difficulties in studies on the control of sodium excretion is that of deciding whether or not a significant change in filtration rate has occurred. The error of measurement of filtration rate is at least ±2% in consecutive clearance periods. Alterations in sodium excretion associated with volume regulation are usually less than 2% of the filtered load. It is evident that the variable that one wishes to measure is less than the graduations on the ruler one uses in measurement.

filtration might remain unchanged. Unfortunately, there is no evidence bearing directly on this thesis, so it remains merely an interesting speculation.

HORMONAL MECHANISM. — Since the demonstration by Loeb and Harrop of the abnormalities in renal tubular reabsorption of ions by adrenalectomized animals, a tremendous volume of evidence has accumulated in favor of the views that adrenal salt-retaining steroids are involved in the fine control of sodium balance. One must recognize that adrenal hormones affect the renal tubular reabsorption of a very small, albeit highly significant, fraction of the filtered sodium. However, the bulk of sodium reabsorption is independent of hormonal control. Figure 12–2 illustrates the time course and order of magnitude of steroidal stimulation of sodium reabsorption (13). The experiment was performed on an adrenalectomized dog maintained some 4 days without steroids and on a high-sodium, low-potassium regimen. During the three control clearance periods, 70–80 μEq of sodium per minute were excreted in the urine. As shown at the bottom of the graph, this represented a failure to reabsorb only 2% of the filtered sodium; i.e., reabsorption was 98% complete. However, this minor defect in sodium reabsorption is highly significant. Maintained over a period of several days and in the absence of adequate replacement, the defect would result in serious, perhaps fatal, depletion of extracellular reserves of salt and water. At the break in the graph, 20 ml of whole adrenocortical extract* was administered intravenously. After a lag

---

*This experiment was performed years ago, before aldosterone was discovered. More recently, a similar stimulation of sodium reabsorption by aldosterone was demonstrated. The lag phase is of similar duration. It is, therefore, possible that the effects of whole adrenocortical extract on sodium reabsorption shown in Figure 12–2 were due to its content of aldosterone. This experiment is particularly appropriate, because essentially complete sodium reabsorption occurred, despite an increase in filtration rate and in filtrated sodium load.

Fig. 12–2. — Effects of intravenous administration of whole adrenocortical extract on glomerular filtration rate and reabsorption and excretion of sodium in the adrenalectomized dog. (Adapted from Roemmelt, J. C., Sartorius, O. W., and Pitts, R. F.: Am. J. Physiol. 159:124, 1949.)

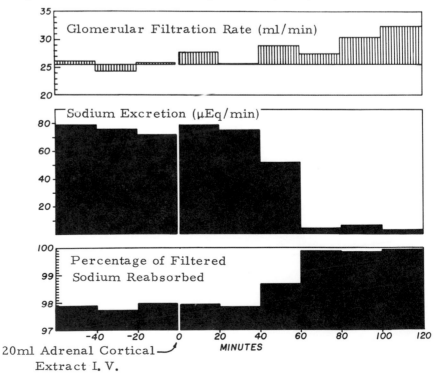

20ml Adrenal Cortical
Extract I. V.

phase of 40 minutes, sodium reabsorption increased, becoming 99.9% complete, and sodium excretion decreased essentially to zero.

Hemorrhage, erect posture, severe restriction of salt intake, partial constriction of the vena cava and other circumstances that presumably stimulate volume receptors and initiate salt conservation cause the secretion of increased quantities of aldosterone. Increased tubular reabsorption and retention of ingested sodium is compensatory and, over a period of time, restores extracellular reserves. In contrast, high salt intake, which expands extracellular volume, reduces the secretion of aldosterone. Renal tubular reabsorption is less complete, and increased excretion restores extracellular sodium to normal.

Two facts make it difficult to explain compensatory salt retention in response to an actual or apparent reduction in extracellular volume entirely in terms of increased secretion of aldosterone. First, increased reabsorption of sodium in response to erect posture, bleeding or trapping of blood in the limbs is prompt: the adrenal steroids, given intravenously, stimulate sodium reabsorption after a lag phase of 40–60 minutes. Second, adrenalectomized patients and patients with Addison's disease, on maintenance doses of adrenal steroids, increase sodium reabsorption in a normal manner in response to bleeding, assumption of erect posture and compression of the thighs. Control of sodium reabsorption by alterations in the rate of aldosterone secretion seems suited to the day-to-day balancing of sodium intake and output. Control of sodium reabsorption by alterations in the rate of glomerular filtration and by redistribution of filtrate among nephrons seems better suited to acute compensation of volume depletion and expansion.

CELLULAR ACTION OF ALDOSTERONE. — Concepts of the cellular action of aldosterone are largely based on studies on the toad bladder, a bilobed sac composed of a single layer of epithelial cells supported externally by a loose framework of smooth muscle, collagen fibers and capillaries. In life, bladder urine is hypotonic and serves as a reservoir for both sodium and water. Crabbé was the first to demonstrate the response of the bladder epithelium to aldosterone: an increase in active transport of sodium from bladder contents to body fluids. If the bladder is isolated, opened and mounted between two chambers filled with isotonic saline solution, a potential difference develops across the membrane — negative on the mucosal or urinary side, positive on the serosal or body fluid side. The application of an equal and opposite potential difference short-circuits the membrane, and the current flow becomes a measure of the active transport of sodium. The addition of aldosterone within concentration limits of 3.3×10^{-10} M and 10^{-7} M to the bathing medium increases the active transport of sodium from the mucosal to the serosal surface in a dose-dependent fashion, without affecting the small passive flux in the reverse direction. Like the kidney, the lag phase of the increase in transport of sodium by the bladder varies from 40 to 120 minutes.

Edelman (14) proposed that aldosterone stimulates sodium transport by interacting with a nuclear receptor to enhance the DNA-directed synthesis of RNA, which codes a specific protein. This protein may serve one of three functions: (1) to control entry of sodium into the mucosal epithelium from the urinary side, (2) to act as the ion carrier of the sodium pump or (3) to regulate the production of ATP enzymatically and thus control the energy supply on which transport depends.

Enhancement of transport of sodium by aldosterone depends on the presence in the medium of specific metabolic substrates, including glucose, oxaloacetate, pyruvate, acetoacetate, and β-hydroxybutyrate. When the steroid is added in the presence of substrate, enhanced sodium transport (i.e., enhanced short-circuit current) begins after an hour or so and increases linearly for 5 hours or more. When the bladder is exposed briefly to steroid and then washed thoroughly to remove excess hormone, no enhancement of transport occurs. If, after several hours, specific substrates are added, enhanced transport occurs at once and without latency. Actinomycin D, which blocks protein synthesis by interfering with DNA-mediated synthesis of messenger RNA, and puromycin, which prevents assembly of amino acids on ribosomes, both block the aldosterone-induced stimulation of sodium transport. These several facts, plus the autoradiographic localization of labeled aldosterone to nuclei of mucosal cells, suggest that aldosterone stimulates sodium transport indirectly by inducing protein synthesis. Further evidence of Edelman (15) suggests that the protein either enhances enzymatic steps between condensing enzyme and α-ketoglutarate dehydrogenase or alters activity of mitochondrial NADH dehydrogenases.

According to Sharp et al. (16) and Sharp and Leaf (17), sodium enters the mucosal epithelium from the urinary side passively and is extruded actively across the basal or serosal side. An increase in cell sodium increases both the rate of sodium transport and the rate of the aerobic metabolism required to drive it. Thus, enzymes involved in energy production are not altered. Amphotericin B and antidiuretic hormone increase sodium transport in a manner analogous to that of the steroid-induced protein, but without delay, by increasing the permeability of the apical surface of the cell to sodium. According to their views, the protein induced by aldosterone is a permease that also acts on the apical surface of the cell.

MECHANISMS BY WHICH RECEPTORS APPRISE THE KIDNEY OF VOLUME ERRORS

In view of the controversy concerning the nature and locus of volume receptors and the significance of the several renal effector mechanisms that control salt and water excretion, it is not surprising that no general agreement exists as to the linkage of the two. If, as seems probable, a number of receptor organs participate in volume regulation, it is highly likely that some portion of the nervous system plays an integrative role. Most investigators place the integrative mechanism in the diencephalon.

CONTROL OF ALDOSTERONE SECRETION. — Aldosterone is secreted by the zona glomerulosa of the adrenal cortex. This portion of the gland retains its functional integrity in hypophysectomized animals and, therefore, is not obligatorily dependent on the presence of pituitary adrenocorticotropic hormone (ACTH). Furthermore, hypophysectomized animals do not exhibit the severe disturbances of electrolyte composition and volume of the body fluids that are characteristic of adrenalectomized animals. Finally, hypophysectomized animals increase their secretion of aldosterone in response to volume depletion much as do normal animals. Although ACTH is known to stimulate aldosterone secretion, alternative mechanisms of control exist. These are probably not directly neural in character, because denervation of the adrenal glands does not alter the nature of the responses.

Bartter and Gann (7) suggest that pulse pressure within the junctions of the thyroid and carotid arteries initiates impulses that are conducted centrally over the vagus nerves and modulate the activity of the integrative center. A decrease in pulse pressure stimulates secretion of aldosterone; an increase in pulse pressure inhibits secretion of aldosterone. Gauer, et al. (8) suggested that the activity of the integrative center is also controlled by the degree of distention of the right atrium. Reduced distention increases aldosterone secretion; increased distention inhibits aldosterone secretion. Other receptors sensitive to volume or flow presumably also deliver regulatory impulses to the integrative center.

Control of aldosterone secretion by the integrative center presumably involves one or more of the following mechanisms:

1. Impulses delivered over the hypothalamic-hypophysial tracts cause the liberation of antidiuretic hormone (ADH) from the median eminence. ADH passes into the portal system supplying the adenohypophysis

and stimulates the secretion of ACTH (18). The latter hormone, in turn, activates the zona glomerulosa of the adrenal cortex and increases the output of aldosterone.

2. ADH (arginine vasopressin), acting directly on the adrenal glands, stimulates the secretion of hydrocortisone and aldosterone (19).

3. Impulses to a presumed diencephalic or pineal neurosecretory system liberate adrenoglomerulotropin, which stimulates the secretion of aldosterone (20).

4. Impulses to sympathetic centers of vascular control are relayed to the kidney and cause vasoconstriction of afferent arterioles. Renin is liberated, and the angiotensin formed in peripheral blood stimulates the secretion of aldosterone (10).

5. Sympathomimetic hormones, liberated from the adrenal medulla, cause the release of ACTH and the stimulation of aldosterone secretion.

The relative significance, or even the existence, of some of these mechanisms has not been definitely established. However, the fact remains that secretion of aldosterone is increased by volume depletion and reduced by volume expansion.

CONTROL OF ANTIDIURETIC HORMONE SECRETION. — Control of the secretion of ADH is undoubtedly mediated over the hypothalamic-hypophysial tracts terminating in the posterior lobe of the pituitary. Volume control is obviously independent of osmoreceptor activity. However, it is well recognized that the ADH system is activated by pain, fear, apprehension and loud sounds and by a variety of centrally acting pharmacologic agents. Impulses from a central integrative mechanism of volume control presumably activate the antidiuretic system as well. According to Gauer et al. (8), the ADH mechanism is especially responsive to impulses arising in stretch receptors of the left atrium and conducted centrally over the vagus nerves. Distention inhibits ADH secretion and results in water diuresis; reduced distention stimulates ADH secretion and results in thirst and antidiuresis.

CONTROL OF GLOMERULAR FILTRATION RATE AND THE DISTRIBUTION OF FILTRATE AMONG NEPHRONS. — Control of the glomerular filtration rate (GFR) and distribution of filtrate among nephrons of varying reabsorptive capacity are probably mediated through sympathetic nerve impulses that control afferent renal arteriolar resistance. Sympathomimetic hormones from the adrenal medulla exert a similar control.

RESPONSE TO SALT DEPLETION AND SALT LOADING. — Normal man tolerates variations in salt intake within a range of 2 – 10 Gm/day with minimal changes in body weight. If the intake is reduced to a few hundred milligrams per day, excretion exceeds the intake for several days and body weight decreases by 1 – 2 kg. Eventually, balance is restored, excretion equaling intake. The GFR may be moderately reduced, and the filtered load of sodium correspondingly diminished. Aldosterone secretion is increased, and sodium is more completely reabsorbed from the tubular urine. Both factors no doubt play some role in the reestablishment of balance on reduced intake.

On the other hand, if some 30 – 40 Gm of sodium chloride are added to the diet each day, body weight increases promptly and stabilizes at a value some 2 – 5 kg or more above normal. The GFR may or may not increase significantly. At best, the increase is small. Aldosterone secretion is reduced, and salt excretion increases until it comes into balance with salt intake. Body weight remains elevated.

In contrast, the volume-receptor – renal-effector mechanism of the dog responds more briskly and more effectively to both salt restriction and salt loading than does that of man. Ladd and Raiz showed that the dog can tolerate as much as 4 Gm of sodium chloride per kilogram per day, drinking copiously after each meal to maintain osmolarity of body fluids and excreting the water and salt in the intervals between meals. Such levels of salt intake correspond to a load of 280 – 300 Gm/day in man — a value far in excess of any that can be tolerated. Although aldosterone secretion is suppressed, the major factor accounting for the dog's high tolerance of sodium is lability of the GFR. Green, Farah, Wesson, Mudge and others have shown that salt loading increases the GFR in the dog as much as 100%. Up to 40% of the filtered load of sodium may be excreted in the urine.

Regulation of Osmolar Concentration of Extracellular Fluid

The osmotic concentration of extracellular fluid of man is maintained within limits of 283 ± 11 mOsm/L, primarily by regulation of the intake and the excretion of water. When the body fluids are diluted by the ingestion of solute-free water, diuresis of hypotonic urine rapidly restores the osmolar concentration of the body fluids to normal. When the body fluids are concentrated by loss of water, oliguria restricts further loss, the elaboration of hypertonic urine permits the excretion of osmotically active solutes without loss of equivalent amounts of water, and thirst drives the person to restore his water deficit. The regulatory mechanism consists of osmoreceptors, which sense the osmolar concentration of the extracellular fluid; a central integrative mechanism; a neurosecretory mechanism, which produces ADH; and a renal effector mechanism, which governs the excretion of water. Regulation of osmolarity is far more clearly defined and understood than is regulation of volume.

OSMOLAR AND WATER CLEARANCE

The major osmotically active constituents of urine are sodium and chloride ions and urea. A person on the usual mixed diet excretes these solutes in amounts of $0.5 - 1$ mOsm/min. The osmolar clearance may be calculated as follows: where U_{Osm} and P_{Osm} represent the osmolarities,

$$C_{Osm} = U_{Osm} \cdot V/P_{Osm}$$

of urine and plasma, respectively, in mil-

liosmoles per milliliter. The osmolar clearance is defined as the milliliters per minute of plasma completely cleared of osmotically active solutes. Customarily, U_{Osm} and P_{Osm} are measured by cryoscopic methods (i.e., by freezing-point depression), and accordingly include the contributions of both electrolytes and nonelectrolytes. The osmolar clearance of the normal fasting person is $2 - 3$ ml/min and is more or less independent of urine flow.

When fluid is restricted, the normal human kidney can elaborate urine some $4 - 5$ times as concentrated as blood plasma. Under such conditions, urine flow may amount to 0.5 ml/min, and

$$C_{Osm} = \frac{1.400 \text{ mOsm/ml} \cdot 0.5 \text{ ml/min}}{0.300 \text{ mOsm/ml}} = 2.33 \text{ ml/min}$$

If a liter or more of water is ingested, urine flow may increase to as much as 20 ml/min, and urine osmolar concentration may decrease to about 0.1 that of plasma; i.e., to 0.035 mOsm/ml.

$$C_{Osm} = \frac{0.035 \text{ mOsm/ml} \cdot 20 \text{ ml/min}}{0.300 \text{ mOsm/ml}} = 2.33 \text{ ml/min}$$

Free-water clearance, C_{H_2O}, is calculated as the difference between the urine flow and the osmolar clearance:

$$C_{H_2O} = V - C_{Osm}$$

In hydropenia, the free-water clearance is negative; and, in the example given above,

$$C_{H_2O} = 0.5 \text{ ml/min} - 2.33 \text{ ml/min} = -1.83 \text{ ml/min}$$

The term "free water" refers to the fact that it is solute-free; and negativity of clearance indicates that the free water is reabsorbed, not excreted. In essence, the excretion of the osmotically active components of 2.33 ml of blood plasma in 0.5 ml of concentrated urine restores to the body 1.83 ml of pure water, to dilute the body fluids.

In water diuresis, the free-water clearance is positive; and, in the example given above,

$$C_{H_2O} = 20 \text{ ml/min} - 2.33 \text{ ml/min} = 17.7 \text{ ml/min}$$

The excretion of the osmotically active components of 2.33 ml of blood plasma in 20 ml of hypotonic urine removes from the body 17.7 ml of pure water, to concentrate the body fluids. It is evident, from these considerations, that the kidney is far more effective in defending the body against dilution than against dehydration. Ultimately, thirst must drive the individual to replace water deficits; the kidney cannot replace them. The elimination or conservation of free water constitutes the means by which the kidneys regulate the osmolarity of the body fluids. These functions are localized in the loops of Henle, the distal convoluted tubules and the collecting ducts.

OSMORECEPTORS

Osmoreceptors are positioned within the zones of distribution of the internal carotid arteries. Verney (21) suggested that they are represented by vesicles in the supraoptic nuclei, which act as tiny osmometers, swelling when their surroundings become hypotonic and shrinking when they become hypertonic. Shrinkage is presumed to stimulate processes of neurons of the supraoptic nuclei, which are applied to their surfaces. Impulses generated in these neurons and conducted over the supraoptic-hypophysial tracts to terminations in the median eminence and neural lobe of the posterior pituitary cause the liberation of ADH. Antidiuresis results. Swelling of vesicles inhibits supraoptic neurons, liberation of hormone ceases and the circulating hormone is rapidly cleared from the blood stream. Water diuresis ensues. The rate of liberation of hormone and urine flow are precisely graded by the osmolarity of the body fluids.

Verney and his colleagues have shown that the injection of minute amounts of hypertonic solutions of sodium chloride into carotid loops of trained, unanesthetized dogs promptly inhibits water diuresis and induces oliguria of hypertonic urine (21, 22). The required dose is small — of such magnitude as to increase the osmotic pressure of carotid blood by only 2%. The same dose injected into a peripheral vein and diluted by distribution in the plasma and extracellular fluid of the whole body has no effect on urine flow.

The injection into a carotid loop of an osmotically equivalent dose of urea, to which the receptors are freely permeable, also has no effect on urine flow. Urea exerts no osmotic effect across vesicle membranes freely permeable to it; accordingly, urea does not stimulate osmoreceptors and does not cause liberation of antidiuretic hormone.

INTEGRATIVE MECHANISM

Antidiuretic hormone is liberated not only in response to an increase in osmotic pressure of the body fluids but also in response to painful stimuli, fear, apprehension, syncope, exercise and smoking. A variety of drugs, including anesthetics (especially ether, morphine and barbiturates), nicotine, adenosine triphosphate (ATP), acetylcholine, epinephrine and histamine, are potent stimulators of ADH secretion. As pointed out earlier, conditions that reduce extracellular volume or which shift fluid from central venous reservoirs to periphery also increase the liberation of ADH. All of these diverse stimuli result in oliguria. On the other hand, the release of ADH is suppressed, and diuresis results, not only in response to the dilution of the body fluids but also in response to the suggestion of water drinking under hypnosis, the development of conditioned reflex diuresis, the ingestion of alcohol and a variety of procedures that expand extracellular volume or increase distention of central venous reservoirs, more specifically the left atrium.

The fact that a variety of stimuli excite and inhibit secretion of ADH implies a central mechanism that receives afferent fibers from many sources, integrates the information transmitted over these pathways and either inhibits or stimulates hormone secretion. Furthermore, the integration of the adrenocortical secretion of aldosterone and of renal vasomotor responses with ADH secretion in the control of extracellular volume implies a central coordinating mechanism. Its location has not been determined, although it is reasonable to infer a hypothalamic site.

RENAL EFFECTOR MECHANISMS

These mechanisms have been discussed in Chapter 7. Antidiuretic hormone exerts three actions on the renal tubule: (*1*) it controls the permeability of distal convoluted tubules and collecting ducts to water, (*2*) it may stimulate the pumping of sodium by the loops of Henle and (*3*) it probably regulates the rate of blood perfusion of medulla and papilla. An increased titer of ADH in circulating blood plasma increases the permeability of the distal tubules to water. Hypotonic fluid entering the distal segments from the loops of Henle rapidly becomes isosmotic with cortical blood plasma. A small volume of isotonic urine (3–7 ml/min) enters the collecting ducts. Water diffuses into the hypertonic medullary and papillary interstitium, and the final urine is reduced in volume and comes into osmotic equilibrium with the interstitial fluid of the tip of the papilla. In the absence of ADH, the hypotonic urine that enters the distal nephron in large volume is further diluted by the reabsorption of solutes in the distal tubules and collecting ducts. Water diuresis ensues. There is some evidence that the hypertonicity of the medullary interstitium is greater in the presence of a high titer of circulating ADH, owing to enhanced pumping of sodium by Henle's loops and to reduced blood flow in the vasa recta. Reduction of blood flow reduces the rate of dissipation of the medullary and papillary osmotic gradient.

OSMOLAR REGULATORY MECHANISM

The operation of the osmolar regulatory mechanism is illustrated in Figure 12–3. If a person drinks 1 L or more of water rapidly, the osmolar concentration of the blood plasma and interstitial fluid begins to decrease at once and reaches a minimum in 30–60 minutes. Reduction of osmolarity is the consequence not only of absorption of water but also of the diffusion of ions into the fluid in the intestine. Urine flow begins to increase within 15–30 minutes and reaches its peak some 15–30 minutes after the minimum of osmolarity of the body fluids. Rapid elimination of a large volume of osmotically dilute urine restores the concentration of the body fluids to normal, and diuresis diminishes (24, 25). The maximum dilution of the body fluids following the ingestion of 1,200 ml of water is 2–3%.

If the subject rapidly ingests the same volume of isotonic saline solution, no dilution of the body fluids occurs, and the diuresis which ensues is moderate and greatly prolonged. A liter of pure water is eliminated in 2–3 hours; a liter of saline solution, in 12–24 hours.

The delay in the onset of diuresis and the

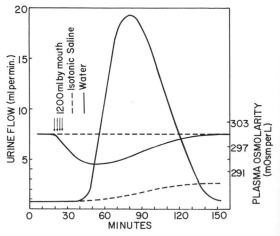

Fig. 12–3. — Relationship of diuresis to dilution of body fluids following the oral ingestion of 1,200 ml of water and of a similar volume of isotonic saline.

displacement of the peak of diuresis relative to dilution of the body fluids are related to the rate of destruction of the circulating ADH. In both the rat and the dog, the liver and kidneys are the major sites of destruction of the circulating ADH. Destruction is much more rapid in the rat than in the dog or man (26).

RATE OF ANTIDIURETIC HORMONE SECRETION

If a person ingests about 2% of his body weight of water and thereafter at intervals takes an amount equivalent to the volume of urine excreted, he achieves and maintains a state of marked overhydration. Urine flow increases to 15–25 ml/min; i.e., to a level that is maximal for that person and that can-

not be increased by more vigorous hydration. Secretion of ADH is completely suppressed; a state of physiologic diabetes insipidus is induced.

Figure 12–4 illustrates the effect of infusion of pitressin in a person so hydrated. It is apparent that the urine flow decreased sharply and the creatinine U/P ratio increased promptly when pitressin was infused at a rate of 7.5 milliunits (mU) per hour. The creatinine U/P concentration ratio is a more sensitive indicator of water conservation at low flows than is urine flow itself. Although absolute changes in urine flow were less striking at higher rates of pitressin infusion, it is evident from the creatinine U/P ratios that graded responses are obtained at infusion rates up to 50 mU/hr. According to Lauson (27), normal man regulates urine flow over

Fig. 12–4. — Effects of the infusion of pitressin on urine flow and on urine/plasma concentration ratios of creatinine in a normal hydrated subject. (Adapted from Lauson, H. D.: Am. J. Med. 11:135, 1951.)

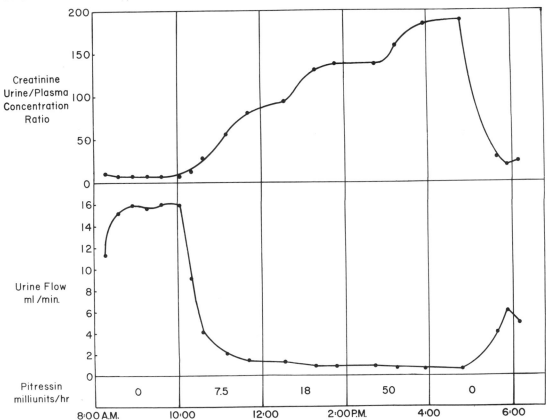

the physiologic range by secreting ADH at rates of 0.1–0.8 mU/kg per hour. Shannon and Verney found that comparable rates of secretion of ADH control urine flow in the dog.

NATURE OF ANTIDIURETIC HORMONE

DuVigneaud synthesized two antidiuretic hormones, derived respectively from beef and hog pituitaries. These are known as arginine vasopressin and lysine vasopressin. Both are octapeptides and consist of a five-membered ring made up of tyrosine, phenylalanine, glutamine, asparagine and cystine and a three-membered side chain made up of proline, either arginine or lysine, and glycinamide. In the structures given below, two molecules of cysteine are joined in disulfide linkage to form a closed ring; i.e., a ring containing one molecule of cystine.

The ring of oxytocin differs from that of vasopressin only in the substitution of isoleucine for phenylalanine. In the fish, the neurohypophysial hormone is also arginine vasotocin, but the hormone is diuretic rather than antidiuretic (28).

NEUROSECRETORY MECHANISM. — Sharrer first proposed that ADH is formed in cells of the supraoptic and paraventricular nuclei and transported to the posterior lobe of the pituitary by protoplasmic flow in axons making up the supraopticohypophysial tracts. The material formed in neurons is thought to be a protein of molecular weight 30,000, to which is bound one molecule of vasopressin and one molecule of oxytocin. The pituicytes of the posterior lobe were once thought to synthesize and secrete the hormone in response to nerve impulses delivered over the supraopticohypophysial tracts. Now the hormone is believed to be liberated from

$$\overline{\text{Cys—Tyr—Phe—Glu}(NH_2)—Asp(NH_2)—Cys}—Pro—Arg—Gly(NH_2)$$

Arginine vasopressin

$$\overline{\text{Cys—Tyr—Phe—Glu}(NH_2)—Asp(NH_2)—Cys}—Pro—Lys—Gly(NH_2)$$

Lysine vasopressin

Arginine vasopressin has been chemically identified in the neurohypophysis of man, cow, sheep and horse. Sound pharmacologic evidence indicates that it is present in the monkey, cat, dog, rabbit, rat, camel and opossum. The pig and the hippopotamus are the only mammals in which the neurohypophysis is known to contain lysine vasopressin (18, 23).

Neither arginine nor lysine vasopressin is found in the neurohypophysis of lower forms of animals. Instead, arginine vasotocin has been tentatively identified as the antidiuretic hormone of chickens, reptiles, frogs and toads. This hormone has the ring structure of oxytocin and the side chain of arginine vasopressin:

nerve terminations of the tracts when they are invaded by nerve impulses. In dog and man, the hormone circulates in plasma as the free (unbound) octapeptide. In the rat, the hormone appears to be largely bound but to dissociate freely; therefore it is subject to rapid clearance from plasma. The plasma concentration of ADH in normal man after overnight dehydration averages 4.6–6.5 μU/ml (29).

CELLULAR ACTION OF ANTIDIURETIC HORMONE

The concepts of cellular action of ADH are largely based on studies made first on frog skin and more recently on toad bladder

$$\overline{\text{Cys—Tyr—Ile—Glu}(NH_2)—Asp(NH_2)—Cys}—Pro—Arg—Gly(NH_2)$$

(30). In life, the bladder serves as a reservoir for water, which is called upon during periods of dehydration to replenish body stores. In hydrated animals, the urine is hypotonic; solutes are present in a concentration of about 50 mOsm/L.

If the bladder is removed and spread out as a membrane separating two chambers containing Ringer's solution, isotopic water (D$_2$O or HTO) diffuses in both directions across the membrane at equal rates. As long as no osmotic gradient exists, no net transfer of water occurs. If, as is shown in Figure 12–5, an osmotic gradient is imposed by dilution of the Ringer's solution on one side, the osmotic flow of water across the untreated membrane is very low. Following the addition of ADH, osmotic flow increases greatly. On the basis of an analysis of diffusional and bulk flow, Leaf has described the operational characteristics of the membrane as follows: The untreated bladder behaves as though it were penetrated by cylindrical pores having a uniform radius of 8 Å. Following the addition of ADH, pore radii increase to 40 Å. The permeability of the membrane to a specific series of solutes of small molecular dimensions is greatly in-

creased by ADH; e.g., permeability to urea is increased some 10-fold.

Antidiuretic hormone also increases the active transport of sodium from the mucosal side (inside) of the bladder to the serosal side (outside). Because the sodium concentration of epithelial cells is always less than that of fluid on the mucosal side, it is probable that sodium pumps are located in the serosal membrane, that they actively extrude sodium from cells into serosal fluid and that sodium diffuses into the cells across their mucosal surface down a concentration gradient. Leaf proposed that increased pumping of sodium following treatment with ADH is the result of increased entry of sodium into the epithelial cells, owing to an increase in permeability, not to stimulation of the pump per se.

Antidiuretic hormone increases permeability of the mucosal surface of the cell to water, to specific organic solutes and to sodium only when it is applied to the serosal cell surface, not when it is applied to the mucosal surface. Accordingly, the hormone may penetrate the serosal surface and exert its action on the inner cytoplasmic side of the mucosal surface. On the other hand, Orloff

Fig. 12–5.—Effects of pitressin on net water flux across the toad bladder exposed to a series of osmotic gradients. (From Leaf, A., and Frazier, H. S.: Prog. Cardiovas. Dis. 4:47, 1961.)

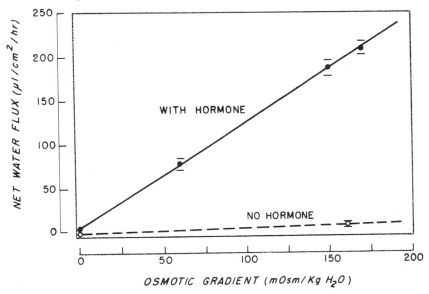

postulated that it attaches to receptors on the serosal surface and liberates cyclic adenosine monophosphate (AMP) into the cytoplasm, which diffuses to the mucosal surface and increases its permeability. This view is based on the observation that cyclic AMP reproduces the effects of ADH in the toad bladder: increased permeability to water and increased transport of sodium.

The conversion of ATP to cyclic 3', 5' AMP is catalyzed by adenyl cyclase, an enzyme present in both kidney tissue and toad bladder and activated by ADH. Inactivation of cyclic 3', 5' AMP is catalyzed by cyclic nucleotide phosphodiesterase to form 5' AMP, a reaction which is inhibited by theophylline. Accordingly, theophylline increases sodium and water transport by the toad bladder much as does ADH. Its diuretic effect on the kidney is possibly related to its greater depression of proximal transport of sodium and water than its stimulation of distal transport. Increased acidity of serosal fluid inhibits the action of adenyl cyclase and reduces the action of ADH on the bladder. Incubation of the bladder with either ADH or theophylline increases greatly the concentration of cyclic nucleotide in the tissue. In an analogous fashion, vasopressin increases the concentration of cyclic nucleotide in homogenates of dog kidney. These facts suggest that cyclic 3', 5' AMP is the mediator of ADH action on both toad bladder and kidney (31).

Schwartz et al. (32) proposed that the hormone acts directly on both toad bladder and kidney. They postulated that ADH binds at a minimum of two sites, the most important being a covalent linkage between the -S-S-bridge of the octapeptide and free -SH groups of the membrane. They suggested that disulfide-sulfydryl interchanges induce separation of fibrillar elements of the membrane or in some other fashion open channels through which water flows. This view is largely speculative, and the concept of an indirect action of the hormone mediated by cyclic nucleotide is better substantiated.

Thirst

Thirst is an important factor in the regulation of volume and osmotic concentration of the body fluids. As a subjective sensation, it may be studied only in man; in terms of drinking, one may infer its presence in experimental animals. The sensation in man seems to be primarily associated with dryness of the mouth and upper respiratory tract—hence, with inadequacy of secretion of fluid by the salivary and mucosal glands. It is temporarily relieved by moistening of these mucosal surfaces, although the water content of the body is unchanged. Because a pebble or a small volume of dilute acid in the mouth stimulates salivary flow, it is evident that fluid secretion is inhibited centrally by factors that induce thirst, not by effects of dehydration or reduced extracellular volume per se on the secretory glands. A sufficiently intense afferent input can break through the inhibition and reflexly excite secretion and temporarily relieve thirst (33).

Not only fluid restriction, but also the infusion of hypertonic salt solutions, causes thirst and stimulates drinking in experimental animals (34). Both procedures increase the osmolarity of body fluids. However, hemorrhage, which has no effect on osmolar concentration, also induces thirst and stimulates drinking (35). All three procedures inhibit the secretion of salivary, buccal and respiratory tract glands. Obviously, some central integrative mechanism must receive afferent impulses from volume receptors and osmoreceptors and control the reflex activity of the fluid secretory mechanisms. If volume is reduced or osmolarity is increased, secretion is inhibited, thirst develops and drinking is stimulated.

If 50 ml of a 10% sodium chloride solution is injected intravenously into a dog, thirst results, and the animal rapidly ingests a volume of water roughly equivalent to that needed to dilute the salt solution to 300 mOsm/L. Then the animal stops drinking, although little or none of the water has yet been absorbed. Satiety apparently is a consequence of moistening of mucous membranes, of some mystical metering of volume drunk and of the degree of distention of the stomach (36). If the animal has an esophageal fistula, so that the ingested water is lost to the outside, thirst is relieved only temporarily. The integrative mechanism must, accordingly, receive afferent impulses from a variety of esophageal and gastric receptors.

Just how this integrative mechanism is organized is uncertain. Some significant portion of it is localized in the hypothalamus: Anderson and McCann (37) found that the injection of minute amounts of hypertonic saline solution into the hypothalamus lateral to the third ventricle or electrical stimulation of that locus induces drinking in goats. With electrical stimulation, the animal begins to drink shortly after stimulation is begun, and it ceases drinking immediately on interruption of the stimulus. Such drinking is obviously independent of inhibition of salivary flow and the afferent impulses that lead to the sensation of thirst. Whether the hypothalamic integrative mechanism is on the afferent or efferent side of the cerebrocortical mechanisms of conscious perception of dryness and of motor initiation of drinking is unknown.

Summary

The volume of the extracellular fluid compartment is largely determined by the compartment's sodium content; the osmolar concentration, by its water content relative to the ion content. Volume and osmolarity are regulated by mechanisms that, although basically independent, are nevertheless interrelated.

The volume regulatory mechanism consists of (1) receptors that sense extracellular or plasma volume, some derivative of volume, such as pressure or distention, or blood flow; (2) an integrative mechanism; and (3) a neurohumoral effector mechanism that controls the excretion of sodium. Under normal conditions, the rate of excretion of sodium precisely balances the intake; volume is kept constant. The rate of excretion of sodium is dependent on the rate at which it is filtered and on the capacity of the tubules to reabsorb sodium from the filtrate. Control of excretion is effected by the vasomotor nerves, which determine the magnitude of the filtered load and its distribution among nephrons of varying reabsorptive capacity, and by the rate of secretion of aldosterone, which exerts a fine control over tubular reabsorption. Other mechanisms, less precisely defined, may also affect the excretion of sodium.

The osmolar regulatory mechanism consists of (1) osmoreceptors, located within the zone of distribution of the internal carotid artery and responsive to changes in osmolarity of blood plasma of the order of $\pm 2\%$; (2) an integrative center; (3) a neurosecretory mechanism, which releases ADH in amounts related to the need for conserving water; and (4) a renal effector mechanism, which responds to the titer of circulating ADH by varying the rate of excretion or conservation of free water. Overhydration inhibits the secretion of ADH; the distal tubules and collecting ducts become impermeable to water, and a large volume of dilute urine is excreted. Dehydration stimulates the secretion of ADH; distal tubules and collecting ducts become permeable to water, and a small volume of urine with an osmolar concentration some $4-5$ times that of the blood plasma is formed; thirst is induced and, as a consequence of increased intake of water, osmolarity is restored to normal.

REFERENCES

1. Smith, H. W.: Salt and water volume receptors: An exercise in physiologic apologetics, Am. J. Med. 23:623, 1957.
2. Welt, L.: *Clinical Disorders of Hydration and Acid Base Equilibrium* (Boston: Little, Brown & Company, 1955).
3. Welt, R. G.: Volume receptors, Circulation 21:1002, 1960.
4. Viar, W. N., Oliver, B. B., Eisenberg, S., Lombardo, T. A., Willis, K., and Harrison, T. R.: The effect of posture and of compression of the neck on the excretion of electrolytes

and glomerular filtration: Further studies, Circulation 3:105, 1951.

5. Strauss, M. B.: *Body Water in Man* (Boston: Little, Brown & Company, 1957).

6. Epstein, F. H.: Renal excretion of sodium and the concept of a volume receptor, Yale J. Biol. & Med. 29:282, 1956.

7. Bartter, F. C., and Gann, D. S.: On the hemodynamic regulation of the secretion of aldosterone, Circulation 21:1016, 1960.

8. Gauer, O. H., Henry, J. P., and Sieker, H. O.: Cardiac receptors and fluid volume control, Prog. Cardiovas. Dis. 4:1, 1961.

9. Borst, J. G. G.: The Characteristic Renal Excretion Patterns Associated with Excessive or Inadequate Circulation, in *Ciba Foundation Symposium on the Kidney* (London: J. & A. Churchill, Ltd., 1954).

10. Davis, J. O.: A critical evaluation of the role of receptors in the control of aldosterone secretion and sodium excretion, Prog. Cardiovas. Dis. 4:27, 1961.

11. Thompson, D. D., and Pitts, R. F.: Effects of alterations of renal arterial pressure on sodium and water excretion, Am. J. Physiol. 168:490, 1952.

12. Goodyer, A. V. N., and Jaeger, C. A.: Renal response to nonshocking hemorrhage: Role of the autonomic nervous system and of the renal circulation, Am. J. Physiol. 180:69, 1955.

13. Roemmelt, J. C., Sartorius, O. W., and Pitts, R. F.: Excretion and reabsorption of sodium and water in the adrenalectomized dog, Am. J. Physiol. 159:154, 1949.

14. Edelman, I. S.: Relationship of protein synthesis to ion transport in mammalian systems, Proc. XXIII Internat. Physiol. Congr., Tokyo 4:587, 1965.

15. Edelman, I. S.: Action of aldosterone on sodium transport, Abstr., III Internat. Congr. Nephrology, Washington, D. C., 1966, p. 67.

16. Sharp, G. W. G., Coggino, C. H., Lichtenstein, N. S., and Leaf, A.: Evidence for a mucosal effect of aldosterone on sodium transport in the toad bladder, J. Clin. Invest. 45:1640, 1966.

17. Sharp, G. W. G., and Leaf, A.: Mechanism of action of aldosterone, Physiol. Rev. 46:593, 1966.

18. Sawyer, W. H., Munsick, R. A., and Van Dyke, H. B.: Antidiuretic hormones, Circulation 21:1027, 1960.

19. Hilton, J. G.: Adrenocorticotropic action of antidiuretic hormone, Circulation 21:1038, 1960.

20. Farrell, G.: Adrenoglomerulotropin, Circulation 21:1009, 1960.

21. Verney, E. B.: Water diuresis, Irish J. M. Sc. 345:377, 1954.

22. Pickford, M.: Antidiuretic substances, Pharmacol. Rev. 4:254, 1952.

23. Thorn, N. A.: Mammalian antidiuretic hormone, Physiol. Rev. 38:169, 1958.

24. Baldes, E. J., and Smirk, F. H.: The effect of water drinking, mineral starvation and salt administration on the total osmotic pressure of the blood of man, chiefly in relation to the problems of water absorption and water diuresis, J. Physiol. 82:62, 1934.

25. Rioch, D. M.: Experiments on water and salt diuresis, Arch. Int. Med. 40:743, 1927.

26. Lauson, H. D.: Vasopressin and Oxytocin in the Plasma of Man and Other Mammals, in Antoniades, H. N. (ed.): *Hormones in Human Plasma* (Boston: Little, Brown & Company, 1960).

27. Lauson, H. D.: The problem of estimating rate of secretion of antidiuretic hormones in man, Am. J. Med. 11:135, 1951.

28. Sawyer, W. H.: Evolution of antidiuretic hormones and their functions, Am. J. Med. 42:678, 1967.

29. Lauson, H. D.: Metabolism of antidiuretic hormones, Am. J. Med. 42:713, 1967.

30. Leaf, A., and Frazier, H. S.: Some recent studies on the action of neurohypophyseal hormones, Prog. Cardiovas. Dis. 4:47, 1961.

31. Orloff, J., and Handler, J.: The role of adenosine 3', 5'-phosphate in the action of antidiuretic hormone, Am. J. Med. 42:757, 1967.

32. Schwartz, I. L., Rasmussen, H., Schoessler, M. A., Silver, L., and Fong, C. T. O.: Relation of chemical attachment to physiological action of vasopressin, Proc. Nat. Acad. Sc. 46:1288, 1960.

33. Cannon, W. B.: The physiological basis of thirst, Proc. Roy. Soc. 90B:283, 1918.

34. Gilman, A.: The relation between blood osmotic pressure, fluid distribution and voluntary water intake, Am. J. Physiol. 120:323, 1937.

35. Gesell, R.: Studies on submaxillary gland: IV. A comparison of the effects of hemorrhage and of tissue abuse in relation to secondary shock, Am. J. Physiol. 47:468, 1918–19.

36. Towbin, E. J.: Gastric distention as a factor in the satiation of thirst in esophagostomized dogs, Am. J. Physiol. 159:533, 1949.

37. Anderson, B., and McCann, S. M.: A further study of polydipsia evoked by hypothalamic stimulation in the goat, Acta physiol. scandinav. 33:333, 1955.

13

Metabolism of the Kidney

IT WAS POINTED OUT on p. 161 that renal blood flow is high relative to organ mass or metabolic demand, no doubt in consequence of the fact that regulatory functions of the kidney necessitate the processing of large volumes of blood. This does not mean that the metabolic cost of renal function is low; it is not. The two kidneys of man, which average 0.5% of body weight, consume 8% of the oxygen used per minute by the body at rest. However, high flow relative to metabolic cost does mean that the renal arteriovenous oxygen difference is low: on average, it is 1.7 ml of oxygen per 100 ml of blood, in comparison with 4–6 ml of oxygen per 100 ml in the mixed venous blood entering the right side of the heart.

Some years ago, Van Slyke et al. (1) demonstrated anomalous behavior of the kidney with respect to its extraction of oxygen from blood. When renal blood flow is reduced by partial clamping of the renal artery, the arteriovenous oxygen difference tends to remain relatively low and constant. In contrast, when flow to other organs is compromised, arteriovenous oxygen difference increases, most notably in heart, skeletal muscle and skin. The cause of this anomalous behavior of the renal circulation became evident when it was recognized that reduction in renal blood flow is accompanied by reduction of glomerular filtration rate. The volume and ionic content of the fluid presented to the renal tubules for reabsorption are propor-

tionally reduced. Thus, reabsorptive work is lessened.

The energy cost of reabsorption of sodium in the kidney of the dog is estimated to be 1 micromole (μM) of oxygen for each 20–28 microequivalents (μEq) of sodium. The oxygen consumption of the normally functioning kidney is 4–6 μM of oxygen per minute per gram. Thus, if we estimate that an 18-kg dog has a total kidney weight of 100 Gm, an oxygen consumption of 5 μM/Gm per minute, a glomerular filtration rate of 80 ml/min and a plasma sodium concentration of 140 μEq/ml, and if the kidney reabsorbs essentially all of the filtered sodium, then the amount of filtered and reabsorbed sodium is 11,200 μEq/min and oxygen consumption is 500 μM/min — a ratio of O_2:Na of slightly more than 1:22.

It seems doubtful that all of the energy consumption of the kidney is derived from oxidative processes or that all is concerned with reabsorption of sodium. In an attempt to correct for non-sodium active transport, filtration rate has been reduced to zero by lowering renal artery pressure. At best, this is only a gross and misleading correction, for there is reason to believe that, in the absence of filtration, passive back flow of sodium from blood to lumen occurs and is accompanied by active transport from lumen to blood. Furthermore, cessation of renewal of tubular contents must severely limit active transport of glucose, amino acids, hydrogen ions and

259

other energy-requiring tubular processes. In any event, abolishing glomerular filtration reduces oxygen consumption to one fifth or one sixth of normal.

The metabolism of the medulla and papillae of the kidney has been described as largely anaerobic and glycolytic (2–5), whereas that of the cortex has been ascribed to the aerobic oxidation of glucose, lactate, pyruvate, citrate and the free fatty acid palmitate (6–9). Partial anaerobiosis of the medulla and papilla are in accord with observations of Kramer *et al.* (10) on regional blood flow. Thus, flow through the cortex averages 4–5 ml/Gm per minute; through the medulla, 0.7–1 ml/Gm per minute; and through the papillae, 0.2–0.25 ml/Gm per minute. Furthermore, the oxygen tension of cortical urine is no doubt high (proximal and distal tubular fluid), whereas that of the final urine is low (11). This observation, first made in 1859, was explained by Kramer *et al.* (12) as a consequence of high diffusibility of oxygen, countercurrent flow of blood through the vasa recta, and the shunting of oxygen across the top of the vascular loops from blood flowing into and out of the papillae. The oxygen tension of the final urine is in diffusion equilibrium with the low tension of the blood at the tips of the papillae.

Most of the studies on substrate use by the kidney have been biochemically oriented and have been performed on slices or homogenates. They have been concerned with biochemical cycles and with possible or probable enzymes, reactions, intermediates or products. The author does not wish to denigrate such studies; they have provided a rich background of information, which constitutes the starting point for studies on the intact, functioning kidney. However, slices or homogenates have no blood flow and form no glomerular filtrate; therefore, they are inadequate for definitive studies of the metabolic reactions that ultimately power the processes of tubular reabsorption or secretion. Furthermore, slices, homogenates or purified enzyme preparations lack normal hormonal and neural control. Single substrates are usually added as the sole source of energy and in high concentration; thus, the questions that can be asked are relatively limited.

For metabolic studies to have true physiologic relevance (i.e., describe conditions as they exist in vivo), two criteria must be met: (1) they must be performed on the intact, functioning kidney of the living animal and (2) they must be performed at endogenous blood concentrations of all normal renal metabolites. Such experimental constrictions do place limits on the questions that can be asked at present and on the precision of the answers that can be expected. Ultimately, as new and more precise methods of study become available, the ultimate goal of the renal physiologist should be to define normal metabolic activities in vivo, and the goal of the functionally oriented nephrologist should be to define abnormalities that occur in disease.

Within limits, one can at present approach these goals in studies on CO_2 production from known renal substrates in the dog. One can measure glomerular filtration rate by the creatinine clearance and true renal blood flow by the clearance and extraction of *p*-aminohippurate. Renal venous blood samples, which are necessary for the measurement of extraction in quantifying true renal blood flow as well as extraction of metabolites, can be collected through a catheter passed into the right renal vein from the femoral vein, under fluoroscopic observation. Urine can be collected from the right kidney by catheterizing the right ureter through a low abdominal incision. Thus, the experiments must be performed under light anesthesia; and, to this extent, conditions are somewhat abnormal. Also, the data are limited to the right kidney; this means that they must be doubled for a description of total renal metabolism. Total renal oxidative metabolism can be measured by the product of true renal blood flow (milliliters per minute) and differences in renal arteriovenous carbon dioxide content (micromoles per milliliter), yielding micromoles per minute of total CO_2 produced.

To measure the contribution of any single substrate to total CO_2 production, it is necessary to infuse a ^{14}C-labeled isotope of that substrate at a constant rate prior to and during the course of an experiment. The product of true renal blood flow and the arteriovenous [14]CO_2 difference, in counts per minute per milliliter (cpm/ml), gives the rate of production of counts in [14]CO_2 derived from the isotopic substrate. If one divides [14]CO_2 cpm/min produced by the specific activity (counts per minute per micromole) of substrate extracted, the quotient equals the number of micromoles per minute of substrate oxidized to CO_2. In essence, one wraps up the [14]CO_2 activity into packages equal to the number of micromoles of substrate extracted. Multiplying micromoles of substrate oxidized to CO_2 per minute by the number of carbons in each molecule yields micromoles of CO_2 produced from substrate per minute. There are several hidden assumptions in this method; the major ones are that (1) the pool of intrarenal substrate is small and turns over rapidly and (2) the pool is in equilibrium with arterial blood substrate and that, for each isotopic molecule extracted, one is oxidized to CO_2. These assumptions seem to be valid for glutamine, lactate, glucose and citrate, and possibly for free fatty acids also. It must be emphasized that the infusion of isotopic substrate of high specific activity at the low rates involved in tracer studies does not appreciably increase the concentration of the normally occurring, nonisotopic substrate.

Metabolism of Glutamine

The method described above was first applied in testing the thesis of Goodman *et al.* (13) and Alleyne and Scullard (14) that the increased production of ammonia by the kidney in acidosis is due to induction of the enzyme phosphoenolpyruvate carboxykinase

and to consequent increase in gluconeogenesis from glutamine. For this reason, the metabolism of glutamine was compared in acidosis and alkalosis in the intact, functioning kidney of the dog (15, 16). Figure 13–1 shows that glomerular filtration rates, renal blood flow and arterial blood concentrations of glutamine were not significantly different in five dogs in acidosis and five dogs in alkalosis. These data describe mean functions of one kidney (the right one). Arterial glutamine concentrations were well within the range of normal, despite the infusion of tracer amounts of uniformly labeled glutamine. However, as would be expected, the renal extraction of glutamine in the acidotic series of dogs greatly exceeded that in the alkalotic series. Only insignificant amounts of extracted glutamine were added to renal venous blood as glutamate or aspartate; the major fraction was converted to α-ketoglutarate and ammonia. The ammonia was in large part excreted in the urine, in acidosis, to buffer excess protons. The minor fraction was added to renal venous blood. The α-ketoglutarate disappeared: the major part (80%)

Fig. 13–1.—Comparison of glomerular filtration rate, renal blood flow, arterial blood glutamine concentration, and renal extraction of glutamine in one kidney of five dogs in acidosis and five dogs in alkalosis. (From Pitts, R. F.: Kidney Internat. 1:295, 1972.)

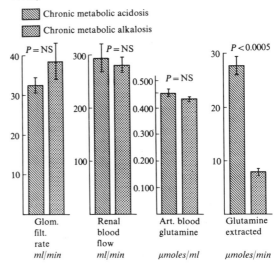

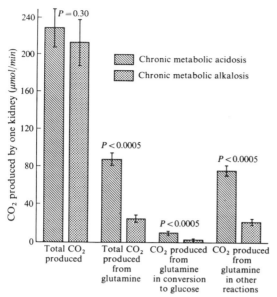

Fig. 13–2.—Comparison of total renal CO_2 production and CO_2 produced in conversion of glutamine to glucose and in other reactions in one kidney of five dogs in acidosis and five dogs in alkalosis. (From Pitts, R. F.: Kidney Internat. 1:297, 1972.)

was oxidized to CO_2, and the minor part (20%) was converted to glucose.

Figure 13–2 illustrates the fact that the total oxidative metabolism of all substrates (first pair of columns) does not differ in acidosis and alkalosis. This is reasonable if most of the energy expenditure of the kidney is concerned with the active reabsorption of sodium from the glomerular filtrate. Plasma sodium concentration and filtration rate do not differ significantly in these two acid-base states. However, the proportion of the total energy that is derived from glutamine is much greater in acidosis (40%) than in alkalosis (14.5%) (second pair of columns). Again, this is reasonable, for the renal extraction of glutamine is far greater in acidosis (27.7 $\mu M/min$) than in alkalosis (8.04 $\mu M/min$); accordingly, α-ketoglutarate production is much higher. Although for every 2 mol of glutamine converted to glucose, 4 mol of CO_2 and 4 mol of ammonia are formed, the proportion of glutamine completely oxidized to CO_2, relative to that converted to glucose, is roughly 5:1 (third and fourth

pairs of columns). The fact that total substrate oxidation is the same in acidosis and alkalosis, yet the contribution of glutamine is much greater in acidosis, has two consequences: (1) some other substrate or substrates must replace glutamine in alkalosis; and (2) there is no obligatory fuel for sodium reabsorption; i.e., glutamine or other fuels may be interchanged in isocaloric amounts. These observations suggested a study of lactate metabolism as a possible source of the deficit of glutamine energy production in alkalosis. Pyruvate as a source was discarded because of its very low plasma concentration.

Metabolism of Lactate

Studies similar to those described above were performed on six dogs in acidosis and six dogs in alkalosis during the infusion of ^{14}C-uniformly labeled lactate in tracer

Fig. 13–3.—Total renal CO_2 production and percentage of total CO_2 derived from lactate in six dogs in acidosis and six dogs in alkalosis. (From Leal-Pinto, E., Park, H. C., MacLeod, M. B., and Pitts, R. F.: Am. J. Physiol. 224:1463, 1973.)

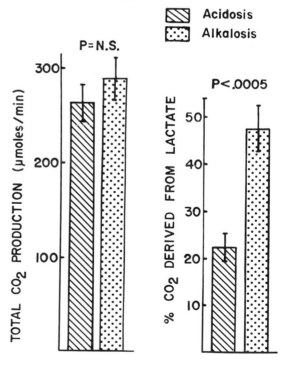

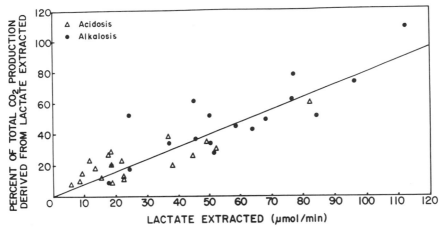

Fig. 13—4.—Percentage of total renal CO_2 produced from lactate as a function of lactate extracted in six dogs in acidosis and six dogs in alkalosis. (From Leal-Pinto, E., Park, H. C., MacLeod, M. B., and Pitts, R. F.: Am. J. Physiol. 224:1463, 1973.)

amounts (17, 18). In contrast to the glutamine studies, the arterial blood concentration of lactate was low in acidosis (1.14 μM/ml) and significantly higher in alkalosis (2.02 μM/ml). However, glomerular filtration rates were essentially the same in acidosis (41.2 ml/min) and alkalosis (43.4 ml/min). Renal blood flows were also nearly the same (281 ml/min in acidosis and 305 ml/min in alkalosis). Because no lactate was excreted in acidosis or alkalosis, it is evident that all that was filtered was reabsorbed. As in the glutamine study, the total oxidative metabolism of all substrates did not differ significantly in acidosis and alkalosis. This is shown in the first pair of columns of Figure 13–3. However, the percentage derived from the oxidation of lactate was essentially twice as great in alkalosis (47.4%) as in acidosis (22.4%). These percentages for lactate metabolism were roughly the reverse of those for glutamine. Summing the percentages in acidosis yielded 62.4% of the total; summing them in alkalosis yielded 61.9% of the total.

The percentage of CO_2 derived from lactate was a direct linear function of extracted lactate (Fig. 13–4). For the most part, low extractions of lactate and low percentages of lactate oxidized to CO_2 were observed in acidotic animals in which plasma concentrations are low. The reverse was true in alkalosis. Thus, the higher the plasma concentration of lactate, the greater the percentage extracted and oxidized to CO_2. The association of increased blood lactate and alkalosis has been repeatedly noted. It has recently been postulated to be due to an increase in the rate of glycolysis by acceleration of the phosphofructokinase step, as a consequence of decreased cellular H^+ ion concentration.

The Metabolism of Free Fatty Acids

Free Fatty Acids (FFAs) have been considered to be metabolic fuels of the kidney of major importance. According to Gold and Spitzer (6), Hohenleitner and Spitzer (19), and Nieth and Schollmeyer (8), FFAs account for 65% or more of the oxygen consumed by the kidney. However, this value, if added to the oxygen utilized in the metabolism of glutamine and lactate, considerably exceeds total oxygen consumption of the kidney. Gold and Spitzer (6) and most who have followed them (8, 20–22) have assumed that palmitate is the only FFA that contributes appreciably to the powering of renal functions. In contrast, recent work (23, 24) casts doubt both on the preponderant role of FFAs and the special prominence of palmitate as a fuel of respiration.

A number of problems complicate the study of energy production from fatty acids. Several are methodologic; one or more are physiologic. Modern gas chromatography permits the duplicate analysis of long-chain fatty acids in single extracted and methylated samples of plasma with an error of ±1.0% or less. However, duplicate extractions and methylations may deviate ±5.0% or more. If one adds to each plasma sample a known amount of a long-chain FFA not present in dog plasma, then extracts and methylates the sample, one can correct errors. Heneicosanoic acid, containing 21 carbons in the chain, is not present in plasma and can be used for correction of errors of extraction and methylation. Since mean renal extractions of individual FFAs from plasma are 8% or less and since uncorrected variations in final analytic values may be as great as ±5%, it is evident that possible errors of renal extraction may approach 100%.

However, it is a truism that the $^{14}CO_2$ produced by the kidney from a labeled fatty acid, expressed in counts per minute per minute, may be factored either by the specific activity of the fatty acid extracted or by the specific activity of the fatty acid in arterial plasma, to obtain the micromoles of fatty acid oxidized to CO_2. This is a consequence of the fact that the ratio of labeled to unlabeled fatty acid molecules in the arterial plasma presented to the kidney must be the same as the ratio of labeled to unlabeled fatty acid extracted by the kidney. This is a basic premise of the use of all ^{14}C-labeled metabolites in any tracer capacity; namely, that an organ does not distinguish between a labeled and an unlabeled molecule of any compound. Use of specific activity of plasma further reduces error.

A practical methodologic problem in such experiments is cost of uniformly labeled free fatty acids, necessitating use of ^{14}C-1-labeled acids. This use is justified by the following statement of Green (25); namely, that once a FFA molecule enters a mitochondrion, each two-carbon fragment that results from

successive beta oxidations is coupled to an oxaloacetate and enters the citric acid cycle to be completely oxidized. Acetoacetate is formed in significant amounts only in the liver. Of course all 16 carbons of palmitate and all 18 of stearate and oleate must enter the final calculation although only one is labeled.

The second type of problem, a physiologic one, concerns the utilization of endogenous neutral lipids as fuels of respiration during the course of an experiment. All experiments were performed from 20 to 24 hours following the last feeding of the dog. It is probable that at this time neutral labile lipids of renal tubular cells have been reduced in amount to such an extent that the equilibrium has been shifted from hydrolysis of neutral tubular lipids to form FFAs for tubular oxidation to one of hydrolysis of neutral lipids of adipose tissue to provide FFA for both oxidation by tubular cells and partial restoration of labile cellular lipids.

A line of evidence that this may be true is shown in Table 13–1. The specific activities (counts per minute per micromole) of palmitate, stearate and oleate entering the kidney in the arterial plasma are essentially identical to the specific activities of these same FFAs leaving the kidney in the renal venous blood. If hydrolysis of stored labile neutral lipid were occurring, one might expect cellular FFAs (unlabeled) to exchange to some degree with renal venous FFAs (labeled) and reduce specific activity

TABLE 13-1.—IDENTITY OF SPECIFIC ACTIVITY OF FAAs IN ARTERIAL AND RENAL VENOUS PLASMA IN ACIDOSIS AND ALKALOSIS*

	MEAN	STANDARD DEVIATION	STANDARD ERROR	SAMPLES
Palmitate				
Acidosis	1.0014	± 0.0454	± 0.0130	(12)
Alkalosis	1.0172	± 0.0611	± 0.0176	(12)
Stearate				
Acidosis	1.0178	± 0.0463	± 0.0130	(12)
Alkalosis	1.0345	± 0.1064	± 0.0306	(12)
Oleate				
Acidosis	0.9961	± 0.0420	± 0.0138	(9)
Alkalosis	0.9971	± 0.0475	± 0.0158	(9)

*From Park, H. C., Leal-Pinto, E., MacLeod, M. B., and Pitts, R. F.: Am. J. Physiol. (in press).

to a value below that of arterial activity. Since this does not occur, it suggests that stored labile neutral lipids of tubular cells are not being hydrolyzed. Equality of specific activity of arterial and renal venous plasma does not negate extraction of FFAs by the kidney. It merely indicates that the micromoles per milliliter and counts per minute per milliliter are extracted proportionately, a fact demanded by use of any labeled compound as a tracer.

These experiments were begun 40 minutes after the start of infusion of the tracer, either palmitate, stearate or oleate. Infusion was continued for the 45 minute duration of three 15 minute clearance periods. The abscissae of the three panels of Figure 13–5 reflect these latter times. This figure also adds confirmatory evidence that a steady state exists for uptake of plasma FFAs and oxidation of FFAs, unperturbed by hydrolysis and utilization of stored tubular cell lipids.

Figure 13–5 (left-hand panel) shows that the specific activities of oleate in arterial plasma in three three-period experiments in acidosis and a similar number in alkalosis exhibit a slight trend upward. This is also true of specific activity of arterial plasma in

four three-period experiments with both palmitate and stearate in acidosis and in similar numbers in alkalosis. The increase in specific activity with time was due to a slight increase in counts per minute per milliliter; micromoles per milliliter remained constant. This indicates that the rate of infusion of tracer amounts of labeled isotopic FFAs slightly exceeded the rate of addition of non-labeled FFAs from adipose tissue. Labeled and non-labeled FFAs were taken up by all tissues of the body, including the kidney, in proportion to their concentrations in arterial plasma.

The middle panel of Figure 13–5 demonstrates that, within fairly wide limits of experimental error, the percent of the total CO_2 produced by the kidney from each of these three FFAs was independent of time in both acidosis and alkalosis. If the specific activity of the CO_2 produced (right-hand panel of Figure 13–5) increases with time in proportion to the increase in specific activity of the FFA from which it originates (left-hand panel), then percent of CO_2 derived from arterial FFAs must be constant (middle panel). I interpret these three graphs to be consonant with these views. In addi-

Fig. 13–5. — Specific activity of arterial plasma FFAs (**A**), percentages of total CO_2 derived from arterial FFAs (**B**) and specific activity of CO_2 produced by the kidney in acidosis and alkalosis (**C**).

Open symbols, acidosis; *closed symbols,* alkalosis. (From Park, H. C., Leal-Pinto, E., MacLeod, M. B., and Pitts, R. F.: Am. J. Physiol. [in press].)

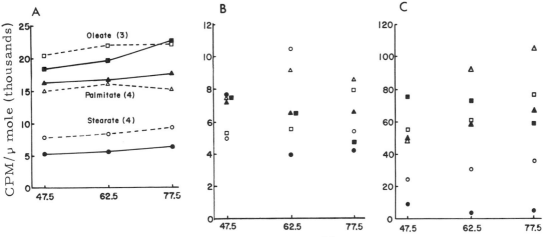

Time in minutes after start of ^{14}C- F.F.A. Infusion

tion, the fact that specific activity does not change (Table 13 – 1) as plasma perfuses the kidney suggests strongly that (1) neutral lipid stored within tubular cells is not hydrolyzed to FFAs during the course of the experiment and that (2) all FFAs oxidized to CO_2 by the kidney are extracted from arterial plasma.

What do these two conclusions really mean? My interpretation is that 20 – 24 hours after the last meal, there are two discrete lipid pools within tubular cells. One takes up FFAs from arterial plasma and disposes of them by oxidation to CO_2. The other pool takes up FFAs and synthesizes them into neutral lipids. In contrast, during the lipemic phase immediately following a meal, FFAs may be taken up by both pools. A few hours later, neutral lipid, stored in tubular cells in some labile form, may be hydrolyzed to FFAs. In part they might be oxidized as a fuel of respiration; in part they might spill over into renal venous blood. Twenty to twenty-four hours after a meal, arterial plasma FFAs are all supplied from adipose tissue, flux of FFAs is all into the cell, and communication between the oxidative pool and the lipid synthesis pool is interrupted. This view is highly speculative and may not be true; however, it does explain the facts outlined in Figure 13 – 5 and Table 13 – 1.

Figure 13 – 6 summarizes the percentage of total renal CO_2 production derived from palmitate, stearate and oleate in 22 three-period experiments: 11 in acidosis, 11 in alkalosis. Standard errors of the means are quite large and P-values indicate that differences are not significant. The three series in acidosis account for 21.7% of total CO_2 production. The three series in alkalosis account for 16.3% of total CO_2 production. It is doubtful that these two means are significantly different.

Three conclusions can be drawn from these experiments: (1) fatty acids are not the predominant fuels of respiration of the kidney; (2) palmitate is not the only fatty acid oxidized; (3) fatty acids are not the

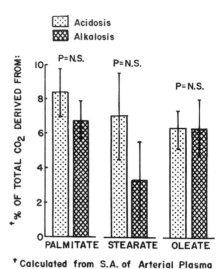

† Calculated from S.A. of Arterial Plasma

Fig. 13 – 6. — Total renal CO_2 production and percentages derived from palmitate, stearate and oleate in 11 dogs in acidosis and 11 dogs in alkalosis. (From Park, H. C., Leal-Pinto, E., MacLeod, M. B., and Pitts, R. F.: Am. J. Physiol. [in press].)

predominant source of energy for reabsorption of sodium in the intact functioning kidney.

The Metabolism of Citrate

Recent studies (26) have shown that citrate extracted from plasma provides a small but significant proportion of the energy supply of the kidney. These experiments of Balagura-Baruch and her associates were performed in an identical fashion on dogs in comparable states of acidosis and alkalosis and at comparable times after the last meal to those previously described in this chapter. As in these earlier studies, renal blood flows, glomerular filtration rates and urine flows were similar in acidosis and alkalosis. Since arterial whole blood CO_2 concentrations and rates of excretion of ammonia were similar to those already described, acid-base states were comparable.

These experiments demonstrated that the rates of total CO_2 production by the kidney from all metabolites were similar in acidosis and alkalosis; i.e., total oxidative metabolism was essentially the same in these two acid-base states. Thus total CO_2 production averaged 217 μmols/min in acidosis and 195 μmols/min in alkalosis, differences that were not statistically significant. The proportion of total renal CO_2 derived from citrate in acidosis amounted to 10.8%, and in alkalosis to 13.8%. These differences were statistically significant.

The Metabolism of Glucose

The final study in this series (27) has shown that glucose is a significant contributor to the fuels of respiration of the kidney. Twelve three-period experiments were performed during infusion of uniformly labeled ^{14}C-glucose, six in acidosis, six in alkalosis. All experimental parameters were exactly the same as in the previous studies. These experiments demonstrated that glucose contributes 19.8% in acidosis and 26.2% in alkalosis of the total CO_2 produced by the kidney. This study (27) is the only one of the five similar studies (15–18, 23, 26, 27) in which a statistically significant difference was observed in total CO_2 production by the kidney in acidosis and alkalosis. A P-value of 0.05 is borderline. Since in the other four studies, total CO_2 production varied slightly, but insignificantly, above and below equality, I interpret this as a chance rather than a significant deviation. It is therefore possible that the difference in percent CO_2 derived from glucose in acidosis and alkalosis is also a chance difference.

Other Fuels of Respiration of the Kidney

The concentrations of other possible fuels of respiration are in general so low that their complete extraction from arterial blood and oxidation to CO_2 would provide little energy for the kidney. Thus concentrations of arterial pyruvate, α-ketoglutarate and intermediates of the Krebs' cycle other than citrate are very low. The concentration of palmitoleate is also low, while utilization of linoleate and arachidonate seem more

related to synthesis of structural lipid than to provision of energy (28). It must be remembered that the approach described above is one of a "black box" nature. α-Ketoglutarate is a major fuel of the kidney in acidosis, but it is extracted as glutamine from arterial blood, not as α-ketoglutarate per se.

The Sum of the Contributions of the Several Fuels to Total CO_2 Production by the Kidney

Table 13–2 summarizes the contributions of the major fuels of respiration of the intact functioning kidney in acidosis and alkalosis. The sum of their contributions in acidosis is 115% and in alkalosis is 118%. The experiments on which these values are based were carried out on 66 dogs over a period of 3 years. These experiments consisted of 198 clearance periods, 99 in acidosis, 99 in alkalosis. Some deviation from 100% is therefore acceptable.

There is at least one error that results in overestimation of the contribution of at least some fuels. All of the $^{14}CO_2$ as well as the total CO_2, measured as arterial-renal venous CO_2 difference times true renal blood flow, is actually produced in the kidney. All of the $^{14}CO_2$ measured ultimately is derived from the labeled substrate. However, if some fraction of the labeled substrate not measured yet in arterial and renal venous blood is converted to some labeled compound as it circulates through other tissues and is oxidized by the kidney, $^{14}CO_2$ produced in the kidney will be overestimated. Factoring total $^{14}CO_2$ production (counts

TABLE 13-2.—Percentages of Total Renal CO_2 Derived from Various Metabolites

Substrate	Acidosis (%)	Alkalosis (%)
Glutamine	40.0	14.5
Lactate	22.4	47.4
Palmitate	8.4	6.8
Stearate	7.0	3.3
Oleate	6.3	6.2
Citrate	10.8	13.8
Glucose	19.8	26.2
Total	114.7	118.2

per minute per minute) by the specific activity of the original labeled substrate extracted or present in arterial blood will yield a figure too high by the $^{14}CO_2$ produced from converted substrate. This is probably the major cause of the excess over 100%.

Summary

It is generally believed that a relatively large proportion of the oxidative metabolism of the kidney is concerned with the reabsorption of sodium from the glomerular filtrate. If one wishes to identify the specific substrates responsible for energizing this and other active tubular processes, one must perform measurements on the intact functioning kidney at normal endogenous concentrations of substrates. To do this, isotopic methods must be employed. In acidotic dogs, approximately 40% of oxidative metabolism is supported by glutamine, 22% by lactate, 22% by fatty acids, 11% by citrate and 20% by glucose. In alkalotic dogs, approximately 15% of oxidative metabolism is supported by glutamine, 47% by lactate, 16% by fatty acids, 14% by citrate and 26% by glucose. Thus, in both acid-base states, somewhat more than 100% of oxidative metabolism has been accounted for. Since the reabsorption of sodium is not significantly different in the acidotic and alkalotic dog, it is evident that a number of metabolites can be utilized interchangeably to power the sodium pumps of the renal tubules. It is obvious that no single fuel is preferentially used by the kidney. Its tastes are catholic and not especially different from other tissues, except its use of glutamine in acidosis, related to the regulation of acid-base balance, and of lactate in alkalosis, related to the available supply.

REFERENCES

1. Van Slyke, D. D., Rhoades, C. P., Hiller, A., and Alving, A. S.: Relationship between urea excretion, renal blood flow, renal oxygen consumption and diuresis: The mechanics of urea excretion, Am. J. Physiol. 109:336, 1934.
2. Dell, R. B., and Winter, R. W.: Lactate gradients in the kidney of the dog, Am. J. Physiol. 213:301, 1967.
3. Kean, E. L., Adams, P. H., Davies, H. C., Winters, R. W., and Davies, R. E.: Energy metabolism of the renal medulla, Biochim. et biophys. acta 54:474, 1961.
4. Lee, J. B., and Peter, H. M.: Effect of oxygen tension on glucose metabolism in rabbit kidney cortex and medulla, Am. J. Physiol. 217:1464, 1969.
5. Lee, J. B., Vance, V. K., and Cahill, G. F.: Metabolism of C^{14}-labeled substrates by rabbit kidney cortex and medulla, Am. J. Physiol. 203:37, 1962.
6. Gold, M., and Spitzer, J. J.: Metabolism of free fatty acids by myocardium and kidney, Am. J. Physiol. 206:153, 1964.
7. Levy, M. N.: Uptake of lactate and pyruvate by intact kidney of the dog, Am. J. Physiol. 202:302, 1962.
8. Nieth, H., and Schollmeyer, P.: Substrate utilization of the human kidney, Nature, London 209:1244, 1966.
9. Weidemann, M. J., and Krebs, H. A.: The fuel of respiration of rat kidney cortex, Biochem. J. 112:149, 1969.
10. Kramer, K., Thurau, K., and Deetjen, P.: Hämodynamik des Nierenmarks, Pflüger's Arch. ges. Physiol. 271:782, 1960.
11. Planer, J.: Über die Gase des Harnes und der Transsudate, Ztschr. K. K. ges. Arzte Wein. 30:25, 1859.
12. Kramer, K., Deetjen, P., and Brechtelsbauer, H.: Gegenstromdiffusion des Sauerstoffs in Nierenmark, Arch. ges. Physiol. 274:63, 1961.
13. Goodman, A. D., Fuisz, R. E., and Cahill, G. F.: Renal gluconeogenesis in acidosis, alkalosis and potassium deficiency. Its possible role in regulation of renal ammonia production, J. Clin. Invest. 45:612, 1966.
14. Alleyne, G. A. O., and Scullard, G. H.: Renal metabolic response to acid-base changes. I. Enzymatic control of ammoniagenesis in the rat, J. Clin. Invest. 48:364, 1969.
15. Pitts, R. F., Pilkington, L. A., MacLeod, M. B., and Leal-Pinto, E.: Metabolism of glutamine by the intact functioning kidney of the dog, J. Clin. Invest. 51:557, 1972.
16. Pitts, R. F.: Control of renal production of ammonia, Kidney Internat. 1:297, 1972.
17. Leal-Pinto, E., Park, H. C., King, V. F., MacLeod, M. B., and Pitts, R. F.: The metabolism of lactate by the intact functioning kidney of the dog. Am. J. Physiol. 224:1463, 1973.

18. Pitts, R. F.: Metabolic Fuels of the Kidney, *Proceedings of the 5th International Congress on Nephrology*, (Basel: Karger, 1974) (in press).

19. Hohenleitner, F. J., and Spitzer, J. J.: Changes in plasma free fatty acid concentrations on passage through the dog kidney, Am. J. Physiol. 200:1095, 1961.

20. Barac-Nieto, M., and Cohen, J. J.: Non-esterified fatty acid uptake by dog kidney: Effects of probenecid and chlorothiazide, Am. J. Physiol. 215:93, 1968.

21. Barac-Nieto, M., and Cohen, J. J.: The metabolic fate of palmitate in the dog kidney in vivo, Nephron 8:488, 1971.

22. Dies, F., Herrera, J., Matos, M., Avelar, E., and Ramos, G.: Substrate uptake by the dog kidney, Am. J. Physiol. 218:405, 1970.

23. Pitts, R. F., Park, H. C., Leal-Pinto, E., and MacLeod, M. B.: Renal oxidation of free fatty acids, Fed. Proc. April, 1973.

24. Park, H. C., Leal-Pinto, E., and MacLeod, M. B., and Pitts, R. F.: Oxidation of free fatty acids by the intact functioning kidney, Am. J. Physiol. (in press).

25. Green, D. E.: Fatty acid oxidation in soluble systems of animal tissues, Biol. Rev. 29:330, 1954.

26. Balagura-Baruch, S., Kim, C. M., King, V. F., Pitts, R. F.: Oxidation of citrate by the intact functioning kidney, Unpublished work.

27. Pitts, R. F., and MacLeod, M. B.: Oxidation of glucose by the intact functioning kidney of the dog, Unpublished work.

28. Spector, A.: Metabolism of free fatty acids, Prog. Biochem. Pharmacol. 6:130, 1971.

14

Renal Function in Renal Disease

MEASUREMENTS OF glomerular filtration rate (C_{in}), minimum effective renal plasma flow (C_{PAH}) and functional tubular mass (Tm_G and Tm_{PAH}) have contributed to an understanding of the functional pathology of renal diseases. Certain derived data—e.g., filtration fraction (C_{in}/C_{PAH}), renal plasma flow per unit of functional tubular mass (C_{PAH}/Tm_G and C_{PAH}/Tm_{PAH}), and rate of glomerular filtration per unit of tubular mass, i.e., relative glomerulotubular balance (C_{in}/Tm_G and C_{in}/Tm_{PAH})—have helped to distinguish the various renal disorders. The mean values for these parameters of renal function in young adult men and women are given in Table 14–1; the range for each datum is at least ±15%.

A simplified classification of the major medical diseases of the kidney is given in Table 14–2. The description of these disorders in a textbook of physiology must, of necessity, be superficial. Here the intention is

TABLE 14–2.—SIMPLIFIED CLASSIFICATION OF RENAL DISEASES

I. Nephritides (bilateral inflammatory diseases of the kidney)
  A. Glomerulonephritis
    1. Acute
    2. Chronic
  B. Pyelonephritis
II. Nephroses (bilateral degenerative diseases of the kidney)
  A. Lipoid nephrosis (the nephrotic syndrome)
  B. Tubular necrosis
III. Nephroscleroses (arteriolar diseases)
  A. Benign
  B. Malignant
IV. Toxemia of pregnancy
V. Congenital disorders
  A. Polycystic disease
  B. Inborn defects of tubular transport

merely to illustrate the way in which functional information can contribute to an understanding of renal disease.

Nephritis

GLOMERULONEPHRITIS

Glomerulonephritis is initially and primarily an inflammatory disease affecting the glomerular capillary tuft. However, with progress of the disease, all elements of the nephron are affected. Fibrosis with obliteration of glomeruli is accompanied by degeneration and disappearance of tubules. Some of the glomeruli enlarge, and their tubules undergo hypertrophy and hyperplasia. In the end stage of chronic nephritis, the kidney is

TABLE 14–1.—RENAL FUNCTION IN NORMAL MAN (Mean Values; Range of Normal ±15%; All per 1.73 m² Surface Area)

	MALES	FEMALES
C_{in} (ml/min)	125	110
C_{PAH} (ml/min)	655	570
Tm_G (mg/min)	375	303
Tm_{PAH} (mg/min)	80	77
C_{in}/C_{PAH}	0.19	0.19
C_{PAH}/Tm_G	1.75	1.88
C_{PAH}/Tm_{PAH}	8.19	7.40
C_{in}/Tm_G	0.33	0.36
C_{in}/Tm_{PAH}	1.56	1.43

converted into a shriveled, contracted mass of scar tissue, in which are embedded atrophic remnants of glomeruli and tubules. Scattered islands of hypertrophic nephrons and more or less normal nephrons account for residual function (1).

ACUTE GLOMERULONEPHRITIS. — Acute glomerulonephritis classically has an abrupt onset a few days to 3 weeks after an attack of pharyngitis or scarlatina. The patient awakes one morning to find his face and hands puffy and the urine blood-tinged and reduced in volume. Examination reveals albuminuria, hypertension and elevated blood urea nitrogen. The causative organism is most commonly the group A, β-hemolytic streptococcus, but the disease is not a bacterial infection of the kidney; rather, it appears to be a manifestation of some obscure antigen-antibody reaction that damages the glomerular capillaries. Acute poststreptococcal glomerulonephritis resembles acute serum sickness nephritis, which is induced by administration of large doses of heterologous serum proteins. In both diseases, onset follows insult with comparable delay, deposition of immunoglobulin in the glomerular capillaries occurs, and serum complement is markedly depressed. It has been observed that mixtures of large amounts of antibody and small amounts of antigen form insoluble and unreactive complexes; the inverse proportions of antibody and antigen form soluble macromolecular complexes, which on intravenous administration tend to localize in glomeruli. In both diseases, γ-globulin and $\beta_1 C$-globulin are deposited in a fine nodular pattern adjacent to the basement membranes of glomerular capillaries. For these several reasons, it is believed that acute poststreptococcal nephritis is an expression of damage resulting from antigen-antibody complexes; but the antigen has not been defined.

In acute glomerulonephritis, the glomeruli are diffusely involved: the capillary lumens are partially or completely obstructed by proliferating endothelial cells and by the deposition of hyalin fibers; the loops are compressed from without by crescents of epithelial cells, which pile up within the cleft between Bowman's capsule and the glomerular tuft. Polymorphonuclear leukocytes invade the tuft, and the basement membrane thickens. In those cases seen at autopsy, many glomeruli are bloodless and apparently nonfunctional. Relatively little change in tubular morphology is evident, although the cells may exhibit moderate derangements of function.

All who have studied renal function in acute glomerulonephritis have observed that the filtration rate is reduced. PAH and Diodrast clearances are also commonly reduced, but not in proportion to the reduction of filtration rate. Accordingly, filtration fraction is depressed (2). In those instances in which renal extraction of PAH has been measured, it has been found to be subnormal. Calculations of true renal plasma flow and true renal blood flow, corrected for reduced extraction, have demonstrated an absolute renal hyperemia in a number of instances (3); i.e., an actual increase in renal blood flow above normal. Relative hyperemia — i.e., high blood flow per unit of functional tubular mass (C_{PAH}/Tm_{PAH}) — has been observed routinely. The finding of renal hyperemia is in accord with the viewpoint that glomerulonephritis is an inflammatory disease. Filtration rate is determined by (1) the area of the capillary filtering surface, (2) the effective filtration pressure and (3) the permeability of the capillary membranes. A major cause of reduced filtration rate in acute glomerulonephritis is the reduction of the filtering surface, owing to the proliferation and piling-up of endothelial and epithelial cells. Many capillaries are completely blocked; others, by cell overgrowth, are rendered ineffective as filters. The latter might well be considered less than normally permeable. However, most of the patent capillaries must be excessively permeable, because they permit increased filtration of protein. Some capillaries rupture and allow red blood cells to escape into Bowman's capsule. Filtration rate may also decrease, in consequence of a reduction in effective filtration pressure caused by afferent arteriolar spasm. The azotemia of acute nephritis seems adequately explained by the reduction in filtration rate; the hematuria, by rupture of occasional glomerular capillaries; and the proteinuria, by increased permeability of those glomerular capillaries that remain patent and functional.

At least moderate involvement of tubular function in acute glomerulonephritis is indicated by reduced extraction and by moderate to marked reduction in maximum transport capacities for Diodrast and PAH (2, 3). However, the reduction of tubular function is not as severe as that of glomerular function. The C_{in}/Tm_{PAH} ratio is low, and glomerulotubular imbalance with tubular preponderance exists. Oliguria, retention of salt and water, and edema are expressions of glomerulotubular imbalance — in part a consequence of reduced filtration rate. The delivery of less than normal volumes of filtrate into tubules with nearly normal reabsorptive capacities results in over-reabsorption of salt and water. However, glomerulotubular imbalance may also be a consequence of enhanced tubular reabsorption of salt and water, stimulated by hypersecretion of aldosterone. Some investigators have found evidence of a generalized vasculitis, which finds its most significant expression in the glomerular capillaries but which results in leakage of protein and fluid through capillaries in other parts of the body, characteristically in periorbital tissue. However, edematous fluid in nephritis is not unusually rich in protein. Others have claimed that congestive heart failure is a common, if not a general, complication of acute glomerulonephritis, but studies of cardiac output in glomerulonephritis have failed to confirm this view (4).

The cause of hypertension in acute glomerulonephritis is not known. Renal ischemia is probably not a major factor, for neither absolute renal blood flow nor blood flow per unit of tubular mass (C_{PAH}/Tm_{PAH}) correlates significantly with the degree of hypertension (3, 4). Reduced excretion of, or reduced renal destruction of, some pressor factor or reduced formation of a neutralizing factor might account more adequately for hypertension.

In a majority of instances, signs of healing of the acute lesions of glomerulonephritis are evident within 3 weeks or less. Most of the patients recover completely and regain normal renal function. However, a few die in the initial episode; others progress into a subacute or progressive chronic stage of the disease with repeated acute exacerbations and remissions, ending in uremia and death.

SUBACUTE AND CHRONIC GLOMERULONEPHRITIS. — The term "subacute glomerulonephritis" is a misnomer. It refers to a chronic form of the disease, the cardial features of which are massive proteinuria, hypoproteinemia, hypercholesterolemia and edema. This stage of glomerulonephritis is functionally so much like lipoid nephrosis that both conditions will be discussed under the heading Nephrotic Syndrome (p. 275).

As a result of repeated acute exacerbations or gradual progression of chronic glomerulonephritis, glomeruli and tubules are destroyed in increasing numbers; in turn, this results in fibrosis and scarring. The remaining nephrons exhibit an amazing diversity of structure and, undoubtedly, of function as well. Some tubules hypertrophy; others atrophy. Some glomeruli are completely obliterated; others consist of only a few patent capillary loops; still others hypertrophy. Gross morphologic glomerulotubular imbalance results. The renal vascular bed is much reduced. Arterioles become thickened, and direct arterial connections with tubular capillaries develop. The kidney is no longer a kidney in the usual sense (5).

The renal functional measurements of glomerular filtration rate and minimum effective renal plasma flow become suspect under such circumstances — the latter more so than the former. Actually, the clearance of inulin and of mannitol agree within ±10%, even when absolute values are quite low. If increased back diffusion through sick but intact tubular cells were a significant factor, then one would expect poor agreement, for mannitol is a much smaller and more diffusible molecule than inulin. However, the clearance of PAH certainly has a different significance in patients with severe chronic renal disease than in normal subjects. The renal arteriovenous extraction of PAH may be as low as 14% in terminal glomerulonephritis, whereas it averages 91% normally. When extraction ratios are determined, renal plasma flow and renal blood flow are found to be far greater than clearance measurements alone would indicate (3). Relative renal hyperemia is observed when true renal blood flow is measured, even when the filtration rate is reduced to a small fraction of its normal value.

In the course of chronic glomerulonephritis, the glomerular filtration rate progressively falls. Azotemia of moderate but significant proportions develops when the glomerular filtration rate declines to less than half of normal; i.e., to less than 60 ml/min. Patients who exhibit azotemia have, on average, kidneys that weigh less than half of normal, because of extensive loss of nephrons. Nitrogen retention and elevation of blood levels of phosphate, sulfate, urate, creatinine, etc., are adequately explained by a reduction in filtration rate, due to total obliteration of some glomeruli and to reduction in numbers of patent capillary loops of others.

When true renal plasma and blood flows are determined, the filtration fraction is found to be low, much as it is in the acute phase of the disease. Certain tubular functions, however, suffer greater reduction than filtration rate in terminal azotemic glomerulonephritis. PAH extraction and Tm_{PAH} are both very low, and the ratio C_{in}/Tm_{PAH} increases above normal. This is probably, in part, a result of specific depression of the PAH transport mechanism, for C_{in}/Tm_G ratios remain normal, although splay of the titration curve increases. Glucosuria and aminoaciduria do not occur in terminal glomerulonephritis; therefore, the glomerular filtration rate and the transport capacities for glucose and amino acids decrease more or less proportionally.

However, glomerulotubular imbalance with glomerular preponderance does develop with respect to salt and water reabsorption. In the absence of frank congestive failure, excessive salt and water loss rather than salt and water retention is a significant problem. Any severe restriction of the intake of salt and water, or any abnormal loss by the azotemic patient, leads to negative balance, reduction in extracellular fluid volume, further reduction in filtration rate and the precipitation of frank uremia.

Hypertension is a significant feature of chronic glomerulonephritis. In view of relative hyperemia — i.e., high true renal blood flow per unit of functional tubular mass — ischemia may not be the major factor. However, the degree of hypertension does correlate reasonably well with the reduction in Tm_{PAH} (functional tubular mass) when the latter decreases below 40% of normal. Again, hypertension may be more closely related to loss of a pressor excretory or neutralizing function than to reduced blood perfusion per se.

Proteinuria in chronic glomerulonephritis is much less severe than in the nephrotic syndrome; and it tends to decrease as filtration rate declines. Edema is not a problem when congestive heart failure is absent. To a major degree, diminished filtration of protein can be ascribed to the reduction in filtration rate. However, in comparison with the massive protein loss of the nephrotic stage of nephritis, reduced loss in chronic azotemic glomerulonephritis may also indicate that the few remaining functional glomeruli regain more normal permeability relationships.

Metabolic acidosis is a characteristic feature of the azotemic stage of chronic glomerulonephritis, although the urine may be quite acidic until the end stage of the disease. Accordingly, no specific inability to reabsorb bicarbonate and to develop a relatively high concentration of hydrogen ions across the epithelium of the collecting ducts exists. However, the secretion of ammonia is markedly reduced. Because ammonia secretion enables the kidney to eliminate acid anions and to restore sodium to the body as sodium bicarbonate, the loss of secretory capacity results in acidosis; i.e., the bicarbonate concentration and the pH of extracellular fluid decrease. Kussmaul breathing (hyperpnea of extreme degree) is characteristic of terminal uremia and is a sign of partial respiratory compensation for the severe metabolic acidosis. Plasma concentrations of phosphate and sulfate increase, these two anions displacing equivalent amounts of bicarbonate. Hyperphosphatemia and hypersulfatemia are consequences of low glomerular filtration rate; plasma concentrations increase until the filtered loads approach normal values.

Potassium retention is not a significant factor in chronic glomerulonephritis until terminal uremia supervenes. Apparently, the potassium secretory mechanism remains relatively intact in functional tubules until the reduction in their numbers compromises maintenance of proper blood levels. This occurs when other elements of uremia develop.

PYELONEPHRITIS

Chronic pyelonephritis of some degree is a common finding in routine autopsies; in two series, the incidence was 6% (6, 7). Because symptoms are minimal and variable in many persons, the diagnosis is often missed during life. In far-advanced disease, with attendant hypertension and azotemia, there is no means of distinguishing pyelonephritis from glomerulonephritis and nephrosclerosis.

Pyelonephritis is a manifestation of bacterial infection of the kidneys. Causal organisms are most frequently *Escherichia coli* and staphylococci. The renal lesion consists of interstitial infiltrates of leukocytes or tiny abscesses, restricted for the most part to the renal medulla. The infection is patchy in distribution, and great differences exist in the extent of inflammation and destruction in the two kidneys and in different parts of the same kidney. Tubular destruction is followed by scarring; atrophic and cystic remnants of tubules are embedded in the scars. The glomeruli retain their normal structure much

longer, being destroyed only when the infection breaks through Bowman's capsule. Pyelonephritis is commonly associated with obstructive lesions in and infections of the lower urinary tract and with the presence of stones in the renal pelvis or the bladder. Because the disease is so frequently unrecognized until late in its course, functional studies in the early stages are few.

Localization of the lesions in the medulla suggests that the major, and perhaps primary, disturbances in function might be expected to involve activities of the collecting ducts and the loops of Henle (8). According to Brod (7), the most sensitive diagnostic test of pyelonephritis is impairment of the maximum concentrating ability of the kidney when fluid intake is restricted. Kaitz (9) showed that the concentrating power is reduced in pregnant women who exhibit asymptomatic bacteriuria without other evidence of renal disease; presumably this is the earliest stage of pyelonephritis. One may infer that inflammatory foci reduce the ability of the loops of Henle to establish the hypertonicity of the medullary interstitium on which urinary concentration depends.

Acidosis in chronic pyelonephritis is also a characteristic finding, which may be ascribed to depression of collecting-duct function. More specifically, renal tubular acidosis is occasionally associated with chronic pyelonephritis, although its basis is frequently genetic (10). The cardinal features of renal tubular acidosis in pyelonephritis are hyperchloremia; inability to form a highly acid urine; absence of significant glomerular insufficiency; excessive urinary excretion of calcium, phosphate, potassium and bicarbonate ions; and the development of osteomalacia. Milkman's syndrome—bone pain with radiographic evidence of osteomalacia and pseudofractures—may be the first evidence of pyelonephritis. The fundamental disturbance seems to be a reduced capacity to establish and maintain a high gradient of hydrogen ions across the epithelium of the collecting ducts. Reduced exchange of hydrogen for sodium ions results in the excretion of alkaline urine, loss of bicarbonate ions, enhanced exchange of potassium for sodium ions and depletion of body potassium stores. Reabsorption of calcium, also in part a function of the distal nephron, is depressed, leading to hypercalciuria and osteomalacia. Ammonia excretion is reduced, but whether the deficiency is one of ammonia production or one of secretion of ammonia into less than normally acid urine is unknown.

As destruction of the renal parenchyma progresses, the glomerular filtration rate, renal plasma flow, Tm_{PAH} PAH extraction and renal blood flow decrease (3, 6). Filtration rate is reduced less than is renal blood flow; hence, filtration fraction increases. The reduction in filtration rate may be more a function of destruction of attached tubules than of loss of glomeruli. The reduction of Tm_{PAH} no doubt represent, in part, a loss of tubular tissue and, in part, a depression of the transport mechanism of marginally functional cells. Reduction in Tm_{PAH} is greater than in blood flow when the latter is corrected for incomplete extraction.

Nephrosis

The term "nephrosis" is variously applied to a variety of dissimilar renal diseases characterized by alterations in tubular structure, presumably of a degenerative nature, It includes the subacute or nephrotic stage of glomerulonephritis, lipoid nephrosis, and tubular necrosis induced by nephrotoxic chemicals and by intense renal ischemia and anoxia. In the nephrotic stage of glomerulonephritis and in lipoid nephrosis, the primary lesion is glomerular, not tubular, and the clinical and physiologic manifestations issue chiefly from this defect. The glomeruli are abnormally permeable to protein; tubular changes are, in large part, secondary to excessive protein reabsorption and to altered lipid metabolism. Chemical necrosis of tubular cells is induced by mercury, lead, uranium, bismuth, oxalate, tartrate, bichromate, elemental phosphorus, carbon tetrachloride,

bacterial toxins, etc. Ischemic anoxic necrosis of tubular cells occurs following transfusions of incompatible blood, hemolytic crises, prolonged peripheral circulatory failure and massive trauma (hemorrhagic and surgical shock). Nephrotoxic chemicals not only act as tubular protoplasmic poisons but may also induce intense renal vasoconstriction and ischemic necrosis.

NEPHROTIC SYNDROME

The nephrotic syndrome includes massive albuminuria, hypoalbuminemia, generalized edema, and hyperlipemia characterized by a marked elevation of plasma cholesterol. It occurs in the course of glomerulonephritis in some, but not all, patients; in amyloid disease; and in intercapillary glomerulosclerosis. In children, the nephrotic syndrome occurs in lipoid nephrosis, often in the absence of evidence of glomerulonephritis. Whether lipoid nephrosis is a distinct disease entity or an expression of one form of juvenile glomerulonephritis is uncertain. In some patients, the disease progresses and culminates in renal failure, which is indistinguishable from that of chronic glomerulonephritis. Many recover completely without exhibiting, at any time, hematuria, hypertension and azotemia and with no recognized preceding streptococcal infection.

The major functional defect in the nephrotic syndrome, whatever its cause, is a marked increase in the permeability of glomerular capillaries to protein. According to Richards et al. the protein concentration of glomerular filtrate is normally less than 30 mg/100 ml. If one assumes no reabsorption and no secretion of protein, the minimum concentration of protein in the filtrate (11) is given by the following equation:

$$F_p = \frac{U_p \cdot V}{GFR}$$

where F_p is the minimum concentration of protein in the filtrate (milligrams per milliliter); U_p, the concentration of protein in the urine (milligrams per milliliter); V, the urine volume (milliliters per minute); and GFR, the filtration rate (milliliters per minute).

In the nephrotic syndrome, the calculated minimum concentration of protein in the filtrate exceeds 30 mg/100 ml, except when the plasma albumin is very low; and it may attain a value as high as 200 mg/100 ml when the plasma albumin is raised toward normal (11). There is no evidence that proteinuria results from diminished tubular reabsorption of albumin; indeed, reabsorption in nephrosis is no doubt increased as a result of the increased filtered load.

Light microscopy often reveals little change in glomerular structure. However, electron microscopy has shown that the glomerular membranes are strikingly altered. Pedicels of epithelial cells are lost; their cytoplasm flattens out into an undifferentiated layer covering the basement membrane; and slit pores disappear. The basement membrane exhibits degenerative changes, including swelling and a punched-out or moth-eaten appearance. Increased permeability to protein has been variously ascribed to changes in the dimensions of slit pores and to alterations in the structure of the basement membranes, depending on the bias of the investigator.

The massive edema and ascites which characterize the full-blown nephrotic syndrome are undoubtedly worsened by hypoalbuminemia, which in turn is the consequence of albuminuria. However, the basic abnormality must be enhanced tubular reabsorption of salt and water. A circulating plasma volume of 3.5 L obviously cannot support the formation of 20 L or more of edematous and ascitic fluid. Water and salt must be retained in the body. In the nephrotic syndrome as it develops in the course of chronic glomerulonephritis, filtration rate is often reduced, and this may contribute to glomerulotubular imbalance. However, in classic lipoid nephrosis without evidence of nephritis, the filtration rate is often greater than normal. Glomerulotubular imbalance must, in these instances, be an expression of enhanced tubular reabsorption of salt and wa-

ter, not of reduced filtration. Increased secretion of aldosterone undoubtedly is a major cause of edema in the nephrotic syndrome. Hypoalbuminemia, of course, favors filtration and restricts the reabsorption of fluid in all capillary beds, but especially in those of the splanchnic regions and of dependent parts of the body.

The tubular changes that have so impressed pathologists in the past are probably in large part a consequence of the reabsorption of excessive amounts of protein and of alterations in lipid metabolism. The kidneys are large and pale; the cortex is greasy and putty-like. The tubular cells are loaded with hyalin and lipid droplets and doubly refractile bodies containing cholesterol esters. In comparison with the marked morphologic changes, functional alterations, except for proteinuria and salt and water retention, are remarkably few in the absence of evidence of nephritis. In so-called true lipoid nephrosis, glomerular filtration rate and renal plasma flow are either normal or somewhat increased. Hypertension and azotemia are rare. When the nephrotic syndrome is associated with nephritis, the changes are those of the early chronic stages of the disease.

TUBULAR NECROSIS

Both nephrotoxic agents and prolonged renal ischemia and anoxia cause necrosis of the renal tubular epithelium. Tubular necrosis, independent of causation, results in acute renal failure: anuria or severe oliguria and rapidly developing uremia (12, 13). Nephrotoxic chemicals, such as bichloride of mercury and carbon tetrachloride, affect primarily the proximal tubule. Because these agents are blood-borne, involvement is diffuse. The epithelium shows cloudy swelling, vacuolation, nuclear fragmentation and dissolution of the brush border. Cells slough into the tubular lumen. Glomeruli are not involved, and the basement membranes of the tubules remain intact. Oliver (14) referred to this type of lesion as nephrotoxic necrosis.

Ischemic injury differs both in nature and

in distribution. It is observed in classic form in hemorrhagic shock and in the reaction to a mismatched blood transfusion. Necrosis is patchy, rather than diffuse, and may involve any segment of the nephron, except that the collecting duct seems resistant to damage. A small portion of the nephron may be involved, with intact and presumably functional epithelium on either side. The lesion itself consists in localized destruction of the epithelium with occasional rupture of the basement membrane. Oliver (14) referred to this lesion as tubulorhexis. Its distribution is patchy because the ischemia is irregular in distribution, some areas suffering a greater reduction in blood flow than others. The distribution and nature of these lesions were determined by the painstaking process of teasing whole nephrons from blocks of acid-fixed and macerated kidneys under binocular magnification.

Fortunately, the kidney has the capacity to regenerate such damaged tubular epithelium within a period of 2 – 3 weeks, provided conservative management or dialysis can prevent the development of fatal changes in the composition and volume of the body fluids. In nephrotoxic necrosis, tubular regeneration begins in scattered islands of viable cells. Because the basement membrane remains intact, a framework exists for the orderly spread of newborn cells to reconstitute the tubule. The epithelium is at first atypical: the cells are flattened with irregular borders, inclusions are sparse and the brush border is absent. At first the regenerating tubules can probably do little more than serve as conduits for filtrate. Eventually the cytologic picture of normal renal tissue is restored. In tubulorhexis, the basement membrane may be locally destroyed and the tubule invaded by granulation tissue. Restoration of the tubular conduit under these conditions may be impossible. However, because the lesion is patchy and rupture of the basement membrane is by no means universal, the epithelial integrity of most of the tubules can be restored.

Because anuria or extreme oliguria is the rule, clearance methods cannot be used as means of studying the early stages of the disease. The effective rate of glomerular filtration is zero. However, some investigators infer from the normal appearance of glomeruli that filtration continues and that the filtrate is reabsorbed in its entirety through damaged epithelium. Brun *et al.* (15), using renal arteriovenous differences and the renal uptake of radioactive krypton (^{85}Kr), showed that blood flow during the anuric phase is low but by no means zero. In the diuretic phase, which develops early in the stage of functional recovery, the glomerular filtration rate, extraction of PAH, and tubular reabsorptive and secretory capacities are all extremely low. Blood flow is low even when corrected for incomplete extraction. Months may be required to restore all of the renal functions to normal.

Glomerulotubular imbalance with relative glomerular preponderance is evident in the early diuretic phase of recovery from acute renal failure. High urine flow, inability to concentrate the urine if fluid intake is inadequate, and salt loss are hazards of the early recovery phase. Although diureses in these days of more enlightened therapy are not so profound as in the early days of excessive hydration, loss of salt and water may complicate recovery.

Nephrosclerosis

Essential hypertension is a relatively common disease if one accepts, as minimum criteria, a systolic blood pressure consistently above 140 mm Hg and, more important, a diastolic blood pressure consistently above 90 mm Hg. So defined, the disease is common, affecting about 25% of the population above the age of 40 years. Obviously, the condition, en masse, is relatively benign; i.e., compatible with many years of active life. Of those who die of their hypertensive disease, about two thirds succumb to heart disease (i.e., congestive failure or coronary thrombosis); about one quarter, to cerebral vascular accidents; and the remaining one tenth or so, to chronic renal disease. Benign nephrosclerosis describes the renal manifestations of essential hypertension. The name "benign nephrosclerosis" derives from the spotty scarring of the renal parenchyma commonly observed at autopsy in patients with hypertension of long duration. Obviously, the renal damage is not of serious proportions in the vast majority of cases. Malignant nephrosclerosis is a fulminating form of hypertensive disease characterized by rapidly progressing renal insufficiency and death in uremia if the patient is spared an earlier cardiac or cerebrovascular climax.

The primary histologic changes in the kidneys in hypertensive disease are observed in the arterioles and small arteries. In benign nephrosclerosis, the vascular lesion consists in proliferation of the intima, subintimal deposition of lipoid and hyalin materials and hypertrophy of the media. Glomerular involvement is not remarkable, degeneration apparently following tubular atrophy. Scattered tubules atrophy, presumably in consequence of vascular insufficiency, and scarring results. Arteriolar lesions are probably a consequence of long-standing hypertension due to humoral or neural vasoconstriction, rather than a primary expression of an arteriolar disease that, of itself, results in hypertension. In malignant nephrosclerosis, the vascular lesion is a necrotizing arteriolitis with widespread subintimal hyalinization and collagenous intimal thickening. The necrotic lesions in arteriolar walls are commonly associated with thrombosis. Atrophy of tubules varies considerably, depending on the duration of the disease. In contrast to minimal functional derangements in benign nephrosclerosis, those in malignant nephrosclerosis may be catastrophic.

Many young people with essential hypertension have measurements of renal blood flow and renal extraction within normal ranges. However, in a group of hypertensive patients without regard to age, the renal blood flow is reduced both in absolute terms and relative to glucose and Diodrast Tm. The kidneys are, thus, relatively ischemic.

Glomerular filtration rate is well maintained despite the reduction in blood flow and Tm values (16). Filtration fraction is, therefore, higher than normal. Hypertensive disease causes a greater reduction in $Tm_{Diodrast}$ than in Tm_G. Accordingly, only a part of the reduction in transport capacity can be assigned to the destruction and fibrosis of tubules; a part must be due to a specific depression of the secretory transport mechanisms (17). Pyrogens, which cause renal hyperemia and lowering of filtration fraction in normal persons, also induce the same changes in hypertensive patients. This indicates that the increased renal vascular resistance is at least partly functional; i.e., due to vasoconstriction rather than to arteriolar obstruction.

In malignant nephrosclerosis, functional changes are more dramatic. Renal blood flow, Tm_{PAH} and PAH extraction are all reduced. Secretory Tm values are more markedly depressed than blood flow; and blood flow, in turn, is more depressed than filtration rate. Because elevated blood pressure in both benign and malignant nephrosclerosis sustains the filtration rate to a greater extent than blood flow, at least some fraction of the increase in resistance must be postglomerular.

Toxemia of Pregnancy

Toxemia of pregnancy is characterized by hypertension, proteinuria and edema, all developing within the last 5 months of pregnancy. Its cause is unknown, although some investigators have speculated that an antigen-antibody reaction somewhat akin to that of glomerulonephritis is the basic abnormality. Edema (gain in weight) and proteinuria precede the hypertension; azotemia and hematuria are rare, except in severe cases. Characteristically, the disturbances clear rapidly following delivery; however, in some patients, hypertension and evidence of renal disease persist.

The most characteristic lesion is that of the glomeruli, which are diffusely involved. The glomeruli are bloodless, swollen and excessively cellular. Epithelial and endo-thelial cells are enlarged and are increased in numbers. The basement membranes are swollen, and the capillary lumens are reduced in diameter. The rather solid-looking glomeruli have a foamy or reticulated appearance. Fatty and hyalin droplets are numerous in the tubular cells.

Glomerular filtration rate and renal blood flow increase progressively over the first 8 months of normal pregnancy but return toward control values during the final month before delivery. In toxemia, filtration rate and renal blood flow are moderately reduced below normal levels of nonpregnant controls, the extent of the reduction varying with the severity of the toxemia. However, in comparison with values for normal pregnant controls, the reductions in filtration rate and renal blood flow in toxemia are more remarkable. Plasma urate concentration is elevated in toxemia, in association with a reduction in urate clearance, to a value about half of normal. Plasma urea concentration is not significantly altered. Proteinuria and reduced rate of glomerular filtration are adequately explained by the changes in glomerular structure and perfusion. Edema must be a result of glomerulotubular imbalance, which in large part probably is due to enhanced secretion of aldosterone (3, 18).

Congenital Disorders

Congenital disorders of renal function fall into two groups: disorders related to structural malformations and those arising from inborn defects in mechanisms of tubular transport.

POLYCYSTIC DISEASE

Polycystic disease is perhaps the commonest of the disorders of the structural type. The infant form, in which failure of union of glomerular and tubular anlagen is widespread, often results in early death from uremia. The so-called adult form of the disease may be an expression of the same type of structural defect existing at birth but involving fewer units. Numerous tiny cysts are formed; these grow larger as the years pass, enlarging the entire kidney and compressing and ultimately destroying normal nephrons. According to Lambert (19), cysts also arise from dysplastic alterations of tubules; in some instances, the walls balloon out and pinch off as cysts, and in other instances the cystic dilations retain their continuity with the remainder of the nephron. Serious functional abnormalities may not arise until the third or fourth decade of life. Lambert injected inulin into patients with polycystic disease shortly before death and observed inulin in cystic fluid in higher concentration than in blood plasma—an indication of continuing glomerular filtration and reabsorption of water. Accordingly, even markedly malformed nephrons may perform useful renal work. This may explain why patients frequently do well for years despite significant azotemia. Functional studies on polycystic disease are few. Glomerular filtration rate and tubular transport capacities are reduced. Diagnosis is usually made on the basis of azotemia, palpably enlarged kidneys and radiographic findings.

INBORN DEFECTS OF TUBULAR TRANSPORT

Within the past two decades, a number of syndromes characterized by one or more defects in tubular transport have been described. For the most part, these defects are congenital; however, some of them may be closely mimicked, if not actually duplicated, in acquired renal disease. A number have been shown to have a genetic basis. Although relatively rare, inborn errors of tubular transport are of interest for several reasons. First, a number of the defects can be very adequately compensated by long-term replacement therapy. Second, the syndromes offer a unique opportunity for the study of the nature and interrelationships of specific tubular transport mechanisms. Third, this group of disorders is of major interest to medical geneticists, because surveys of families, and even large population groups, can frequently be made on the basis of relatively simple laboratory examinations of blood and urine (10, 19). Two such disorders have already been considered: benign renal glucosuria and uricosuria in the Dalmatian dog. The latter disorder is transmitted by a single recessive gene.

NEPHROGENIC DIABETES INSIPIDUS. — This condition is characterized by polyuria, inability to concentrate the urine on fluid restriction and a lack of responsiveness to large doses of pitressin, despite normal renal function in all other respects. In infants, the condition is likely to be associated with severe dehydration, hyperosmolarity of the body fluids, fever without evidence of infection, and retarded growth and mental development. If fluid intake is high, the infant thrives, especially if salt intake is restricted to reduce the total daily solute load (10). Glomerular filtration rate and all tubular functions other than that of urinary concentration are within normal limits. No evidence of pituitary dysfunction exists, and histologic studies of the kidneys have revealed no obvious lesion. The condition is familial and at one time was thought to be a sex-linked recessive trait. However, more recently it has been observed in females and is probably incompletely recessive, in view of the fact that mothers and grandmothers of affected infants may exhibit an impaired concentrating ability.

RENAL TUBULAR ACIDOSIS. — Renal tubular acidosis (RTA) has been described in some detail on page 209. Two types are recognized: one proximal, the other distal in origin. Either type may be idiopathic or acquired. Of course acidosis in renal disease is always tubular in origin, but RTA is distinguished from the acidosis of chronic end-stage renal disease as occurring in individuals with essentially normal glomerular filtration rates and without signs of azotemia and uremia.

Proximal RTA is characterized by a deficiency in proximal secretion of hydrogen ions, thus in proximal reabsorption of bicarbonate. The distal tubules are flooded with bicarbonate and the excess above their limited reabsorptive capacities is excreted in the urine. In contrast, in distal RTA the final urine cannot be acidified to a greater extent than pH 6.6 to 7.0; i.e., to the pH of tubular urine as it leaves the proximal tubule. Abstraction of bicarbonate from the final urine is incomplete and loss in the urine is greater than normal. The functional consequences of both types of RTA, the self-limited nature of the proximal type and the treatment of both types are given on page 210.

RENAL HYPOPHOSPHATEMIA, RENAL HYPERPHOSPHATURIA, AND VITAMIN D-RESISTANT RICKETS. — These conditions all refer to a single syndrome, characterized by continued excretion of phosphate despite reduction in plasma phosphate concentration. The phosphate clearance is, therefore, abnormally high. Phosphate Tm is reduced to about half of the usual value, and, because excretion is significant at very low plasma levels, the titration curve must exhibit abnormal splay. Other renal functions are normal; glucosuria and aminoaciduria do not occur. Renal hypophosphatemia is the commonest cause of rickets in children in areas in which vitamin D intake is adequate (10).

The defect in tubular reabsorption of phosphate is transmitted as a sex-linked dominant trait. The full syndrome occurs in male children of couples of which one or the other parent is hypophosphatemic. When the trait is transmitted by the mother, her hypophosphatemia is asymptomatic; apparently, a normal allele ameliorates the manifestations of the underlying disorder.

GENERALIZED RENAL AMINOACIDURIA. — Generalized renal aminoaciduria occurs in cystinosis, heavy metal poisoning, Wilson's disease, galactosemia, scurvy, Lysol poisoning, multiple myeloma, the Fanconi syndrome and various other conditions. The pattern of amino acid excretion in these conditions is highly variable and is probably more of an expression of nonspecific cell injury than of interference with discrete transport mechanisms. Specific aminoacidurias, including essential cystinuria, glycinuria, β-aminoisobutyric aciduria and Hartnup disease are more definitely related to defects in individual transport mechanisms and, for the most part, have a genetic basis.

ESSENTIAL CYSTINURIA.—This disease is characterized by increased urinary excretion of cystine, lysine, arginine and ornithine. Plasma concentrations are subnormal, indicating that increased metabolic production and overflow are not the cause of enhanced excretion. Filtration rate is commonly normal (22, 23), no glucosuria occurs, the reabsorption of other amino acids is nearly complete, and tubular reabsorption of salt and water is undisturbed.

Cystine is normally reabsorbed to the extent of 95% or more. In essential cystinuria, reabsorption may be nearly zero; and, in an occasional patient, the net secretion of cystine can be demonstrated (24). Reabsorption of cystine is most depressed, reabsorption of arginine and lysine is somewhat less depressed, and reabsorption of ornithine is least depressed.

Studies of essential cystinuria provided the first clear-cut evidence that the four amino acids—cystine, lysine, arginine and ornithine—are reabsorbed by a single mechanism. Attention has been focused on cystine because its low solubility underlies the frequent formation of cystine stones in the urinary tract. Dent and Harris (25) showed that two genetic types of essential cystinuria exist. In one, the defect is transmitted as a typically mendelian recessive gene: in the homozygote, all four amino acids are excreted in excessive amounts; in the heterozygote, none. In the other type, the defect is incompletely recessive. Three classes of cystinuric subjects exist: those with the complete defect, those who excrete increased amounts of cystine and lysine but not of the other two amino acids, and those with no phenotypic defect themselves but who transmit the trait.

SIMPLE GLYCINURIA.—This syndrome is characterized by a single defect in amino acid transport (26). All other discrete renal functions are normal. In three generations of one family, four female subjects were affected, and the inheritance pattern suggests a dominant gene. Renal lithiasis with oxalate stones containing glycine was observed in three of the four siblings.

β-AMINOISOBUTYRIC ACIDURIA.—This common condition affects 5% of the population. No other defects in tubular function are observed, and the condition is of no clinical import. β-Aminoisobutyric acid is normally reabsorbed to the extent of 95% or more. In affected persons, reabsorption may be 25% or less (27).

HARTNUP DISEASE.—Hartnup disease is a complex syndrome best described by the title of the original paper: "Hereditary pellagra-like skin rash with temporary cerebellar ataxia, constant renal aminoaciduria and other bizarre biochemical features" (28). The aminoaciduria differs from that of the so-called generalized category only in the fact that it does not involve any increase in proline excretion and is associated with no other defects in renal tubular function. The syndrome is familial.

FANCONI SYNDROME.—The Fanconi syndrome is a constellation of renal defects, most commonly including renal glucosuria, renal aminoaciduria and renal hypophosphatemia. The last-named may lead to rickets or osteomalacia, depending on the age of the patient. Because many causal factors are involved, the syndrome probably represents merely the summed effects of proximal tubular inadequacy, irrespective of cause. It is, however, significant that reabsorption of salt and water is unimpaired, although the bulk of these components of the filtrate are known to be reabsorbed in the proximal segment. Proximal inadequacy is, therefore, not entirely nonspecific. In addition to the triad of defects noted above, deficiencies in the renal regulation of the plasma concentrations of potassium, hydrogen ion and urate may also develop.

The infant form of the Fanconi syndrome is associated with a disturbance of cystine metabolism known as cystinosis. Cystine crystals are deposited in many organs — most commonly in the cornea, reticuloendothelial system, kidney and bone marrow. The disease is familial and is said to be the expression of a simple mendelian recessive factor. Renal function is normal until about the fifth month of life, when cystine crystals appear in the cornea and aminoaciduria and glucosuria develop.

The adult type of the Fanconi syndrome is similar to the infantile type, except that it occurs in the absence of cystinosis. The disease usually is first recognized with the onset of symptoms of osteomalacia or of potassium depletion. According to Dent and Harris (25), the adult trait is also the expression of a simple mendelian recessive gene.

Heavy metal poisoning with lead, cadmium, mercury or uranium is associated with one or more of the features of the Fanconi syndrome. With recognition of the heavy metal intoxication and adequate treatment, the renal defect may clear completely. Wilson's disease, an inborn error of copper metabolism, is also associated with the Fanconi syndrome — no doubt a result of excessive deposition of copper within the proximal tubular epithelium. Multiple myeloma and glycogen storage disease may also be associated with the syndrome. Darmady and Stranack (29), in a microdissection study of a limited number of kidneys from cases of the Fanconi syndrome, have observed a "gooseneck" atrophy of the first part of the proximal tubule. It is tempting to speculate that atrophy of this portion of the nephron, either for genetic reasons or as a consequence of renal cystinosis or heavy metal intoxication, results in reduced reabsorption of phosphate, glucose and amino acids (10).

Intact Nephron Hypothesis

"A large number of disease entities exhibit predilection for the complete destruction of nephrons. As nephron destruction proceeds and the number of surviving units diminishes, the economy of the human being becomes altered indelibly, until ultimately there evolve the multiple system abnormalities which characterize the uremic state" (Bricker et al. [30]). The "intact nephron hypothesis" of Bricker maintains that nephrons, when diseased, are destroyed in toto. The residual nephrons are essentially normal. Uremia develops in consequence of the destruction of so many nephrons that the composition of the body fluids is irrevocably compromised. Uremia is not a consequence of the regulatory behavior of functionally distorted nephrons; rather, it is merely the result of a reduction in the numbers of nephrons.

In patients who have died of uremia due to end-stage renal disease, microdissection of the kidneys shows marked diversity of structure in the few residual nephrons (1). It is incomprehensible that a mixture of morphologic units — of aglomerular, hypertrophic and hyperplastic tubules and hypertrophic glomeruli joined to atrophic tubules — should not exhibit equivalent heterogeneity of function. It is equally evident that such architectural heterogeneity is compatible with continuing existence, at least for a limited period of time in the absence of stress; thus, remarkable compensations of glomerular and tubular functions must exist in these residual caricatures of nephrons.

A controversy has arisen between proponents of these two views — a controversy that may be more semantic than rational. The term "intact nephron hypothesis" is a misnomer if applied to the residual nephrons in end-stage renal disease, especially if "intact" means "unchanged from normal." However, in support of his hypothesis, Bricker and his associates have shown, in patients with naturally occurring unilateral pyelonephritis, in dogs with induced unilateral pyelonephritis and in dogs with progressive infarction of portions of one kidney, that an equivalent degree of glomerulotubular balance exists in the two kidneys. Furthermore, when the normal kidneys of dogs were removed, in Bricker's laboratory, GFR and a variety of tubular functions of the abnormal kidneys increased, indicating residual adaptive capacity.

Figure 14–1 (upper panel) illustrates the fact that glomerular filtration rates of the two normal kidneys of a dog were equal. When one kidney was experimentally diseased or infarcted and GFR reduced to 35% of the control value, GFR of the normal kidney increased by 11%—an indication of glomerular adaptation. The lower panel illustrates the fact that a series of tubular functions, including secretion of PAH, NH_3, and titratable acid and reabsorption of glucose, phosphate and urate, were equal in the two normal kidneys. When one kidney was experimentally diseased or infarcted, these tubular functions decreased in proportion to the decrease in GFR. Thus, the ratio of tubular and glomerular functions remained constant and equal to that of the control kidney. This has reasonably been interpreted as indicating that, in certain renal diseases or at certain

stages of renal disease, nephrons are deleted one by one and in toto. Loss of a glomerulus is accompanied by loss of its attached tubule, and vice versa. The residual nephrons are essentially normal or retain normal glomerulotubular balance. This, in brief, is the intact nephron hypothesis.

This is certainly not true in the active inflammatory stage of chronic glomerular or tubular disease: note changes from normal in C_{in}/C_{PAH}, C_{in}/Tm_{PAH} in studies on human renal disease. Another point, which is glossed over by Bricker, is that his were not really models of end-stage renal disease. Total glomerular filtration rate in his unilaterally diseased or infarcted dogs was 73% of normal ($[111 + 35]/2 = 73\%$). Even when the normal kidney was removed, the GFR of the remaining diseased or infarcted kidney increased to such an extent that azotemia was minimal. Uremia did not develop.

Bricker has also performed glucose titra-

Fig. 14–1. — Functional relationships between two kidneys of the dog prior to and following induction of unilateral renal disease or infarction. *Upper panel*, change in filtration rate as a consequence of disease or infarction; *lower panel*, ratio of a series of tubular functions to glomerular filtration rate prior to and following induction of renal disease or infarction. (From Bricker, N. S., Klahr, S., Lubowitz, H., and Slatopolsky, E.: Pediat. Clin. N. A. 18:595, 1971.)

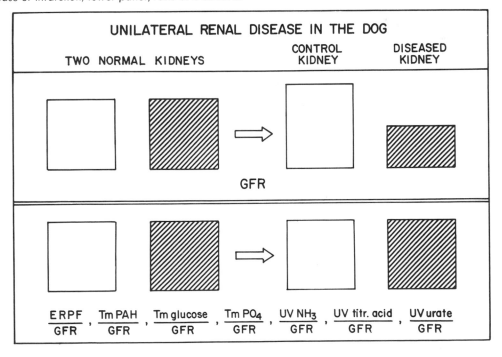

tions on the normal and diseased kidneys of his dogs (see Chapter 6). As might be expected, he found that the splays of the titration curves of normal and diseased kidneys were comparable. He therefore correctly inferred that heterogeneity of glomerular and tubular functions did not exist. However, the same criticism of Bricker's model may be made as before: it was not really one of chronic end-stage renal disease.

The intact nephron hypothesis may be accepted with certain reservations. It is probably true throughout most of the course of chronic renal disease, if one excludes the acute inflammatory phases of progressive active disease. It has not yet been determined when, in the course of chronic renal disease, heterogeneity of glomerular and tubular architecture and function first becomes significant. It certainly becomes significant in end-stage renal disease. Are the heterogeneic changes late terminal events, or do they occur earlier? Are they direct consequences of the disease process itself, or are they in part compensations for or reactions to the changes in composition of body fluids in uremia?

Summary

At onset, renal diseases may affect primarily the function of the glomerular capillary tuft (glomerulonephritis, lipoid nephrosis), the activities of one or another or all segments of the renal tubules (pyelonephritis, tubular necrosis, inborn defects of tubular transport) or the adequacy of blood perfusion of the renal parenchyma (nephrosclerosis). However, if the disease is progressive, functional derangements tend to become generalized. When damage to one element of the nephron leads to its destruction, other elements of the same nephron atrophy and are replaced by scar tissue. The functional mass of the kidney is reduced. However, neither morphologically nor functionally are glomeruli, tubules and blood vessels proportionally affected. Heterogeneity of the remaining nephron population is increased by atrophy of one portion of the nephron and hypertrophy of another, and functional imbalance results. The various symptoms of those renal diseases customarily grouped as chronic Bright's disease, nephritis, pyelonephritis, nephrosclerosis and polycystic disease ultimately converge into a common pattern of absolute renal insufficiency, with death from uremia. Acute tubular necrosis results either in early death from uremia or in more or less complete morphologic regeneration and return of function. A number of the inborn defects of tubular transport are not progressive and, if properly managed, are compatible with a relatively healthy life. Others, associated with cystinosis, renal calcinosis, renal lithiasis and pyelonephritis, may progress to renal insufficiency and death from uremia.

REFERENCES

1. Oliver, J.: *Architecture of the Kidney in Chronic Bright's Disease* (New York: Paul B. Hoeber, Inc., 1939).
2. Earle, D. P., Jr., Taggart, J. V., and Shannon, J. A.: Glomerulonephritis: A survey of the functional organization of the kidney in various stages of diffuse glomerulonephritis, J. Clin. Invest. 23:119, 1944.
3. Bradley, S. E., Bradley, G. P., Tyson, C. I., Curry, J. J., and Blake, W. D.: Renal function in renal diseases, Am. J. Med. 9:766, 1950.
4. Farber, S. J.: Physiologic aspects of glomerulonephritis, J. Chron. Dis. 5:87, 1957.
5. Oliver, J.: When is the kidney not a kidney?, J. Urol. 63:373, 1950.
6. Raaschau, F.: *Studies of Chronic Pyelonephritis with Special Reference to the Kidney Function* (Copenhagen: Ejnar Munksgaards Forlag, 1948).
7. Brod, J.: Chronic pyelonephritis, Lancet 1: 973, 1956.
8. Quinn, E. L., and Kass, E. H. (eds.): *The Biology of Pyelonephritis* (Boston: Little, Brown & Company, 1960).
9. Kaitz, A.: Urinary concentrating ability in pregnant women with asymptomatic bacteriuria, J. Clin. Invest. 40:1323, 1961.
10. Mudge, G.: Clinical patterns of tubular dysfunction, Am. J. Med. 24:785, 1958.
11. Chinard, F. P., Lauson, H. D., Eder, H. A., Greif, R. L., and Hiller, A.: The study of the mechanism of proteinuria in patients with the nephrotic syndrome, J. Clin. Invest. 33:621, 1954.

12. Smith, H. W.: Acute renal failure, Kaiser Found. M. Bull. 6:18, 1958.

13. Breen, C.: *Acute Anuria* (Copenhagen: Ejnar Munksgaards Forlag, 1954).

14. Oliver, J.: The pathogenesis of acute renal failure associated with traumatic and toxic injury: Renal ischemia, nephrotoxic damage and the ischemuric episode, J. Clin. Invest. 30:1305, 1951.

15. Brun, C., Crone, C., Davidsen, H. G., Fabricius, J., Hansen, A. T., Lassen, N. A., and Munck, O.: Renal blood flow in anuric human subjects determined by the use of radioactive krypton 85, Proc. Soc. Exp. Biol. & Med. 89:687, 1955.

16. Goldring, W., Chasis, H., Ranges, H. A., and Smith, H. W.: Effective renal blood flow in subjects with essential hypertension, J. Clin. Invest. 20:637, 1941.

17. Smith, H. W., Goldring, W., Chasis, H., Ranges, H. A., and Bradley, S. E.: The application of saturation methods to the study of glomerular and tubular function in the human kidney, J. Mt. Sinai Hosp., New York 10:59, 1943.

18. Fomon, S. J. (ed.): *Toxemia of Pregnancy: Report of the First Ross Obstetrical Research Conference* (Columbus, Ohio: Ross Laboratories, 1956).

19. Lambert, P. P.: Polycystic disease of the kidney: A review, Arch. Path. 44:34, 1947.

20. Burnett, C. H., and Williams, T. F.: An analysis of some features of renal tubular dysfunction, A.M.A. Arch. Int. Med. 102:881, 1958.

21. Albright, F., and Reifenstein, E. C.: *Parathyroid Glands and Metabolic Bone Disease* (Baltimore: Williams & Wilkins Company, 1948).

22. Dent, C. E., Senior, B., and Walshe, J. M.: The pathogenesis of cystinuria: II. Polarographic studies of the metabolism of sulfur containing amino acids, J. Clin. Invest. 33:1216, 1954.

23. Doolan, P. D., Harper, H. A., Hutchins, M. E., and Alpen, E. L.: Renal clearance of lysine in cystinuria, Am. J. Med. 23:416, 1957.

24. Frimpter, G. W., Horwith, M., Furth, E., Fellows, R. E., and Thompson, D. D.: Inulin and endogenous amino acid renal clearances in cystinuria: Evidence for tubular secretion, J. Clin. Invest. 41:281, 1962.

25. Dent, C. E., and Harris, H.: The genetics of "cystinuria," Ann. Eugenics 16:60, 1957.

26. De Vries, A., Kochwa, S., Lazebnik, J., Frank, M., and Djaldetti, M.: Glycinuria, a hereditary disorder associated with nephrolithiasis, Am. J. Med. 23:408, 1957.

27. Crumpler, H. R., Dent, C. E., Harris, H., and Westall, R. G.: β-Aminoisobutyric acid (α-methyl-β-alanine): A new amino acid obtained from human urine, Nature, London 167:307, 1951.

28. Baron, D. N., Dent, C. E., Harris, H., Hart, E. W., and Jepson, J. B.: Hereditary pellagra-like skin rash with temporary cerebellar ataxia, constant renal aminoaciduria and other bizarre biochemical features, Lancet 2:421, 1956.

29. Darmady, E. M., and Stranack, F.: Microdissection of the nephron in disease, Brit. M. Bull. 13:21, 1957.

30. Bricker, N. S., Klahr, S., Lubowitz, H., and Slatopolsky, E.: On the functional transformations in the residual nephrons with advancing disease, Pediat. Clin. N.A. 18:595, 1971.

15

The Uremic Syndrome

THE TERM "UREMIA" literally means urine in the blood; it was coined in 1840 by Piorry to describe the consequences of retention of excretory products. A more precise definition is that uremia is a complex of symptoms and signs reflecting the dysfunctions of all organ systems as the result of failure of renal regulation of the composition and volume of the body fluids. In the progressive renal diseases grouped as chronic Bright's disease, the onset of uremia is slow and insidious. In acute nephritis, in chemical and ischemic tubular necroses, in acute urinary obstruction and after surgical removal of a single functional kidney, onset is abrupt: the uremic syndrome develops in 2–7 days (1, 2).

Nervous manifestations of the syndrome include apathy, torpor, drowsiness or coma; psychosis or acute mania; muscular weakness and muscular twitching; and headache, vertigo and neuralgic or neuritic pains.

Alimentary tract disturbances include anorexia, nausea and vomiting. In chronic renal disease, emaciation may be extreme. In terminal uremia, stomatitis, ulcerations throughout the gastrointestinal tract and gastrointestinal bleeding are common. An ammoniacal odor of the breath is often present.

Respiratory alterations include the dyspnea of hypertensive heart failure and the Kussmaul breathing of severe metabolic acidosis. Pulmonary edema is a frequent complication of advanced uremia.

Circulatory manifestations are commonly secondary to the hypertension that accompanies renal disease. In fact, congestive failure may precipitate uremia in the patient with marginally adequate renal function. It is often difficult to distinguish circulatory factors specifically related to uremia from those accompanying cardiovascular disease. Some four factors definitely related to uremia may be cited: alterations in rate and rhythm of the heart and in myocardial contractility associated with hyperkalemia; purpura due to capillary fragility and alterations in the clotting mechanism; progressive and often severe anemia; and precordial pain and friction rub resulting from uremic pericarditis.

Skeletal manifestations include osteomalacia in the adult and rickets in the growing child.

The skin is generally pale, dry and of a peculiarly yellow-brown tint in chronic uremia. Pruritis is a common early symptom; urea frost (crystals on the skin) is a late-appearing sign.

General metabolic disturbances probably underlie most of the functional manifestations of uremia. Specific examples include easy fatigability and generalized muscular weakness, susceptibility to infection, retardation of growth and development (in children) and delayed wound healing after trauma or operation.

Pathogenesis of the Uremic Syndrome

The alterations in glomerular and tubular functions and in renal blood flow that underlie the excretory and regulatory deficiencies of kidney disease have been discussed in the preceding chapter. Here we shall consider only the relationships between selected biochemical abnormalities of the body fluids and the symptoms and signs of uremia.

UREA

In a quantitative sense, an increase in urea concentration is the most striking abnormality of the body fluids in uremia, although it is certainly not the most important functionally. When urea is administered to a normal person in amounts sufficient to achieve blood levels comparable to those in uremic patients, it causes thirst and polyuria but none of the other manifestations of uremia. Furthermore, in the treatment of uremic patients by hemodialysis (discussed below), the blood urea can be maintained unchanged by the addition of urea to the dialysis bath. Relief of the signs and symptoms of uremia occurs even though the level of blood urea remains high. The ammoniacal odor of the breath comes from bacterial decomposition of salivary urea. Urea frost is crystallized on the skin from sweat.

POTASSIUM INTOXICATION

Potassium intoxication is a major lethal factor in acute renal failure but is of lesser significance in chronic renal disease, except in the terminal stages. The development of hyperkalemia is hastened in the presence of extensive trauma, severe infections, and bleeding into the gastrointestinal tract, body cavities or tissues. It may develop rapidly, in acute renal failure, or slowly, in the end stages of chronic renal disease. Acidosis favors the loss of potassium from cells; and, because the total intracellular store of this ion is massive, the loss of a relatively small fraction raises the extracellular concentration to lethal levels (8–10 mEq/L). The heart is the most vulnerable organ, and death in acute renal failure can frequently be assigned to the effects of hyperkalemia on the initiation and conduction of the cardiac impulse and on myocardial contractility. Electrocardiographic changes pathognomonic of hyperkalemia include high and peaked T waves, broadened QRS complexes, signs of conduction defects progressing to bundle-branch block and reduced or absent P waves. Hyperkalemia also plays a role in the pathogenesis of central nervous hyperexcitability and muscular weakness. Hypokalemia is also a cause of muscular weakness and may develop in chronic uremia as a sequel to pernicious vomiting and diarrhea.

ELEVATION OF PLASMA SULFATE AND PHOSPHATE AND REDUCTION OF PLASMA BICARBONATE AND pH

These changes are the consequences, respectively, of diminished glomerular filtration and failure of renal regulation of acid-base balance. Because the phosphate and sulfate excreted in the urine enter the renal tubules in the filtrate, a reduction in filtration rate results in increases in the plasma concentrations of these two ions. Plasma concentrations rise until the filtered loads again exceed metabolic production. High plasma phosphate levels depress the solubility and ionized fraction of calcium. Muscular twitching and, less commonly, tetany develop. Acidosis partly counteracts the effects of hyperphosphatemia on the solubility and ionization of calcium. When acidosis is corrected by alkali therapy, frank tetany may occur if calcium is not administered simultaneously. Osteomalacia is in part a consequence of acidosis and in part a result of parathyroid overactivity. Acidosis increases cellular loss of potassium, and, because potassium is poorly excreted, hyperkalemia develops.

Acidosis is common in the uremic stage of chronic renal disease; it develops slowly and insidiously. Its major cause is failure of the diseased kidney to excrete hydrogen ions dissociated by the sulfuric acid and phosphoric acid formed in the metabolism of protein and phospholipid. Buffering of hydrogen ions by ammonia secreted into the urine normally accounts for the elimination of twice the amount of acid excreted in free titratable form. In chronic renal disease, the formation of titratable acid is reduced; however, production of ammonia is even more severely curtailed.

HYPONATREMIA

Hyponatremia most commonly develops in acute renal failure because of excessive administration of water. In chronic renal failure, it is more likely to result from rigid restriction of intake of salt. Because the capacity of the chronically diseased kidney to conserve sodium is limited, restriction of salt intake in the treatment of the associated hypertension may lead to depletion of body sodium stores and dehydration. Renal blood flow and filtration rate decrease, further decreasing renal excretory and regulatory capacities and increasing uremia. Water is retained to restore volume of body fluids, and hyponatremia results. Sodium, potassium and calcium are mutually antagonistic with respect to neuromuscular excitability. The effects of hyperkalemia on the heart, skeletal muscle and nervous system are intensified by hyponatremia and hypocalcemia; conversely, the effects of hyponatremia and hypocalcemia are intensified by hyperkalemia.

UREMIC TOXINS

The symptoms and signs of uremia have in the past been ascribed to some elusive toxic product, whose failure of excretion in chronic renal disease leads to its increased concentration in the body fluids. Possible uremic toxins that have been implicated include guanidinosuccinate, methylguanidine, phenols and catecholamines. Another view suggests that the uremic state is merely the manifestation of the sum of all the abnormalities in the composition of the body fluids that develop in the course of chronic renal disease.

THE TRADE-OFF HYPOTHESIS

A third and intriguing concept developed by Bricker *et al.* (3), is that the various elements that characterize uremia are the consequences of a "trade-off" of, on the one hand, the adaptive and beneficial effects of renal hormones that regulate tubular functions and, on the other hand, the adverse effects of these hormones on extrarenal tissues and organs. Presumably, the concentrations of these hormones increase above normal in response to a fall in glomerular filtration rate.

The trade-off hypothesis is best illustrated in terms of the skeletal abnormalities that result from the secondary hyperparathyroidism observed in chronic renal disease. A normal person ingests about 1 Gm of phosphorus per day. To maintain a normal plasma phosphate concentration (1 mM/L) while excreting that which he ingests, he reabsorbs about 90% of the phosphate filtered through his glomeruli (GFR = 120 ml/min). In contrast, the patient in uremia whose GFR is 2 ml/min must excrete about 90% of filtered phosphate to maintain phosphorus balance. Even with markedly reduced reabsorption, plasma and filtrate concentrations of phosphate are increased. The concentration of ionized calcium is reciprocally reduced. Reduction of ionized calcium stimulates the parathyroid glands, leads to their hypertrophy and increases their rate of secretion of parathyroid hormone. This has the beneficial effect of reducing tubular reabsorption of phosphate; but the trade-off is the adverse effect of hyperparathyroidism on the integrity of the skeleton.

Figure 15–1 illustrates the effects of sequential reductions of glomerular filtration rate by progressive ligation of branches of the renal arteries of dogs, carried out over a period of months. The solid circles represent a group of dogs maintained on a 1,200-mg/day phosphorus intake. The hollow circles represent a group of dogs maintained on a vanishing low-phosphorus intake. In the dogs on high phosphate intake progressive reduction of GFR from a normal of 70 ml/min to 10 ml/min was accompanied by a decrease in tubular reabsorption of phosphate (TRP) from more than 95% of filtered phosphate to about 40%. This occurred in

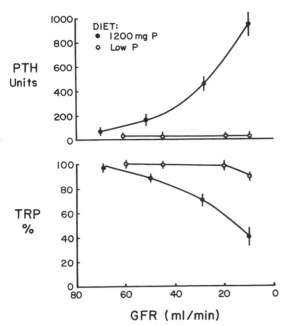

Fig. 15—1. — Influence of phosphate intake on the evolution of secondary hyperparathyroidism in the dog as a consequence of progressive reduction of glomerular filtration rate by successive ligation of intrarenal branches of the renal arteries. *TRP*, tubular reabsorption of phosphate; *PTH*, radioimmunoassayable parathyroid hormone. (From Bricker, N. S.: N. Engl. J. Med. 286:1093, 1972.)

association with, and presumably in response to, an increase in concentration of plasma parathyroid hormone from about 75 to 950 units/ml (measured by radioimmunoassay). In contrast, in dogs maintained on a low-phosphorus intake, TRP decreased only to 90% of that filtered, and radioimmunoassayable parathyroid hormone concentration changed not at all.

These findings suggest an appropriate form of preventive therapy of bone disease in developing chronic renal disease. If phosphorus intake were reduced in proportion to the reduction of GFR, there should be no increase in plasma phosphate, no decrease in plasma ionized calcium, no increase in parathyroid hormone secretion and no necessity for depression of tubular reabsorption of phosphate. The bony changes of secondary hyperparathyroidism would be avoided. Such fine control of phosphorus intake in man is difficult. Some phosphate-binding gel, such as Amphogel, is effective in preventing absorption of phosphate by the gut. This concept is not opposed to a role for vitamin D resistance or chronic acidosis in the pathogenesis of uremic osteodystrophy.

The trade-off hypothesis may well have broader application to the signs and symptoms of uremia than merely those of osteodystrophy. In a normal person, more than 99% of filtered sodium must be reabsorbed (i.e., less than 1% excreted) to maintain sodium balance on a 7-Gm intake of sodium chloride. As filtration rate declines in chronic renal disease, a greater proportion of filtered sodium must be excreted (i.e., less reabsorbed) than in the normal person. Preliminary evidence from Bricker's group suggests that a hormone is secreted in response to a fall in GFR—a hormone that inhibits renal tubular reabsorption of sodium. It is, presumably, a polypeptide of molecular weight of 500 – 1,000. It may act on tissue cells in general to block extrusion of sodium; if so, this would explain changes in neuromuscular excitability in uremia. This concept is supported by the isolation from uremic serum of a fraction that blocks sodium transport across epithelial tissues, such as frog skin and the renal tubular epithelium of the rat. This fraction is absent from normal serum or else is present in much-reduced amounts. Other hormones may be responsible for some of the remaining abnormalities of uremia. One virtue of Bricker's hypothesis is that it shifts emphasis from the uremic toxin to adaptive changes in tubular transport associated with declining filtration rates. To date, search for a renal toxin has been rather sterile.

Renal Control of Erythropoiesis

Three stimuli have long been known to increase the rate of production of erythrocytes: anemia, reduction in inspired oxygen pressure (Po_2) and the administration of salts of cobalt. For many years, it was thought that erythroid tissue responded directly to hypoxia—anemia inducing anemic hypoxia, reduced Po_2 inducing hypoxic hypoxia and cobalt salts inducing histotoxic hypoxia. Reissmann (4), in 1950, provided clear-cut evidence of the intermediation of a humoral factor by exposing one of a pair of parabiotic rats to low Po_2. Both rats became polycythemic. Subsequently, it was demonstrated that an erythrocyte-stimulating factor (ESF, or hemopoietine) appears in the peripheral blood in response to hypoxia and that this humoral agent stimulates erythrocyte production. Plasma containing this factor, when administered to a normal animal, increases the rate of disappearance of protein-bound radioactive iron (^{59}Fe) administered intravenously, increases the rate of incorporation of ^{59}Fe into circulating red cells, causes the proliferation of erythroblasts in bone marrow and induces reticulocytosis of peripheral blood. If given repeatedly, it produces polycythemia (5).

The regular occurrence of anemia in chronic renal disease and the occasional association of polycythemia with renal tumors suggested that the kidney might be involved in the production of hemopoietine (5). Jacobson et al. (6) observed that nephrectomized rabbits and rats fail to produce hemopoietine when subjected to reduced barometric pressure or to acute hemorrhage or when treated with cobalt salts. Erslev (7) and others have claimed that nephrectomized animals fail to respond to the hemopoietic stimulus with increased red cell production and fail to produce hemopoietine because of metabolic depression of the marrow by accumulated toxic products of uremia, not because of absence of the kidneys.

Naets (8), Suki and Grollman (9) and others have provided strong evidence that hemopoietine is produced in the kidney. Thus, in nephrectomized dogs, anemia may appear before azotemia becomes significant. Anemia is not prevented by repeated peritoneal dialysis, which reduces azotemia to a minimum. Anemic uremic dogs respond to exogenous hemopoietine with an increase in red cell production; hence, their marrow is

not metabolically depressed. In animals with ureterovenous anastomoses and marked uremia, anemia does not develop. Such animals produce hemopoietine in response to bleeding. Finally, kidney extracts stimulate the production of erythrocytes (9).

With respect to hemopoietine production, ureteral ligation is not as benign a procedure as is ureterovenous anastomosis, although the two are comparable as far as production of uremia is concerned. Ureteral ligation results in hydronephrosis, which appears to interfere with the renal production of hemopoietine. Ureteral section, which permits drainage of urine into the peritoneum, does not interfere to the same degree; thus, animals with sectioned ureters are essentially as responsive to hypoxic stimulation as are those with ureterovenous anastomosis.

Hemopoietine is rapidly formed and liberated into the blood stream in response to hypoxic stimulation. It is also rapidly cleared from the blood: its half-life has been variously estimated as 3–7 hours. Perhaps 10% of hemopoietine cleared from the blood is excreted in the urine; however, the liver accounts for the removal and destruction of the major fraction of circulating hemopoietine.

The blood plasma of anoxic or anemic patients is a potent source of hemopoietine and has been widely used in the characterization of the properties of this hormone. The substance is nondialyzable, resistant to boiling in dilute acid and precipitable by 70–80% saturation with ammonium sulfate or 60–80% ethanol. It is destroyed by incubation with trypsin, chymotrypsin or pepsin. It contains sialic acid and exhibits the electrophoretic properties of an α-globulin. Some believe that hemopoietine is a low-molecular-weight glycoprotein with, possibly, an associated active polypeptide side chain. The humoral agent apparently acts to increase both the rate of red cell production in, and the rate of release of red cells from, the bone marrow and spleen (5).

There is no information as to where within the kidney hemopoietine is produced. Indeed, not all investigators agree that the kidney is the sole, or even the major, source of the hormone. However, recent evidence inclines the author to the belief that the kidney is at least one source of the hormone.

The anemia of chronic renal disease is of a normocytic, normochromic type. The clearance of radioiron from blood plasma is slow; incorporation into erythrocytes is delayed. A major cause of anemia is thus the reduced replacement of worn-out erythrocytes. However, a variety of evidence suggests that a hemolytic factor may also play some role, especially in those patients in whom anemia develops precipitously. Red cells from such an anemic nephritic patient are abnormally fragile when tested in the patient's plasma, but they have a normal life span when infused into a normal person. Furthermore, red cells from a normal donor have a short life span when infused into a uremic recipient. Accordingly, the hemolytic factor must be extracorpuscular and associated with the plasma. Gastrointestinal bleeding may contribute to anemia, especially in terminal uremia (10). Anemia, like azotemia, has an insidious onset and develops slowly in chronic renal disease. Both can be correlated with reduced renal mass. In acute renal failure, anemia develops rapidly, owing not only to deficient production of hemopoietine by damaged tubular cells but also to the accumulation of a hemolytic factor in the plasma.

Treatment of the Uremic Syndrome

Treatment of the patient with either acute or chronic renal failure should begin with attention to those elements of the renal disease that are amenable to prompt correction, such as obstruction, infection, circulatory insufficiency and the action of nephrotoxins. Further therapy is directed toward reduction of the excretory load, use of extrarenal routes of excretion and compensation for regulatory inadequacies. The first of these aspects of therapy is outside the scope of the text of physiology, and only a cursory treatment of the latter can be justified here. Sev-

eral monographs cover the entire subject in detail (1, 2).

DIET

Dietary treatment of acute renal failure differs in principle from that of chronic renal failure. Because the former condition is self-limited and of relatively brief duration, restrictions of intake can be more drastic. Protein is completely eliminated from the diet during the anuric and oliguric phases of acute renal failure, in order to reduce not only the rate of rise of blood nonprotein nitrogen but also that of phosphate, sulfate and potassium. Theoretically, pure carbohydrate and fat should be administered orally in amounts adequate to cover caloric requirements, to prevent loss of weight and to reduce to a minimum endogenous protein catabolism. Practically, these ends are rarely attainable, because nausea and vomiting often occur early in acute renal failure and, at best, a high-fat diet is unpalatable. Glucose is tolerated orally far better than is fat, reduces protein catabolism and prevents ketosis. Although fruit and vegetable juices are good sources of glucose, they must be absolutely proscribed because of their high potassium content. In the presence of nausea and vomiting, glucose must be given intravenously. Anuria or severe oliguria introduces the additional requirement that water must be limited, to avoid overhydration. Therefore, conventional glucose infusions cannot be given. However, as much as 200 Gm of glucose can be given each day in 400 ml of water if it is administered slowly by intravenous drip through a catheter passed into a central vein. When infused into a peripheral vein, concentrated glucose solutions are painful and cause thrombosis. Although the 800 Cal derived from 200 Gm of glucose by no means supplies the calories expended, endogenous protein metabolism is reduced and ketosis is prevented. The average patient has large-enough fat depots to supply the additional calories needed for a period of several weeks.

The problem of dietary management in chronic renal failure is more difficult. Again, protein is restricted, but severe limitation of intake over prolonged periods of time is undesirable because of tissue wastage due to catabolism of body proteins. For the adult, the diet should contain 0.5 Gm/kg of body weight per day of protein of high biologic value; e.g., meat, fish, poultry, eggs or milk. For the growing child, perhaps twice this amount should be provided. Ample calories in the form of fat and carbohydrate permit the achievement of nitrogen balance despite minimum protein intake. Except in terminal renal failure, potassium intoxication is not a problem, so a more varied diet is permissible. However, anorexia makes difficult the preparation of a diet adequate in calories.

The keto acid analogues of the essential amino acids can be administered orally to reduce nitrogen intake still further. These keto acids are transaminated to form the essential amino acids, thus reducing catabolism of tissue proteins and maintaining nitrogen balance on a lower intake. The drawback of this regimen is cost.

PHOSPHORUS AND SULFUR

Unfortunately, phosphorus and sulfur are present in relatively large quantities in proteins of high biologic value. Because of exceptionally high phosphorus content, large quantities of milk should be avoided. Aluminum hydroxide gels, by binding phosphate in the gastrointestinal tract, decrease the absorption of dietary phosphate and promote the excretion of phosphate secreted into the intestine.

CALCIUM

Calcium, administered orally, together with vitamin D, may slow or prevent the advance of the bone lesions of chronic renal failure (osteomalacia and rickets) if they are significant. Such therapy has little effect on muscle twitching and other signs of central nervous system hyperexcitability. Accord-ingly, most patients with chronic renal failure do not profit from calcium therapy. In acute renal failure, intravenous calcium gluconate is used mainly in the emergency treatment of hyperkalemia.

WATER

In acute renal failure, water should be administered only in amounts sufficient to correct existing deficits and to replace current losses. Because of oliguria or anuria, excesses are not excreted; overhydration and hyponatremia contribute to rapid deterioration, not to restoration of renal function. As much as 400–500 ml of water are produced in the body each day in the metabolism of endogenous fat and protein and of administered glucose. This metabolic water plus the 400 ml/day required as a vehicle for glucose provide for the basal evaporative losses from lungs and skin. Little additional water is needed in the absence of vomiting, diarrhea and sweating. Of course, water equal to urine output, if any, and gastrointestinal losses must be supplied. Accurate daily weights provide the simplest guide to adequacy of intake. An expected weight loss of 0.3–0.4 kg/day should be permitted. No weight loss, or a gain once optimum hydration is established, indicates overhydration; conversely, excessive weight loss indicates dehydration.

In chronic renal failure, water intake should be sufficient to provide for a daily urine volume of about 3 L. Although relatively large volumes of water can be tolerated, no advantage accrues from excessive intake. However, inadequate intake leads to increasing azotemia, hyperkalemia and an exacerbation of symptoms and signs of uremia.

HYPERKALEMIA

Hyperkalemia is a serious threat in acute renal failure. Even though intake is zero, potassium, liberated from metabolized tissues and lost from cells in consequence of increasing acidosis, may accumulate rapidly in extracellular fluid. Mounting plasma level is an indication for immediate hemodialysis or peritoneal dialysis, the only effective means of treating the condition. If immediate dialysis is impossible, two palliative measures will temporarily halt an alarming rate of increase of plasma concentration: (1) The infusion of glucose and insulin and the infusion of sodium bicarbonate or lactate often improve the patient's condition dramatically by favoring the uptake of potassium by cells. The improvement is only temporary, and the potassium again leaks out into the extracellular fluid within a few hours. (2) Intravenous administration of calcium gluconate and hypertonic sodium chloride by ionic antagonism may also improve conditions temporarily. At best, these procedures provide only a few hours' grace in which to initiate more effective therapy. Gastric or intestinal lavage, although less effective than hemodialysis and peritoneal dialysis, can be used to remove significant amounts of potassium from the body if initiated before critical hyperkalemia develops. Fortunately, many patients, anuric or oliguric for 10 days or more, recover renal function without developing serious hyperkalemia.

In chronic renal failure, hyperkalemia is not a serious problem until late in the course of renal disease, provided the fluid intake and output are adequate and serious acidosis is avoided or corrected. Sodium-cycle exchange resins given orally and gastric or intestinal lavage may help in the hyperkalemia of terminal renal failure.

ACIDOSIS

In both acute and chronic renal failure, acidosis develops from retention of phosphate and sulfate, from loss of sodium or gain of water and from failure of mechanisms of excretion of anions as titratable acid or in combination with ammonia. An absolute or relative excess of hydrogen ions exists in the extracellular fluid. Hyperpnea, which in severe acidosis becomes so marked as to merit the special designation of Kussmaul breathing, is a respiratory compensation for acidosis. Buffering of hydrogen ions reduces the extracellular concentration of bicarbonate. Compensatory hyperpnea reduces the P_{CO_2} and carbonic acid concentration and lessens the increase in hydrogen ion concentration that would otherwise occur. Additionally, hydrogen ions enter cells in exchange for potassium ions and are bound by cellular buffers. Correction of extracellular acidosis by the administration of sodium bicarbonate reverses this exchange; potassium ions reenter cells, and the extruded hydrogen ions are buffered by extracellular bicarbonate. However, in acute renal failure, the amount of bicarbonate that can be administered is limited by the patient's inability to excrete sodium and fixed anions. Retention of these ions and of equivalent quantities of water expands extracellular volume and poses the threat of congestive failure and pulmonary edema. In any event, it is unwise to attempt to restore a normal bicarbonate concentration by the administration of bicarbonate. Because of low serum calcium levels, tetany may be precipitated. Because elevation of bicarbonate alone does not correct the elevated phosphate and sulfate concentrations, the ionic structure of the body fluids cannot be restored to normal. However, partial correction of acidosis by the administration of sodium bicarbonate often leads to dramatic symptomatic improvement, clearing of the sensorium and alleviation of hyperpnea. Complete restoration of the ionic pattern of the extracellular fluid can only be achieved by removal of phosphate and sulfate at the same time that bicarbonate is replaced. Hemodialysis and peritoneal dialysis are the only effective means of achieving these ends.

SODIUM

In acute renal failure, the sodium intake should be limited to replacement of losses, once optimal hydration is established. In the absence of vomiting, diarrhea and sweating, sodium intake should be zero throughout the anuric and severely oliguric phases. The administration of sodium bicarbonate is justified only for the correction of severe acidosis and for the emergency treatment of hyperkalemia. In the diuretic phase of recovery from acute renal failure, excessive salt loss is possible, and an adequate intake must be provided.

In chronic renal failure, restriction of salt intake can be calamitous. There is a common, and unfortunate, belief that salt should be restricted in all stages of renal disease. Although this is reasonable in acute nephritis and in the nephrotic stage of chronic renal disease, restriction of salt is unwise in the azotemic patient in the absence of frank edema. Although the blood pressure of the azotemic hypertensive patient can be lowered by severe limitation of salt, filtration rate and renal blood flow are reduced and uremia precipitated at the same time. Adequate hydration by a generous intake of salt and water preserves a maximum of renal excretory and regulatory ability. The treatment of congestive failure in the patient with severely impaired renal function by either salt restriction or the administration of diuretics should be conservative and with full appreciation of the hazard of impending uremia.

ANEMIA

At the present time, anemia in renal disease can be treated only by blood transfusion. Active preparations of hemopoietine are not available commercially.

HEMODIALYSIS—THE ARTIFICIAL KIDNEY

Considering the complexity of its function, it is surprising that the kidney was the first organ for which man devised an adequate, although temporary, replacement. Despite the fact that its principles of operation are different from those of the natural organ, the artificial kidney performs most of the basic excretory and regulatory operations necessary to sustain life. An important use is in self-limited renal diseases that result in acute renal failure and in which return of function can be expected in a few weeks. Developments in technic have encouraged the extended treatment of patients in chronic renal failure. Other uses of dialysis are the improvement of the patient's condition preparatory to transplantation and the rapid removal of toxic doses of certain dialyzable drugs from the body.

PRINCIPLES OF OPERATION.—The artificial kidney is a continuous-flow dialysis system of large surface area. A stream of blood from a cannulated artery spreads out in a film over a thin cellophane membrane in contact with a balanced salt solution. Exchange of all diffusible components of the two fluids occurs across the semipermeable membrane. The blood returns to the body through a venous catheter; the dialyzing medium is rapidly renewed from a large reservoir.

Any substance* present in higher concentration in the blood diffuses into the dialysis fluid. Conversely, any substance present in higher concentration in the dialysis fluid diffuses into the blood. Accordingly, the artificial kidney can be used either to extract substances from the blood, including waste products or toxic chemicals and drugs, or to add substances to the blood, such as bicarbonate ions in acidosis.

The rate at which any component is added to or subtracted from the blood is determined by the area of the dialyzing membrane, by its permeability to the component (related to thickness, pore diameter and total pore area) and by the difference in concentration of the component in the blood and the dialysis fluid. In the course of a 6-hour dialysis, 50–250 Gm of urea can be removed from a patient by any of the artificial kidneys in use today. One may calculate the urea clearance of the artificial kidney in much the same manner that one calculates the urea clearance of the normal kidney. Rate of removal of urea in milligrams per minute divided by plasma

---

*The substance, of course, must be diffusible through cellophane; plasma proteins and substances strongly bound to proteins are not diffusible.

concentration in milligrams per milliliter equals clearance. At zero time, when the concentration of urea in the patient's blood is high and that in the dialysis fluid is zero, the urea clearance of the artificial kidney is high: 150–250 ml/min,* which greatly exceeds the urea clearance of normal kidneys. As urea accumulates in the dialysis fluid and concentration rises, clearance decreases, to reach zero when the urea concentrations of the two fluid phases become equal. Wolf *et al.* (11) therefore suggested the use of the expression "dialysance" (D), which, in simplest terms, is rate of removal (R) of a substance per unit difference in concentration between blood (B) and dialysis fluid (DF):

$$D = R/(B - DF)$$

Relative dialysance of any component is its dialysance divided by that of urea. Chloride and urea dialyze faster than amino acids and glucose; sulfate and phosphate dialyze more slowly.

TECHNICS. — Able *et al.* (12) devised the first artificial kidney in 1913 and used it in a series of experiments on dogs. These investigators suggested that the procedure, which they called vividiffusion, might be useful for the removal of toxic materials from the

---

*Such clearances are obtained with a dialyzing membrane of minimal thickness and about 2 m² of surface area, blood flows of 200–400 ml/min and flows of dialysis fluid that are high in proportion to blood flow.

blood in uremia and in drug poisoning.

The first clinical use of the artificial kidney was described by Kolff and Berk (13) in 1944. In the succeeding years, apparatus and technics have undergone extensive modification and improvement in the hands of Kolff, Merrill, Skeggs, Leonards, Alwall and Scribner. The first Kolff kidney was a cumbersome affair, consisting of a large horizontal drum around which cellophane sausage casing was wound in a spiral. The cylinder dipped into a shallow tank; its rotation carried the blood from the point of arterial inflow to that of venous outflow and exposed it as a thin film to an equally thin film of dialysis fluid.

Two types of apparatus in common use today are the Skeggs-Leonards (14) and the Kolff twin-coil kidneys (15), illustrated in Figure 15–2. These two apparatuses are stationary; blood is pumped from an arterial cannula or large venous catheter into the apparatus and pumped from the apparatus back into the patient through a venous cannula. By varying inflow and outflow pressures, ultrafiltration can be controlled, either to remove fluid if the patient is edematous or to maintain constancy of weight if extracellular fluid volume is normal. However, except for water, the mechanism of removal of substances from blood is diffusion, not ultrafiltration.

Fig. 15–2. — The artificial kidney. **A**, Kolff twin-coil kidney. **B**, Skeggs-Leonards kidney.

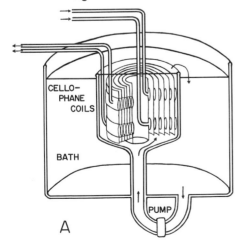

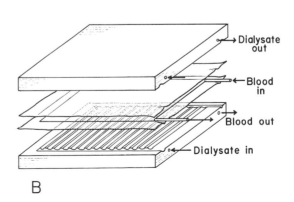

The Skeggs-Leonards kidney is composed of flat sheets of cellophane clamped between ridged plates. Blood flows in the channels between the cellophane sheets. Dialysis fluid flows in the grooves between the cellophane sheets and the plates. The flow of blood is countercurrent to the flow of dialysis solution. The twin-coil kidney is composed of two cellophane tubes, each 10 m in length, connected in parallel and sewed between two layers of Fiberglas net for support. The twin coil is wound around a cylindrical core and completely fills the container. The dialysis fluid flows into the bottom of the container and overflows the top.

Both kidneys use a large reservoir of dialysis fluid, amounting to some 100–300 L. Fortunately, it does not need to be kept bacteriologically sterile during dialysis runs of 4–6 hours. The composition of the dialysis fluid used by Kolff (14) is given in Table 15–1. It can be modified, depending on the specific end to be achieved. For example, in hyperkalemia, potassium is reduced in concentration or omitted from the bath. If alkalosis exists, the bicarbonate is reduced and the chloride increased. In acidosis, the reverse alterations are made.

The blood must be kept from clotting in the extracorporeal circuit. Heparin is introduced by constant drip just distal to the arterial cannula; a heparin antagonist, such as protamine, is added just proximal to the venous cannula. This avoids excessive administration of heparin, with its attendant danger of internal bleeding.

Dialysis requires a good deal of technical skill, whether it is carried out by a hospital team or is self-administered by the patient in his home. Granted these skills, two factors limit the repeated use of the procedure in the long-term treatment of protracted acute or chronic renal insufficiency. The first and most obvious factor is the limited number of blood vessels available for cannulation. The development of scar tissue at the site of cutdown often prevents the repeated use of a given vessel. The second factor is the volume of bank blood required to charge the kidney and its connecting lines prior to use.* Repeated transfusions of such volumes result in the formation of multiple antibodies, which render subsequent typing and matching difficult or impossible. Scribner and his co-workers (16–18) have modified the procedure in such a way that repeated dialyses over a long period of time are now feasible. The radial artery and a peripheral vein are catheterized in the forearm with Teflon catheters. The catheters are bent upon themselves, are run through subcutaneous tunnels to a site some distance from that of cannulation and are brought out through stab wounds. An arteriovenous fistula is created by attaching a connecting loop to the two ends of the catheters, to prevent clotting in the intervals between dialyses. Because of the nature of Teflon, the catheters cause no tissue reaction; and, because Teflon is unwettable, clots are less likely to form. A Skeggs-Leonards kidney is used because of its low internal volume. Blood pumps do not have to be used; the patient's arterial pressure is sufficient to cause a volume flow of 40–70 ml of blood per minute through the artificial kidney and its connecting tubes. To prevent clotting within the kidney, the blood is cooled to 0° C before entering the kidney, and minute amounts of heparin are added by a constant drip just distal to the arterial cannula. The blood is warmed to body temperature before entering the vein. The dialysis fluid, chilled to 0° C, is pumped

TABLE 15–1.—COMPOSITION OF DIALYZING FLUID*

	mEq/L
Sodium	133
Potassium	5
Calcium	5
Magnesium	3
Chloride	110
Bicarbonate	36

*From Kolff, W. J., and Watschinger, B.: J. Lab. & Clin. Med. 47:969, 1956.

*From 300 to 800 ml of blood is needed to prime the various artificial kidneys.

through the kidney at a rate of 600 ml/min. Used in this fashion, the Skeggs-Leonards kidney has a relatively low clearance value, but the dialysis time can be proportionally lengthened. With pumps to increase blood flow and with higher rates of flow of dialysis fluid, the process can be hastened. Using such a system, biweekly or weekly dialyses over prolonged periods of time are feasible. Scribner and others have used repeated dialysis as a means of keeping patients with chronic Bright's disease alive and in reasonably good health despite nearly zero renal function.

Experience with hemodialysis in recent years has encouraged groups in Boston and Seattle to introduce it as a home therapeutic procedure in those instances where husband or wife is intelligent, responsible and psychologically suited to supervise it. Such patients welcome the independence that home dialysis affords. Furthermore, home dialysis maintains the patient with end-stage kidney disease until such time as transplantation can be performed without crowding the dialysis facilities of the research hospital (19).

BENEFITS OF HEMODIALYSIS. — The artificial kidney is remarkably effective in removing urea from the body of the uremic patient and in lowering the blood urea concentration. However, removal of urea is of relatively little significance, for the compound is unusually benign. A number of investigators have added urea to the dialysis fluid in sufficient concentration to prevent its removal from the body and have observed that the beneficial effects of dialysis are unaltered.

Hyperkalemia, which may develop rapidly in acute renal failure, especially if tissues have been extensively traumatized or if acidosis is severe, can be corrected promptly by dialysis. In fact, hypokalemia and depletion of cellular potassium stores may develop if dialysis is prolonged and the bath contains no potassium. Plasma sulfate and phosphate can be reduced and acidosis corrected by proper adjustment of the composition of the dialysis fluid. Creatinine and uric acid are also removed with reasonable rapidity. If the patient is edematous as a result of injudicious water and electrolyte therapy, fluid can be removed by ultrafiltration; i.e., by increasing the outflow resistance and raising the hydrostatic pressure within the blood circuit or, conversely, by lowering the hydrostatic pressure in the dialysis fluid circuit.

Some of the major benefits of hemodialysis have not been characterized biochemically. Restlessness, muscular fibrillation, vomiting and confusion or coma are often relieved dramatically within the first few hours of dialysis. Some substance or substances accounting for these elements of the uremic syndrome are diffusible and removed by the artificial kidney. Their nature is unknown.

Those who have had the greatest experience in the use of the artificial kidney agree that dialysis should be performed before the condition of the patient becomes critical. There is, of course, a hazard inherent in the procedure; furthermore, many patients in acute renal failure respond well to conservative management. When to use dialysis is a difficult question, ultimately to be decided on the basis of the physician's experience and clinical acumen. It is also generally agreed that the hyponatremic, acidotic and hyperkalemic patient should not be precipitously restored to biochemical normality. The biochemical abnormalities have developed gradually, and the tissues have become more or less adapted to their abnormal extracellular environment. Rapid and too complete correction may cause a worsening of the patient's condition.

USE OF HEMODIALYSIS IN DRUG INTOXICATION. — The artificial kidney also may be used in the treatment of drug intoxication if the drug is diffusible and present in the circulating plasma in significant concentration. It is actually far more effective in the removal from the body of toxic amounts of bromide and thiocyanate than is the kidney itself, because these two substances are highly reabsorbed by the renal tubules. Dialysis has been used successfully in the treatment of barbiturate and salicylate intoxication and in the removal of various other drugs as well (20).

OTHER MEANS OF DIALYSIS

In the absence of the trained personnel and apparatus needed for successful hemodialysis, peritoneal, gastric or intestinal dialysis can be performed to achieve somewhat the same ends.

To perform peritoneal dialysis, some 2–4 L of a sterile inorganic salt solution containing sufficient glucose to bring osmolar concentration to 450 mOsm/L is introduced into the peritoneum through a large-bore needle. After 1 hour, a trocar is introduced in the midline and a sterile polyvinyl catheter is inserted. The fluid is drained with change in the patient's position and abdominal massage, to insure complete collection. Broadscale antibiotics are added to the dialysis fluid to reduce the hazard of peritonitis. The procedure is repeated frequently over a period of 12–20 hours, during which time 40–60 L of dialysis fluid are passed through the peritoneum. Peritoneal dialysis has been used successfully in the treatment of the hyperkalemia and azotemia of acute renal failure. The hazard of peritonitis and the lesser efficiency of peritoneal dialysis, compared with hemodialysis, render this the method of second choice if facilities for hemodialysis are available (21, 22). Chronic peritoneal dialysis, like hemodialysis, has been introduced as a home procedure. Since infection is much less common by the repeated peritoneal puncture technic than by the use of in-dwelling peritoneal access devices, the services of a physician to introduce trocar and catheter are needed at the start of each dialysis (23).

Even less efficient are the methods of gastric and intestinal lavage. However, they are inherently less hazardous; and, if vomiting and ileus do not complicate the picture of uremia, they may be used to remove significant amounts of potassium from the body. Removal of urea, phosphate, sulfate and creatinine by gastric or intestinal dialysis is far less complete than by peritoneal dialysis or hemodialysis. The isolation and exteriorization of a loop of bowel has been performed in a few patients with chronic renal disease. Daily lavage of this loop by the patient at home has been used to remove small but significant quantities of wastes (21, 23).

RENAL TRANSPLANTATION

The conventional treatment of chronic renal failure is palliative rather than curative. Effective regeneration of tissue destroyed by chronic renal disease does not occur. Restoration of function in a patient with diseased kidneys by transplantation of a normal organ from a healthy donor has, until recently, been feasible only between identical twins — an operation that has been successfully performed in several instances (24, 25). However, such instances constitute a minute and statistically insignificant fraction of the total number of cases of chronic renal failure. Transplantation of kidneys between genetically dissimilar persons fails because the transplanted kidney behaves in the host as a foreign body, which stimulates the production of antibodies against itself. Initially, the transplant may function; but, sooner or later, it is rejected and destroyed by the host.

Recent advances in knowledge and control of tissue immune responses have increased the number of successful transplants and the duration of their function. Because there is less genetic difference among father, mother and offspring than between unrelated persons, the ideal donor of the normal kidney should be as closely related as possible. Pre- and post-treatment with immunosuppressive agents, thymectomy and splenectomy, prednisone, actinomycin C and local irradiation of the graft are used as needed to control rejection of the transplanted kidney. Because transplantation is still an experimental procedure and because the degree and duration of rehabilitation are unpredictable, the obtaining of a suitable donor is frequently difficult. Experience with transplantation of cadaver kidneys is increasing, and, although results are far less satisfactory than transplantation from a closely related living donor, this may develop into the procedure of choice (26, 27).

Summary

The uremic syndrome is a constellation of symptoms and signs arising from failure of renal regulation of the composition and volume of body fluids. Although the increase in concentration of urea nitrogen is quantitatively the most striking abnormality of the body fluids, it is by no means functionally the most significant. Of greater import are hyperkalemia, hyperphosphatemia, hypersulfatemia, hypocalcemia, hyponatremia, metabolic acidosis and the retention of uncharacterized products of protein catabolism that affect central nervous excitability. In addition, significant elements of control of erythropoiesis, blood pressure and volume of the body fluids are inadequate in uremia. The ability of the kidney to compensate for inadequate or excessive intake of water and electrolytes is greatly reduced.

The treatment of uremia is directed toward correction of reversible elements of the renal disease. Further therapy is directed toward reduction of excretory load, compensation for regulatory inadequacies and the use of extrarenal routes of excretion. In the future, treatment may more frequently involve organ transplantation.

REFERENCES

1. Fishberg, A. M.: *Hypertension and Nephritis* (5th ed.; New York: Lea & Febiger, 1954).
2. Merrill, J. P.: *The Treatment of Renal Failure* (New York: Grune & Stratton, Inc., 1955).
3. Bricker, N S.: On the pathogenesis of the uremic state. An exposition of the "trade-off" hypothesis, N. Engl. J. Med. 296:1093, 1972.
4. Reissmann, K. R.: Studies on the mechanism of erythropoietic stimulation in parabiotic rats during hypoxia, Blood 5:372, 1950.
5. Gordon, A. S.: Hemopoietine, Physiol. Rev. 39:1, 1959.
6. Jacobson, L. O., Goldwasser, E., Fried, W., and Plzak, L. F.: Role of the kidney in erythropoiesis, Nature, London 179:633, 1957.
7. Erslev, A. J.: Erythropoietic function in uremic rabbits, Arch. Int. Med. 101:407, 1958.
8. Naets, J. P.: The role of the kidney in the production of erythropoietic factor, Blood 16:1770, 1960.
9. Suki, W., and Grollman, A.: Role of the kidney in erythropoiesis, Am. J. Physiol. 100:629, 1960.
10. Loge, J. P., Lange, R. D., and Moore, C. V.: Characterization of the anemia associated with chronic renal insufficiency, Am. J. Med. 24:4, 1958.
11. Wolf, A. V., Remp, D. G., Kiley, J. E., and Currie, G. D.: Artificial kidney function: Kinetics of hemodialysis, J. Clin. Invest. 30:1062, 1951.
12. Able, J. J., Rowntree, L. G., and Turner, B. B.: The removal of diffusible substances from the circulating blood by means of dialysis, Tr. A. Am. Physicians 28:51, 1913.
13. Kolff, W. J., and Berk, H. T. J.: The artificial kidney: A dialyzer with a great area, Acta med. scandinav. 117:121, 1944.
14. Merrill, J. P.: The artificial kidney, Scient. Am. 205:56, 1961.
15. Kolff, W. J., and Watschinger, B.: Further development of coil kidney: Disposable artificial kidney, J. Lab. & Clin. Med. 47:969, 1956.
16. Quinton, W., Dillard, D., and Scribner, B. H.: Cannulation of blood vessels for prolonged hemodialysis, Tr. Am. Soc. Artif. Int. Organs 6:104, 1960.
17. Scribner, B. H., Caner, J. E. Z., Buri, R., and Quinton, W.: The technique of continuous hemodialysis, Tr. Am. Soc. Artif. Int. Organs 6:88, 1960.
18. Scribner, B. H., Buri, R., Caner, J. E. Z., Hegstrom, R., and Burnell, J. M.: The treatment of chronic uremia by means of intermittent hemodialysis: A preliminary report, Tr. Am. Soc. Artif. Int. Organs 6:116, 1960.
19. Hampers, C. L., Merrill, J. P., and Cameron, E.: Hemodialysis in the home — A family affair, Tr. Am. Soc. Artif, Int. Org. 11:3, 1965.
20. Maher, J. F., and Schreiner, G. E.: The clinical dialysis of poisons, Tr. Am. Soc. Artif. Int. Org. 12:349, 1966.
21. Schloerb, P. B.: Peritoneal dialysis and newer methods of intestinal perfusion in renal failure, Arch. Int. Med. 102:914, 1958.
22. Grollman, A.: *Acute Renal Failure* (Springfield, Ill.: Charles C Thomas, Publisher, 1954).
23. Tenkhoff, H., Shilipetor, G., and Boen, S. T.:

One year's experience with home peritoneal dialysis, Tr. Am. Soc. Artif. Int. Org. 11:11, 1965.

24. Merrill. J. R.: Current and future problems in the management of renal failure, Arch. Int. Med. 102:891, 1958.

25. Merrill, J. R.: Transplantation of normal tissues, Physiol. Rev. 39:860, 1959.

26. Bower, J. D., and Hume, D. M.: Experience with the Seattle hemodialysis system in renal homotransplantation, Tr. Am. Soc. Artif. Int. Org. 11:225, 1965.

27. Khastagir, B., Shibagaki, M., Willbrandt, R., Montandon, A., Nakamoto, S., and Kolff, W. J.: Further experiences with cadaver kidney transplantation, Tr. Am. Soc. Artif. Int. Org. 12:239, 1966.

16

Functions of Ureters and Bladder

Ureters

THE URETERS serve merely as conduits connecting the renal pelves with the urinary bladder. They traverse the lower part of the posterior wall of the bladder obliquely and open into its cavity 1 – 2 cm above and to the sides of the urethral orifice. The two ureteral openings are connected by a low transverse elevation to form a triangular area, the trigone, at each angle of which is located one of the openings. Each ureteral orifice is closed by a flaplike fold of mucous membrane. The oblique course of the ureters through the muscular wall, as well as the mucosal valves at their openings, prevent reflux of urine during contraction of the bladder.

The ureters are lined with transitional epithelium, and their walls are formed of a submucous layer of connective tissue and inner longitudinal and outer circular layers of smooth muscle. Peristaltic waves originating in the pelves force urine along the ureters and into the bladder in a series of jets at frequencies that vary from 1 per 2 – 3 minutes to 5 or 6 per minute. Normally, the pressures developed by ureteral peristaltic waves vary from 2 to 10 cm of water. If outflow is obstructed, pressures as high as 70 cm of water may develop. The ureters are innervated by fibers derived from the aortic, spermatic or ovarian, and hypogastric plexuses. At least a fraction of these fibers are afferent, for the pain that accompanies the violent peristaltic contractions proximal to an obstruction (renal colic) is one of the most severe pains

suffered by man. Denervation of the ureter results in no functional abnormality. On the other hand, if the ureter is sectioned and sutured, peristaltic waves progress only to the suture line. Passage of urine into the lower segment distends it and initiates another peristaltic wave. Whether peristalsis is myogenic in origin or dependent on the intramural autonomic plexus is unknown. However, frequency of peristaltic waves is modified by extrinsic autonomic impulses and by blood-borne hormones, as well as by the degree of distention.

Urinary Bladder

The bladder is a hollow viscus, lined, like the ureter, with transitional epithelium. Three rather poorly defined layers of smooth muscle make up the bulk of its wall. In the trigonal region, at the neck of the bladder, the mural musculature sweeps over, under and around the urethral orifice to form an internal sphincter of smooth muscle. The external sphincter lies distal to the internal sphincter and is made up of striated muscle fibers, which arise from the transverse ligament of the pelvis and from the inferior rami of the pubis and sweep around the membranous portion of the urethra.

NERVE SUPPLY

The nerve supply of the bladder and sphincters is shown diagrammatically in Figure 16 – 1 *(1)*. Sympathetic fibers, arising in

301

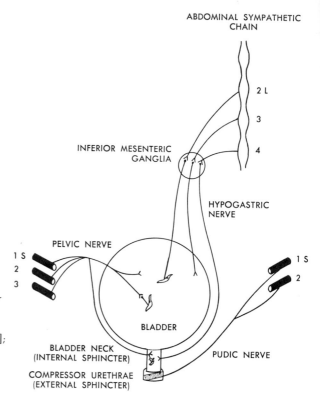

Fig. 16–1. — Innervation of the bladder and urethral sphincters. (From Root, W. S., in Bard, P. [ed.]:*Medical Physiology* [11th ed.; St. Louis: C. V. Mosby Company, 1961]; modified from Learmouth.)

the anterolateral columns of segments *L2 – L4* and traversing the lateral chain ganglia, synapse in the inferior mesenteric ganglion. Postganglionic fibers, forming the hypogastric plexus, are distributed to the body and neck (internal sphincter) of the bladder. Parasympathetic fibers have their origins in segments *S1 – S3* and reach the hypogastric, pelvic and vesical plexuses via the pelvic nerves. Short postganglionic fibers arise in vesical ganglia and supply the body and the neck of the bladder. The external sphincter of the bladder is supplied by the pudendal (pudic) nerves, which are derived from segments *S1* and *S2*, or, according to some investigators, from segments *S1 – S4*.

BLADDER FUNCTION

The function of the bladder is twofold: to serve as a distensible reservoir for urine and to evacuate its contents at suitable intervals. Both functions of the bladder are conven-

iently studied by cystometry. A double-lumen catheter is introduced into the bladder through the urethra. One lumen of the catheter is connected to a calibrated fluid reservoir, the other to a pressure-measuring device. In Figure 16–2, curve *A* illustrates the change in pressure that occurs when the volume of the bladder of the cat is slowly and progressively increased by introducing fluid from the reservoir. The so-called tonus curve exhibits three segments: in segment (*1*) (Fig. 16–2), the pressure rises moderately with the first introduction of fluid; thereafter (*2*) the pressure rises very slowly over a considerable range of volume until (*3*) some critical volume is reached, above which the pressure rises rapidly. The entire cystometrogram can be recorded only if the micturition reflex is abolished; e.g., by acute transection of the spinal cord. The arrow labeled *M* shows the pressure increase that normally occurs as a consequence of reflex contraction of the bladder musculature at some critical volume

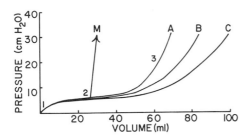

Fig. 16–2. — Cystometrograms of the spinal-sectioned cat, recorded in succession of A, B, and C. M, micturition reflex in same cat prior to spinal section. (Freely adapted from Ruch, T. C.; in Field, J., and Magoun, H. W. [eds.]:*Handbook of Physiology* [Washington, D.C.: American Physiological Society, 1960], Sec. 1, Vol. II, pp. 1207–1223.)

and that results in the expulsion of fluid around the catheter. Similar results are obtained in cystometric studies on the bladder of normal man.

BLADDER TONE

Bladder tone is best defined in terms of the relationship between volume and pressure described by the cystometrogram (2). Tone, so defined, seems to be entirely dependent on the physical state of the smooth muscle making up the bladder wall. It is not a response to a continuous low-frequency discharge of nerve impulses, such as that which underlies skeletal muscle tone.

Segments *1* and *2* of the cystometrogram of a cat lightly anesthetized with pentobarbital is identical with that observed after full anesthesia (with procaine) of the sacral roots or section of those roots. However, the micturition reflex, which is somewhat depressed by light general anesthesia, is completely abolished by anesthetic blockade or section of the sacral roots. Nevertheless, bladder tone up to the volume that initiates micturition is independent of extrinsic bladder innervation. Similar experiments have shown that spinal transection does not alter the tonus curve, nor does treatment of the animal with tetraethylammonium bromide in amounts sufficient to block all peripheral ganglionic activity.

On the other hand, if repeated cystometrograms are recorded following transection of the cord to abolish the micturition reflex, the tonus curve is depressed and considerably extended to the right on successive trials (Fig. 16–2, *B* and *C*). Presumably, stretch has altered the physical state of the bladder wall, rendering it more easily distensible. Because the bladder does not contract actively, it does not return rapidly to its initial state. In contrast, if the ureters are explanted so that the bladder remains empty and contracted, it becomes less distensible with the passage of time and the tonus curve is elevated. Hypertrophy of the bladder similarly elevates the curve. In summary: the tonus curve of the bladder—i.e., the compliance of the bladder ($\Delta V / \Delta P$)—is a function of the viscous elastic properties of the bladder wall, not a function of tonic innervation.

Micturition

The act of micturition involves the coordinated contraction of the detrussor muscle (smooth muscle of the bladder wall), the abdominal wall and muscles of the pelvic floor; fixation of the chest wall and diaphragm; and relaxation of the internal and external urethral sphincters. Accordingly, both autonomic and voluntary activities are involved.

Contraction of the detrussor muscle is reflex: afferent inflow is mainly over the pelvic nerves from tension receptors in the bladder wall; efferent outflow is also over the pelvic nerves to mural smooth muscle. The reflex is both facilitated and inhibited by supraspinal portions of the nervous system and is reinforced by impulses that arise from the urinary tract itself in consequence of the act of micturition. In many respects, the reflex is similar to the myotatic reflex of skeletal muscle. Interference with afferent or efferent limbs of the reflex arc or with afferent or efferent pathways connecting the sacral spinal cord with central facilitatory and inhibitory mechanisms profoundly affects the micturition reflex.

BLADDER AFFERENTS

Normally, man first experiences a desire to void when the bladder volume is about 150 ml, and he becomes uncomfortably aware of bladder distention when volume increases to 350–400 ml. Rapid distention in the course of cystometry induces a desire to void at a lower vesical volume than does slow distention; therefore, it is probable that tension within the bladder wall, rather than length of the elements, is the significant stimulus. In the cat, rapid distention of the bladder initiates impulses in single afferent fibers of the pelvic nerve at frequencies of 20–30/sec. When fluid inflow ceases, tension within the bladder wall falls as the viscus accommodates to its contents, and the afferent impulse frequency decreases to 3–4/sec at constant volume. At an adapted volume near the micturition threshold, frequency is low: 4–6/sec. Only at large vesical volumes with the wall under high tension can afferent impulses be recorded in the hypogastric nerves.

BLADDER EFFERENTS

When the inflow over vesicle afferents reaches some critical value determined by the excitability of the sacral spinal center, impulses are discharged into motoneurons making up the pelvic nerve; the detrussor muscle then contracts. When intravesical pressure rises to 20–40 cm of water, the internal sphincter relaxes. Tonic outflow of impulses to the striated muscle of the external sphincter is inhibited, and the bladder empties its contents completely.

MICTURITION REFLEX

The micturition reflex is exceptionally long sustained in comparison with other phasic spinal reflexes. The following factors account for prolonged activity:

1. The receptor elements are in series with the contractile elements. Therefore, their afferent discharge is well maintained throughout the phase of bladder contraction.

2. Impulses ascending spinal pathways are "long-circuited" through centers in the pons, hypothalamus and cerebral cortex before relay back to the sacral cord. Each of these circuits may, in addition, exhibit reverberating or re-entry properties and sustain efferent outflow, despite reduction in afferent inflow.

3. The act of micturition, resulting in the flow of fluid through and distention of the urethra, reinforces itself by further relaxation of the external sphincter and enhancement of contraction of the detrussor muscle.

Table 16–1 summarizes the six components of the micturition reflex described by Barrington (3). The stimulus for the first three is distention of the bladder; the afferent fibers course in the pelvic nerves. Two efferent pathways are involved: the pelvic nerves, which cause contraction of the detrussor muscle and relaxation of the internal sphincter, and the pudendal nerves, inhibition of which results in relaxation of the external sphincter. The flow of urine along the urethra excites receptors whose afferent fibers are contained in the pudendal nerves. Within the sacral segments, these impulses reinforce inhibition of the external sphincter and contraction of the detrussor. The existence

TABLE 16–1.—COMPONENTS OF THE MICTURITION REFLEX*

STIMULUS	AFFERENT LIMB	EFFERENT LIMB	RESPONSE
Distention of bladder	Pelvic nerve	Pelvic nerve	Contraction of detrussor
Distention of bladder	Pelvic nerve	Pudendal nerve	Relaxation of external sphincter
Distention of bladder	Pelvic nerve	Pelvic nerve	Relaxation of internal sphincter
Fluid through urethra	Pudendal nerve	Pudendal nerve	Relaxation of external sphincter
Fluid through urethra	Pudendal nerve	Pelvic nerve	Contraction of detrussor
Distention of posterior urethra	Hypogastric nerve	Hypogastric nerve	Contraction of detrussor

*From Barrington, F. J. F.: Brain 54:177, 1931.

of the last reflex, involving distention of the posterior urethra, is doubtful, at least in man.

FACILITATION AND INHIBITION OF MICTURITION REFLEX

The sacral spinal mechanism acutely isolated from descending facilitatory impulses by transection of the spinal cord is reflexly inactive. No matter how distended the bladder becomes, reflex contraction of the detrussor and relaxation of the sphincters do not occur. In contrast, if the neuraxis is transected at an intercollicular level, leaving intact the anterior portion of the pons, the micturition reflex is initiated at a fraction of the normal vesical volume. If a second section is made, a few millimeters caudad, if the pons is locally cooled or if focal pontine lesions are made at appropriate sites, the micturition reflex is lost and bladder function is reduced to the spinal state. Thus, the anterior portion of the pons contains a powerful facilitatory center (Fig. 16–3).

If the brain is transected a few millimeters higher, a midbrain inhibitory mechanism can be defined. The threshold volume initiating the micturition reflex may still be less than normal, yet much greater than that observed when the anterior pontine mechanism alone is intact. A transhypothalamic section, leaving the posterior hypothalamus and other more caudal structures intact, reveals a second powerful facilitatory mechanism. Ob-

viously, the brain rostrad to the posterior hypothalamus must exert a net inhibitory effect. Stimulation of the rostral portions of the brain, including the paracentral lobule, premotor area, posterior cingulate gyrus and posterior pyriform area of the cortex, the amygdala and even the cerebellum, has demonstrated that these areas exert both facilitatory and inhibitory effects on the micturition reflex. The ascending and descending pathways connecting sacrospinal centers with facilitatory and inhibitory mechanisms in the brain are concentrated in the posterolateral part of the cord. The fibers are superficial and just ventral to the posterior horn. Section of the two dorsal quadrants is equivalent to complete transection of the cord.

In the clinical literature, the effects of lesions of the nervous system on threshold volume of micturition have been ascribed most commonly to alterations in bladder tone, based on a presumed state of tonic innervation of the bladder wall. In contrast, experimental studies have demonstrated that alterations in threshold volume initiating micturition are mainly dependent on the excitability of the sacral spinal reflex center. A reduction in facilitatory impulses increases threshold volume, and an increase in facilitatory impulses reduces threshold volume. Bladder tone (related to the physical state of the smooth muscle) and threshold volume (related to the sum of excitatory and inhibitory impulses impinging on the sacrospinal center) are basically independent (2).

Fig. 16–3. — Effects of suprasegmental structures on the activity of the sacral spinal micturition reflex. (From Ruch, T. C., in Field, J., and Magoun, H. W.

[eds.]: Handbook of Physiology [Washington, D.C.: American Physiological Society, 1960], Sec. 1, Vol. II, pp. 1207–1223.)

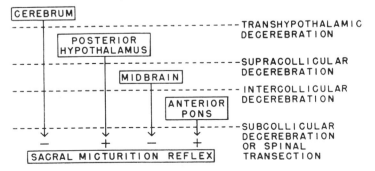

EFFECTS OF NERVE LESIONS ON MICTURITION

If one pelvic nerve of a cat is sectioned, micturition is unimpaired. If both nerves are sectioned, urine is retained for several days, and the bladder becomes grossly distended. The animal exhibits no evidence of discomfort. Manual compression of the bladder through the abdominal wall raises pressure, forces the sphincters and results in partial emptying of the bladder. After a few days, the cat squats and voids small quantities of urine. The residual volume is large, and the bladder hypertrophies.

If the pelvic nerves have been cut, section of the pudendal nerves results in urinary incontinence. Urine drips continuously, and urethral resistance to abdominal pressure is nil. The cat no longer squats. Accordingly, the residual bladder sensation in an animal with pelvic nerves cut is mediated over the pudendals. Section of the pudendal nerves alone results in slight urinary incontinence in the cat but has little effect in man.

Section of the hypogastric nerves increases the frequency of voiding but otherwise has little effect on bladder function.

Division of sacral dorsal roots abolishes the micturition reflex; bladder volume increases 5–10-fold, and overflow incontinence develops. Despite marked bladder distention, pain and discomfort are absent.

Summary

The ureters and bladder serve conduit and temporary storage functions, respectively. Innervation of the ureters is not essential for normal transport of urine from renal pelves to bladder. Neither is innervation essential for the gradual accommodation of the bladder to increasing volume of its contents. However, intermittent and complete evacuation of the bladder depends not only on the integrity of the afferent and efferent nerves and sacrospinal reflex centers but also on the proper balance of facilitatory and inhibitory influences acting on the reflex center from supraspinal levels of the nervous system.

REFERENCES

1. Root, W. S.: Micturition: A Specific Autonomic Function, in Bard P. (ed.): *Medical Physiology* (11th ed.; St. Louis: C. V. Mosby Company, 1961), p. 1174.
2. Ruch, T. C.: Central Control of the Bladder, in Field, J., and Magoun, H. W. (eds.): *Handbook of Physiology* (Washington, D. C.: American Physiological Society, 1960), Sec. 1, Vol. II, p. 1207.
3. Barrington, F. J. F.: The component reflexes of micturition in the cat, Brain 54:177, 1931.

Index